Orthopaedic Examination Techniques

Third Edition

Orthopaedic Examination Techniques

A Practical Guide

Third Edition

Edited by

Fazal Ali
Chesterfield Royal Hospital & Sheffield Children's Hospital

Nick Harris
Spire Hospital, Leeds & Leeds Beckett University

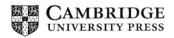

CAMBRIDGE
UNIVERSITY PRESS

University Printing House, Cambridge CB2 8BS, United Kingdom

One Liberty Plaza, 20th Floor, New York, NY 10006, USA

477 Williamstown Road, Port Melbourne, VIC 3207, Australia

314–321, 3rd Floor, Plot 3, Splendor Forum, Jasola District Centre,
New Delhi – 110025, India

103 Penang Road, #05–06/07, Visioncrest Commercial, Singapore 238467

Cambridge University Press is part of the University of Cambridge.

It furthers the University's mission by disseminating knowledge in the pursuit of
education, learning, and research at the highest international levels of excellence.

www.cambridge.org
Information on this title: www.cambridge.org/9781108796705
DOI: 10.1017/9781108859295

First published 2022
Third edition published 2022
Second edition first published 2014
First edition first published 2003

Printed in the United Kingdom by TJ Books Limited, Padstow Cornwall

A catalogue record for this publication is available from the British Library.

ISBN 978-1-108-79670-5 Paperback

Cambridge University Press has no responsibility for the persistence or accuracy of
URLs for external or third-party internet websites referred to in this publication
and does not guarantee that any content on such websites is, or will remain,
accurate or appropriate.

....

Every effort has been made in preparing this book to provide accurate and up-to-date information that is in accord with accepted standards and practice at the time of publication. Although case histories are drawn from actual cases, every effort has been made to disguise the identities of the individuals involved. Nevertheless, the authors, editors, and publishers can make no warranties that the information contained herein is totally free from error, not least because clinical standards are constantly changing through research and regulation. The authors, editors, and publishers therefore disclaim all liability for direct or consequential damages resulting from the use of material contained in this book. Readers are strongly advised to pay careful attention to information provided by the manufacturer of any drugs or equipment that they plan to use.

To Gill, Reza, Sara, for your everlasting support. And my parents for believing in me.

To Becky, Lucy, Rosie, Molly, Jack and our two Ridgebacks Atilla and Odin, a constant source of strength.

Contents

Contributors

Amjid Ali FRCS Tr&Orth
Consultant Orthopaedic Shoulder & Elbow Surgeon
Sheffield Teaching Hospitals, Sheffield, UK

Fazal Ali FRCS (Eng), FRCS Tr&Orth
Consultant Orthopaedic Surgeon
Chesterfield Royal Hospital, Chesterfield, UK

Armughan Azhar FRCS Tr&Orth
Locum Consultant Orthopaedic Surgeon
The Queen Elizabeth Hospital, King's Lynn,
UK

L. Chris Bainbridge FRCS
Consultant Orthopaedic Hand Surgeon
Royal Derby Hospital, Derby, UK

Paul A. Banaszkiewicz FRCS (Tr & Orth)
Consultant Orthopaedic Surgeon & Visiting
Professor, Northumbria University
Queen Elizabeth Hospital and North East
NHS Surgical Centre (NENSC), Gateshead,
UK

Vijay Bhalaik FRCS Tr&Orth
Consultant Hand & Upper Limb Surgeon
Wirral University Teaching Hospital NHS
Foundation Trust, Merseyside, UK

Derek Bickerstaff MD, FRCS
Consultant Knee Surgeon
One Health Group,
Sheffield, UK

Meg Birks FRCS Tr&Orth, Dip Hand Surg
Consultant Orthopaedic Hand Surgeon
Sheffield Teaching Hospitals, Sheffield, UK

Caroline M. Blakey FRCS Tr&Orth
Consultant Paediatric Orthopaedic Surgeon
Sheffield Children's Hospital, Sheffield, UK

Simon Booker FRCS Tr&Orth
Consultant Orthopaedic Surgeon
Sheffield Teaching Hospitals, Sheffield, UK

Stephen Bostock FRCS Orth
Consultant Orthopaedic Hand Surgeon
Sheffield Teaching Hospitals, Sheffield, UK

Kate Brown FRCS Tr&Orth
Consultant Hand and PNI Surgeon
Pulvertaft Hand Centre, Royal Derby Hospital,
Derby, UK

Jeevan Chandrasenan FRCS Tr&Orth
Consultant Orthopaedic Surgeon
Chesterfield Royal Hospital, Chesterfield, UK

Charlene Chin-See DM (Orthopaedics), MBBS,
B.Med.Sci
Senior Resident in Paediatric Orthopaedics
Bustamante Hospital for Children, Kingston,
Jamaica

Neil Chiverton FRCS Tr&Orth
Consultant Orthopaedic Spinal Surgeon
Sheffield Teaching Hospitals, Sheffield, UK

Jonathan A. Clamp FRCS Tr&Orth
Consultant Spinal Surgeon
University Hospitals of Derby and Burton NHS
Foundation Trust, Derby, UK

Daine O. Clarke DM (Orthopaedics), MBBS,
B.Med.Sci
Consultant Orthopaedic and Spinal Surgeon
University Hospital of the West Indies, Kingston,
Jamaica

Ashley Cole FRCS Tr&Orth
Consultant Orthopaedic Spine Surgeon
Sheffield Children's Hospital, Sheffield, UK

James A. Fernandes FRCS Tr&Orth
Consultant Paediatric Orthopaedic Surgeon
Sheffield Children's Hospital, Sheffield, UK

Michael Gale FRCS Tr&Orth
Consultant Orthopaedic Hand Surgeon
Sherwood Forest Hospitals, Nottinghamshire, UK

Joe Garcia FRCS Tr&Orth
Consultant Orthopaedic Hand Surgeon
Chesterfield Royal Hospital, Chesterfield, UK

Nick Harris FRCS Tr&Orth
Consultant Orthopaedic Surgeon,
Professor, Leeds Beckett University
Spire Hospital, Leeds, UK

Antonia Isaacson PhD, FRCS Tr&Orth
Consultant Orthopaedic Spinal Surgeon
James Cook University Hospital, Middlesbrough, UK

Stan Jones FRCS Tr&Orth
Consultant Orthopaedic Surgeon
Al Ahli Hospital, Doha, Qatar

Simon Kay FRCS (Plas)
Professor of Plastic Surgery
Leeds Teaching Hospitals, NHS Foundation Trust,
Leeds, UK

Tom Kurien PhD, MSc, FRCS Tr&Orth
Knee Reconstruction Fellow
Royal Devon and Exeter Hospital, Exeter, UK

David Limb FRCSEd (Orth)
Consultant Orthopaedic Shoulder & Elbow
Surgeon
Leeds Teaching Hospitals, NHS Foundation Trust,
Leeds, UK

A. L. Rex Michael FRCS Tr&Orth
Consultant Orthopaedic Spine Surgeon
Sheffield Teaching Hospitals, Sheffield, UK

Yulanda Myint FRCS Tr&Orth
Consultant Orthopaedic Surgeon
Nottingham University Hospitals NHS Trust,
Nottingham, UK

Jimmy Ng FRCS Tr&Orth
Specialist Registrar
Royal Derby Hospital, Derby, UK

Oghor Obakponovwe FRCS Tr&Orth
Consultant Orthopaedic Surgeon
St Richards Hospital, Chichester, UK

Karen Robinson FRCS Tr&Orth
Consultant Orthopaedic and Trauma Surgeon
Sheffield Teaching Hospitals, Sheffield, UK

Simon J. Robinson FRCS Tr&Orth
Consultant Upper Limb Surgeon
Wirral University Teaching Hospital NHS
Foundation Trust, Merseyside, UK

Shantanu Shahane FRCS Tr&Orth
Consultant Orthopaedic Shoulder & Elbow Surgeon
Chesterfield Royal Hospital, Chesterfield, UK

Ravikumar Holalu Shankarlingegowda MBBS, MS
Orth
Assistant Professor Orthopaedics
Mandya Institute of Medical Sciences, Mandya, India

Faiz Shivji FRCS Tr&Orth
Knee Fellow
University Hospitals Coventry and Warwickshire
NHS Trust, Coventry, UK

David Stanley FRCS
Consultant Shoulder and Elbow Surgeon
Parkhead Consultancy, Sheffield, UK

Ian Stockley MD, FRCS
Emeritus Consultant Orthopaedic Surgeon,
Honorary Professor Sheffield Hallam University
Sheffield Teaching Hospitals, Sheffield, UK

James Tomlinson FRCS Tr&Orth
Consultant Orthopaedic Spinal Surgeon
Sheffield Teaching Hospitals, Sheffield, UK

Shashikanth Vokkaleri MBBS, MS Orth
Consultant Orthopaedic Surgeon
Trust in Hospital, Bangalore India

Shomari Webster-Prince DM (Orthopaedics),
MBBS, B.Med.Sci
Paediatric Orthopaedic Fellow
Sheffield Children's Hospital, Sheffield, UK

John E. D. Wright FRCS Tr&Orth
Consultant Upper Limb Surgeon
Chesterfield Royal Hospital, Chesterfield, UK

Preface to 3rd edition

Since the second edition was published, we have received numerous positive comments and reviews on how this book has helped the reader. There have also been suggestions for improvement, all of which have been taken on board. This has resulted in some distinct changes to the content and layout of this third edition. Despite that, it is essential that this book will continue to teach the reader clinical examination in a systematic manner, which was the strength of the previous edition.

The summary has been brought to the beginning of the chapter to help the more junior reader understand the subject. For other readers an "Advanced Corner" has been added at the end of the chapter. Also, wherever relevant, the anatomical basis of each test has been described within the chapter.

Virtually all the pictures demonstrating clinical examination techniques have been changed, with an emphasis on diversity. More than 50 new illustrations have been included and 5 chapters have been added which comprise more than 80 clinical case examples showing how clinical examination will help in the assessment and management of various conditions. This includes a chapter on orthopaedic conditions in the developing world which we hope will be useful for our international readership.

The Covid-19 pandemic has had both a positive and negative effect on this book. For an entire year it provided me with periods of 'self-isolation' and living apart from the rest of my family where I could dedicate the hundreds and hundreds of hours needed to completely revise this book. Conversely, social distancing made it difficult to obtain the photographs demonstrating the clinical examination techniques. Fortunately, most of these were taken 3 weeks before the first lockdown in the UK. For the remaining photos I had to use members within my own family and work 'bubbles'.

It has been a great honour for me to have Professor Bruce Reider writing the foreword for this edition. I used Bruce's own book when I was training and it was by reading his book that I was inspired to learn and perfect the art of clinical examination. It has been a privilege to have since met Bruce and to be involved in various projects with him.

Orthopaedic Examination Techniques 3 Ed has been a labour of love, but it is the hope of myself, and Nick Harris, that readers continue to find this book user-friendly and informative and that it helps them throughout their career in orthopaedics.

We have both said this may be the last edition before we 'hang up our boots'. But let us see what the future brings. In the meanwhile, the hunt is on for us to pass over the baton to the next generation!

Fazal Ali

Foreword to 2nd edition

I am pleased to be asked to write the foreword for the second edition of *Examination Techniques in Orthopaedics*, coedited by Mr Nick Harris and Mr Fazal Ali. The first edition of this textbook was one of the bestselling orthopaedic books in the United Kingdom for almost a decade. This second edition is likely to at least equal that success. So often in the world of orthopaedic surgery we jump to advanced imaging and forget about the importance of the examination. This is clearly a mistake and has caused many errors in clinical judgement. Therefore, careful review of orthopaedic examination as presented in this textbook is critical for all orthopaedic surgeons, young and old alike. This book provides a complete repository of all examinations, beginning with general principle and proceeding literally from head to toe, to include paediatric examination. This is truly an excellent book and likely will be the gold standard to which examination textbooks are compared. It is my pleasure to write this foreword. I think you will enjoy this textbook and it should stay on your shelf until the third edition is available. I give it my strongest endorsement and look forward to studying it myself.

Mark D. Miller, MD

S. Ward Cassells Professor of Orthopaedic Surgery

Division Head, Sports Medicine

Team Physician, James Madison University

JBJS Deputy Editor for Sports Medicine

Director, Miller Review Course

Charlottesville, VA, USA

Foreword to 3rd edition

Is the orthopaedic physical examination outmoded? Considering the continued refinement of magnetic resonance and other imaging techniques, an orthopaedic surgeon might be tempted to assume that diagnostic methods that require observing, palpating and manipulating the patient are no longer necessary. Indeed, a colleague of mine reports that many patients who come to him for a second opinion are surprised when he examines them, because the 'first opinion' surgeon never did. Apparently, there is a sizable number of practitioners who feel that a modern imaging study is all they need to arrive at a treatment recommendation.

On the contrary, I would propose that the advent of contemporary imaging techniques makes the mundane history and physical examination all the more important. Modern imaging methods are wonderful, but they often uncover findings that may not be clinically relevant. The orthopaedic literature is full of studies that document a plethora of imaging abnormalities in asymptomatic individuals, especially athletes and older folks. In symptomatic patients, multiple imaging abnormalities may be present when only one of them is responsible for the patient's complaint. An accurate history and physical examination are vital for selecting the correct treatment.

Before the actual examination begins, a clinician must take the time to elicit a complete history from the patient. Most orthopaedic problems have a characteristic pattern that can be discerned by listening to the patient. Even when evaluating trauma, the history is important. Patients may reveal areas of injury that might otherwise be overlooked, and their description of the mechanism of the injury may point out the structures most likely to have been damaged. A good history is the prelude to a focused and fruitful physical examination.

This excellent volume, now in its third edition, takes the reader through this process one step at a time. The first portion of the book is organized by body part from top to bottom. Each chapter starts with an outline of the entire examination, then proceeds to a section on the important historical points that will allow the examiner to narrow the diagnostic possibilities before the examination begins. It then continues logically through the examination itself, from inspection to palpation to active and passive motion. Finally, the chapter ends with advanced tests that will be of particular interest to the specialist. Throughout, a profusion of detailed photographs supplements the verbal descriptions in the text. References are provided for the reader who wants to learn more about the evidence behind the various examination manoeuvres.

The second portion of the book includes an outstanding variety of clinical cases to illustrate the pathological findings in many orthopaedic and rheumatological conditions. The authors have taken great pains to collect photographs that dramatically document many common and some uncommon abnormalities that a clinician may encounter in the course of practice. The final chapter, 'Orthopaedic Cases in the Developing World', is a unique contribution that will prove valuable to clinicians wherever they may practice.

The orthopaedic examination is vast and complex. A newcomer to orthopaedics should not expect to assimilate the contents of this comprehensive text in one read. This is a book to be thoroughly studied and then kept handy for ready reference. As experience accumulates, readers will build their own memory bank and begin to appreciate subtleties that recall cases from prior experience.

I would like to congratulate Messrs. Ali and Harris on the completion of this excellent text. Having written a similar book myself, I can readily appreciate the huge amount of work and meticulous attention to detail that goes into such a volume, which can only be accomplished as a labour of love. It is an honour to have been asked to write this foreword. Fazal and Nick, please accept my best wishes for the success of this magnificent volume.

Bruce Reider MD

Professor of Orthopaedic Surgery, Emeritus
University of Chicago
Editor-in-Chief
American Journal of Sports Medicine
Orthopaedic Journal of Sports Medicine.

Chicago, Illinois, USA
January 2022

Acknowledgements

Firstly, we would like to acknowledge the comments about the second edition, both positive and negative, without which the drive to construct a perfect third edition would not have been as crucial. We thank Nick Dunton, now retired, and Katy Nardoni from Cambridge University Press for guiding us through this process.

We would like to thank Jeevan Chandrasenan, organiser of the *Chesterfield, Sheffield and Derby Clinical Examination course* and Paul Banaszkiewicz, organiser of the *Postgraduate Orthopaedics FRCS Revision courses*, for the funds they provided to help pay for the photography session and the illustrations. Without their generosity the production of this edition would have been difficult.

Thank you to Shane Nicoll, Claire Chadwick, Tony Hadfield and Kathryn Whittle for utilising their talents and being our models at the photo shoot. Philip Wagstaff again insisted he modelled for us in his Brachial Plexus chapter. Philip is a legend!

This photo shoot was expertly conducted in our fracture clinic waiting room on a Sunday just before lockdown by Jessica Findlow of *Northern Star Photography*. Jess had to use all her skills to photograph 'models' who were not used to being in front of a camera.

Covid-19 and lockdown meant that because of social distancing rules we were unable to use models for those images we missed on the official photography day. This meant that secretary Leanne Heath within our work bubble had to fill in. In addition, Reza Ali, Sara Ali and friend Louis Govignon were also drafted in. We are hoping that they will all enjoy their new fame!

In this edition we added more than 50 illustrations with the hope that it would enhance the text. For this we thank Surita Devi (www.freelancer.com/u/surita verma) in India who expertly and patiently followed instructions via WhatsApp in order to meet our requirements.

Finally, clinical examination is an acquired skill. Knowledge gained from a textbook is not complete without the guidance of the expert tutor. For this we would like to thank the following consultants and experts in clinical examination who for years have shared their skills and helped refine the techniques in our book. They have lectured and demonstrated these techniques on national courses and throughout the world. This is a great group of highly talented individuals:

Shantanu Shahane, Nick Phillips, Amjid Ali, Ben Gooding, Stephen Bostock, Joe Garcia, Alex Baker, Becky Aspinall, Paul Banaszkiewicz, James Williams, Paul Haslam, Stan Jones, Chris Blundell, John Wright, James Fernandes, Ashley Cole, Sanjeev Madan, Rex Michael, Irwin Lasrado, Simon Royston, Osmond Thomas, Mark Flowers, Steve Giles, Kevin Wembridge, Mick Dennison and Saeed Qaimkhani.

Fazal Ali
Nick Harris

About the authors

Fazal Ali has a special interest in soft tissue knee problems in the child and adult. He is an Honorary Senior Lecturer at the University of Sheffield and Honorary Secretary of BOSTAA (British Orthopaedic Sports Trauma and Arthroscopy Association). He is an accomplished teacher of clinical examination and has published and lectured on his examination techniques worldwide. He has won numerous regional and national awards for training and is a 'Lifetime Trainer of the Year' for South Yorkshire. He is a senior examiner for the UK and International FRCS Tr&Orth examinations. Fazal Ali also serves on the panel of examiners in developing countries with the view that this would help advance the standard of orthopaedic training and care worldwide.

Nick Harris has special interest in Foot & Ankle Surgery, Trauma and Sports Injuries. He is a Visiting Professor of Sports Medicine at Leeds Beckett University. His current research projects include long term function after achilles tendon rupture, novel amino acid supplements, and ankle syndesmotic injuries in athletes. He has produced over 100 original publications and presentations. He was the Orthopaedic Lead Designer of the mobile-bearing Rebalance Total Ankle Replacement. Approximately 3000 have been implanted globally with 90% survivorship on the Swedish Joint Registry. In 2019, Nick Harris was awarded North of England Surgeon of the Year.

General Principles of Orthopaedic Clinical Examination

Oghor Obakponovwe, Stanley Jones and Fazal Ali

Summary of General Orthopaedic Examination Principles

1. Respect your patient and ensure that he or she is comfortable.
2. Give clear instructions on what you want the patient to do.
3. Expose the region to be examined fully yet maintain dignity.
4. Observe not only the region being examined but your patient as a whole.
5. Always compare both limbs.
6. When palpating a region remember to look at the patient's face for signs of pain or discomfort.
7. Assess both active and passive range of movement.
8. Examine the joint above and the joint below and perform a neurovascular assessment.
9. Special tests can be used to help elicit or confirm findings.
10. Do not cause pain.

Clinical examination is an art that has to be learnt, as it does not come naturally. Most clinicians refine their examination routine with experience and practice. All patients must be respected, made to feel at ease and assured of their confidentiality and dignity.

A detailed history should always be taken, followed by an appropriate clinical examination.

It is often assumed that clinical examination begins on the couch. This should not be the case, as significant information can be gained by observing the patient as they enter the room for a consultation or as you approach them.

Consider using a chaperone, especially if examining the shoulder, spine or hip. If the patient is seated, they should be asked to stand as this is usually the first part of any orthopaedic clinical examination, except when the hand is being examined. You will observe

whether the patient is tall, short, obese, thin, ill, well, energetic or lethargic. Observe if there is pain or if there are stigmata of orthopaedic disease such as blue sclera (osteogenesis imperfecta), café-au-lait spots (neurofibromatosis), multiple exostoses (diaphyscal aclasis, Figure 1.1) etc.

In addition to the patient's gait pattern, the presence of limb deformities, the use of walking aids and orthotic braces or prosthetic devices should also be noted. This is particularly relevant when examining the lower limbs and spine.

Examples of gait patterns include:

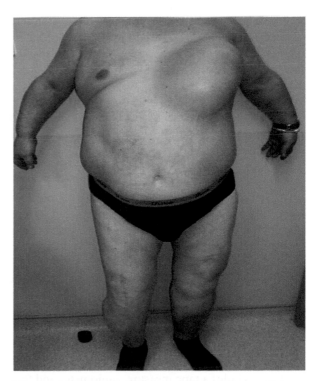

Figure 1.1 Patient with diaphyseal aclasis (hereditary multiple exostosis). Note the short limbs, bowing of the forearm, swellings around the knees and the large tumour in the left pectoral region.

- Antalgic gait caused by pain stemming from the sole of the foot to the hip. The stance phase of the affected limb is shortened, lessening the loading time of the painful limb.
- High stepping gait is seen in patients with hereditary sensorimotor neuropathy or those with a foot drop.
- Shuffling gait is typical of neurological conditions, such as Parkinson's disease, and frequently leads to an increased risk of falls secondary to loss of balance and coordination.

The clinical signs and associated deformities of some clinical conditions, e.g. hallux valgus, may be so characteristic that the diagnosis can be made without a full clinical examination. However, this is not always the case, and an examination carried out in a systematic manner not only instils confidence in the patient but also avoids missing important and salient clinical signs.

The system of *look, feel, move* advocated by Apley[1] is recommend, although when examining the wrist, elbow and foot and ankle *look, move, feel* is advised by the authors.

The part of the musculoskeletal system being examined must be suitably exposed; for example, when examining the shoulder, the patient should be undressed to the waist. The patient's sense of modesty should always be preserved. The use of a strapless garment or appropriate screen to cover sensitive areas should be practised and a chaperone considered for every examination. The patient must be given clear instructions on which clothes to take off. The ease or difficulty of undressing and any associated pain experienced whilst doing so are useful information that help in the assessment. In addition, it is advisable to expose both limbs for comparison even though only one limb may be affected.

Examination of paediatric patients requires skill and flexibility. Children are not small adults. Remember to look at the parents as the patient may be presenting with an inherited clinical condition. Involve the parents as much as possible. Useful information can be acquired by observing and adopting methods of play rather than using a rigid system of examination as previously suggested.

Equipment

The basic equipment required for orthopaedic examination includes a tape measure, goniometer and tendon hammer. In addition, a pen, key and coin are required for assessment of hand function (Figure 1.2).

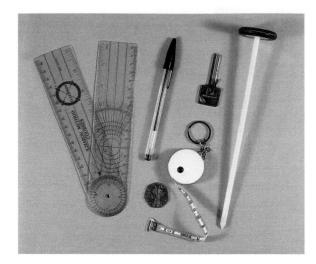

Figure 1.2 Equipment required for examination.

Look

Inspection is an integral part of a physical examination. It begins the sequence and should always be undertaken before palpation and movement. It also forms an important part of palpation and movement.

It is important to look at the part being examined from different angles, e.g. the shoulder joint should be observed from the front, back and side and the axilla must also be inspected. Inspection of the foot is not complete without examining the sole and between the toes. Whilst observing a limb, any scars, skin colour changes, swelling, bruising, muscle wasting and alteration in shape or posture are noted. Skin colour changes may be the result of infection, vascular compromise or pain syndrome.

Scars may be the result of injury or previous surgery or infection and may be a clue to the underlying problem (Figure 1.3).

Swelling may be localised or diffuse. Localised swelling and its location with respect to the underlying anatomical structures usually give a clue as to the possible cause, e.g. a well-defined swelling in the radiovolar aspect of a wrist is likely to be a ganglion, and a swelling on the medial joint line of the knee is likely to be a meniscal cyst.

Diffuse swelling confined to a joint may be the result of:

- Synovial fluid from an inflammatory process such as rheumatoid arthritis or osteoarthritis

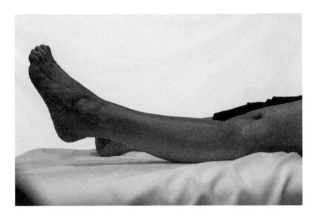

Figure 1.3 The location of scars is a clue to the underlying injury or surgery. This patient has a transverse scar, which may indicate damage to the extensor mechanism. In this case, the patient had a direct impact injury which resulted in a lacerated patella tendon which was repaired and a posterior cruciate ligament (PCL) injury that was untreated. Hence, there is recurvatum as she tries to straight leg raise.

- Blood (haemarthrosis) from a recent injury, blood coagulation defect or medication such as warfarin
- Pus from an infection

Diffuse swelling affecting part or an *entire limb* in a patient with orthopaedic injuries or recent orthopaedic intervention, particularly pelvic and lower limb surgeries, should arouse a differential diagnosis of a venous thromboembolic event, which warrants further investigations.

Bruising is usually the result of trauma to tissues owing to a recent injury or surgery.

Muscle wasting may arise from disuse because of pain, other abnormality or muscle denervation. Muscle wasting is quantified by comparing the affected limb with the normal limb or by measuring the circumference of the limb at a fixed point from a bony landmark.

Alteration in shape or posture may be caused by a congenital anomaly, skeletal dysplasia, joint degeneration or the sequelae of a previous injury.

Finally, inspection should conclude by looking for and describing any orthosis or walking aid.

In clinical examinations at a junior level, it is desirable to describe both positive and negative findings. In more senior examinations, inspection should still be complete, but is performed much more rapidly with only positive and important negative findings expressed. Examiners may become agitated if senior candidates spend too much time on inspection.

Feel

Irrespective of the joint being examined palpation should always be carried out in a systematic manner with reference to the anatomic landmarks. The details of how to carry out a satisfactory palpation of the various joints are discussed in the relevant chapters, but an essential aspect of palpation is that the examiner must not only look at the joint being examined but also look at the patient's face to appreciate any areas of tenderness (Figure 1.4).

Ensure that hands are washed or antiseptic gel is used. Rubbing your hands together to warm them makes palpation more comfortable for the patient.

Some joints, such as the hip, spine and shoulder, are deeper and therefore significant information may not be gained from palpation compared to the more superficial joints such as the hand, elbow, knee, foot and ankle. By knowing the surface anatomy of these joints, tenderness over the relevant areas may lead to the diagnosis. For example, tenderness over the lateral epicondyle of the elbow indicates tennis elbow and tenderness over the medial joint line of the knee may indicate a medial meniscus tear.

If a *bony lump* is felt, there are particular aspects of the lump that must be described: site, size, consistency, margin, tenderness, multiplicity.[1] Each of these features can give particular information with regards to the diagnosis and if benign or malignant. For example, a lump nearer to the joint is more likely to be a tumour compared to a mid-shaft lump; a lump with a well-defined margin is more likely to be benign; a benign tumour is usually hard, whereas a malignant one can give the impression that it can be indented; multiple bony lumps are uncommon, but if present can suggest hereditary multiple exostosis or even Ollier's disease.

Sensory Testing

There are various methods of testing sensory deficit in a peripheral nerve lesion. There is usually overlap between the nerves, but mapping an area of sensory loss is usually determined firstly by light touch. This is usually performed with a piece of cotton wool with the patient closing their eyes (Figure 1.5). A Semmes–Weinstein monofilament can be used for light touch; this is especially useful in the foot, where it has been shown to be a reliable and specific method of assessing protective sensation.[2]

Following light touch, sharp sensation with a pin can be assessed. It should be noted that following

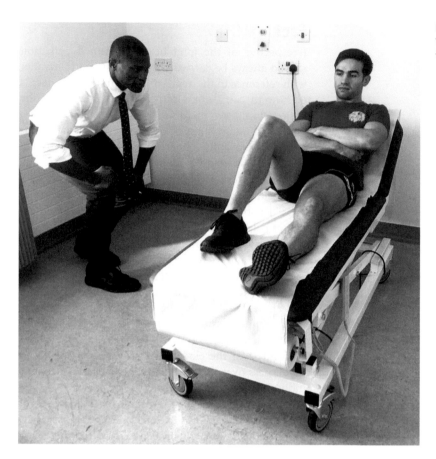

Figure 1.4 Observe the patient closely whilst examining. Look at the joint or limb and always remember to observe the face.

a peripheral nerve injury, pinprick sensation usually returns before light touch.

In the hand, where the tactile ability of the hand is so refined, *two-point discrimination* is a useful way of assessing nerve deficit. Normally someone can differentiate two sharp points placed 5 mm apart. In performing this test, the patient closes his or her eyes and is asked whether they can feel one or two points by randomly pressing one or two tips onto the skin. If the patient is unable to discriminate the two tips placed 5 mm apart, this distance is then increased and the test repeated (Figure 1.6).

Move

Both active and passive range of movement of the joint being examined should be assessed. It is advisable to carry out active range of movement before passive as this gives the examiner an idea of the functional range of movement and any associated pain. The patient must be given clear instruction or a demonstration of the range of movement to be

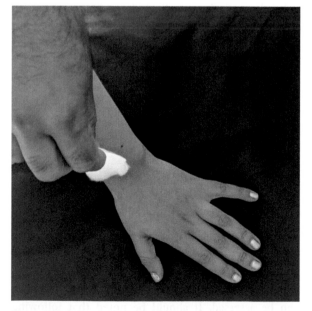

Figure 1.5 Cotton bud used for light touch.

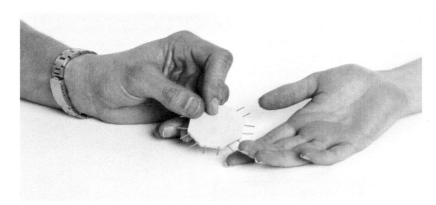

Figure 1.6 Testing two-point discrimination.

assessed. Demonstration is sometimes the best method of communicating to the patient.

It is always advisable to compare the range of movement of the symptomatic with the asymptomatic or normal joint, and the range achieved should be recorded in degrees as measured by a goniometer.

With regards to movement, some points should be noted:

- Sometimes it may not be possible to assess active range of movement in certain situations (such as with a very young child or a patient with cerebral palsy or neurological disturbance.
- Tendon, muscle or nerve injury may preclude active movement, and in these situations only passive movement can be assessed. However, be aware that the patient may use gravity or a trick movement to move the affected joint, thus misleading the examiner.
- In certain conditions, such as following injury or surgery, a tendon may heal at a longer length. Here there may be a difference in active and passive movements. For example, in a chronic quadriceps rupture when the patient is asked to straight leg raise, there may be an extensor lag that is only evident after passive extension of the knee joint is performed.
- Excessive passive joint movement or movement in abnormal planes may be the result of generalised ligamentous laxity or ligament/bony abnormality. Generalised ligamentous laxity can be assessed fully using Beighton's scoring system (Figure 1.7). A total score greater than or equal to 4 indicates hypermobility. In a child, this may be a score of 5 or 6.[3]
- A joint that is grossly degenerate may have limited active or passive range of movement.

- Complete loss of (active and passive) movement may be the result of previous surgery, e.g. in a patient who has had a previous arthrodesis.

Table 1.1 summarises normal joint range of movement and acceptable positions of surgical fusion.[4,5,6]

Power

Muscle strength is an integral part of the neurological assessment and is best carried out in a systematic manner from proximal to distal and recorded using the Muscle Research Council (MRC) scale (Table 1.2). It is important to understand how to differentiate between grade 2 and grade 3 by eliminating gravity (Figures 1.8 and 1.9). In general, this can be accomplished by examining the joint movements in a plane that is 90 degrees from that in which gravity acts.

Correctly identifying the signs of a neurological lesion may be important in helping to distinguish between an upper motor neuron (UMN) lesion and a lower motor neuron (LMN) lesion. In an UMN lesion paralysis affects movement rather than muscle. Muscle wasting is slight and usually due to disuse, whereas in an LMN lesion the wasting is pronounced.

Table 1.3 provides a summary of the differences between the two.

Gait

It is important that normal gait be understood when examining a patient, especially with regards to the lower limb and the spine. It is only then can pathology that affects the gait be picked up.

The prerequisites for normal gait are:

- Stability in stance
- Foot clearance in swing
- Pre-positioning of the ankle in swing

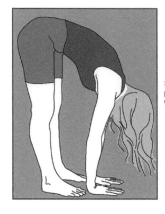

Figure 1.7 Assessing Beighton's score. Note that four pairs of tests are passive and one test is active (spine).

MCP, metacarpophalangeal

Score one point if you bend and place your hands flat on the floor without bending your knees.

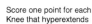

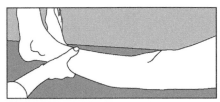

Score one point for each Knee that hyperextends

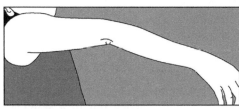

Score one point for each elbow that hyperextends

Score one point for each thumb that will bend back backwards to touch the forearm.

Score one point for each hand when you can bend the little finger MCP joint back beyond 90°

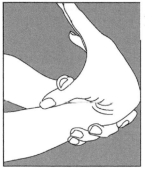

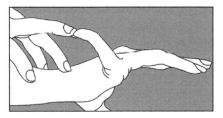

- Adequate step length
- Energy conservation

When describing the gait of a patient, this can only sound proficient if certain definitions are understood. The important ones are explained below. In addition, Figure 1.10 illustrates the varied positions of the parts of the lower limb through the gait cycle.

Gait cycle: Point in time from initial contact of one foot to initial contact of the same foot.

Step: From initial contact of one foot to the initial contact of the contralateral foot.

Stride: Period from initial contact of one foot to initial contact of the same foot. Therefore, there are two steps in a stride.

Cadence: Number of steps per minute.

Stance: Period when the foot is on the ground. It starts with initial contact and finishes with toe off. Stance makes up 60% of the gait cycle.

Swing: Period when the foot is off the ground. It starts at toe off and finishes with initial contact. Swing makes up 40% of the gait cycle.

During stance phase, three foot and ankle rockers can be described in sequence (Figure 1.11). In the first rocker (heel rocker), there is initial contact with heel strike followed by plantarflexion of the ankle. In the second rocker (ankle rocker), there is tibial advancement over the foot achieved by ankle dorsiflexion. In the third rocker (forefoot rocker), there is

Table 1.1 Average range of movement (ROM) of some of the joints in the body. The acceptable positions of surgical fusion for the various joints are also shown.

	Range of motion	Position of surgical fusion
Cervical spine	Flexion: 80° Extension: 50° lateral flexion: 45° rotation: 80°	
Thoraco-lumbar spine	flexion(thoracic): 45° flexion (lumbar): 60° lateral flexion: 30° rotation (thoracic): 40°	
Shoulder	Flexion: 165° Extension: 60° Abduction: 170° internal rotation: 70° external rotation: 100°	20°–25° (30° avg) 15°–20° (30° avg) 40°–50° (30° avg)
Elbow	Flexion: 140° Extension: up to −10° Supination: 80° Pronation: 75°	90° if unilateral, 110° vs 65° if bilateral
Wrist	Dorsiflexion: 75° palmar flexion: 75° radial deviation: 20° ulnar deviation: 35°	10°–20°
Hip *at 90° flexion	Flexion: 120° Extension: 10° Abduction: 45° Adduction: 25° internal rotation*: 45° external rotation* : 50°	20°–30° 0°–5° 5°–10°
Knee	Flexion: 135°	10°–15° (flexion) 0°–7° (valgus)
Ankle	Dorsiflexion: 20° Plantarflexion: 50°	neutral (dorsiflexion) 5° (hindfoot valgus) 5°–10° (external rotation)
Foot	Inversion: 20° Eversion: 10°	
Thumb	IP joint flexion: 80° IP joint extension: 15° MCP joint flexion: 55° opposition- able to touch tip of little finger	15°–30° 20°–25°
Fingers	MCP joint flexion: 90° MPJ passive hyperextension: up to 40° PIP joint flexion: 100° DIP joint flexion: 80°	index 25°, long 30°, ring 35°, small 40° index 40°, long 45°, ring 50°, small 55° 10°
Great toe	MTP joint flexion: 40° MTP joint extension: 70° IP joint flexion: 60° IP joint extension: 0°	 10°–15° dorsiflexion; also slight valgus/neutral rotation

DIP, distal interphalangeal; IP, interphalangeal; MCP, metacarpophalangeal; MTP, metatarsophalangeal; PIP proximal interphalangeal

Table 1.2 MRC grading for motor power

Grade	
0	No muscle contraction
1	Flicker of contraction
2	Movement with gravity eliminated
3	Movement against gravity
4	Movement against gravity and some resistance
5	Full power

heel rise caused by forefoot dorsiflexion and ankle plantarflexion.

In children, there are some differences in gait that are more evident in the younger child:

- Wider base of support
- Flat foot strike instead of heel strike
- Greater knee flexion in stance
- Leg externally rotated in swing
- Cadence higher
- Absence of reciprocal arm swing

As the child gets older, these become more like the adult pattern. For example, heel strike, knee flexion and external rotation become adult pattern by 2 years. Walking base and arm swing by 4 years.

Further Examination

Special Tests

In addition to the triad of *look, feel, move,* other tests specific to the part being examined may be required to enable the examiner to reach a diagnosis, e.g. the anterior draw or Lachman's test for anterior cruciate ligament insufficiency. The various tests will be discussed later in this book in the respective chapters. Each test has a variable sensitivity and specificity. Table 1.4 shows some of these values. It can be seen that very few clinical tests are reliable on their own. A combination of clinical tests may be of greater diagnostic value, e.g. combining Neer's and Hawkins–Kennedy tests to make the diagnosis of subacromial impingement.[18]

The examiner must be prepared to examine the joint above and below the main joint being examined, as the patient may be presenting with referred pain. For example, a patient with a slipped upper femoral epiphysis may present with knee pain, and failure to examine the hip joint will cause the examiner to miss the diagnosis. In addition, pathology in one joint may directly affect adjacent joints.

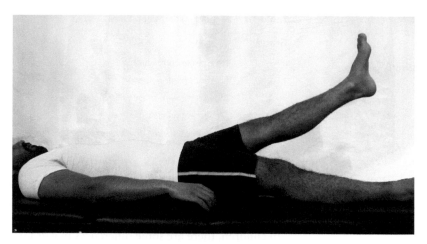

Figure 1.8 Testing MRC grade 3 motor power of the quadriceps.

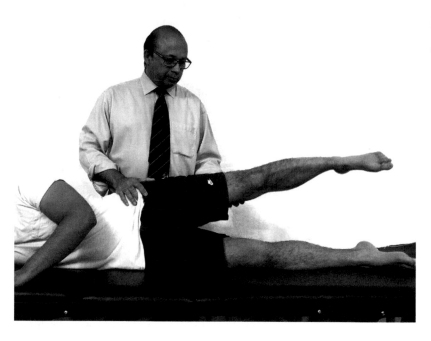

Figure 1.9 Testing MRC grade 2 motor power of the quadriceps with the effect of gravity eliminated.

Neurovascular Assessment

A neurovascular assessment is also an important aspect of any examination. It is important to ascertain if there is a true neurological deficit or if neurological symptoms are mimicking musculoskeletal symptoms. In some instances (e.g. in patients with nerve palsy), it may be necessary to undertake this assessment early on in the examination after inspection.

In the neurological assessment, it is not good enough to assess only power. Tone must also be assessed because it is possible to have reduced power in the presence of either increased or decreased tone.

The tendon reflex is also regarded as a reliable pointer to the segmental level of a dysfunction.

Vascular symptoms such as vascular claudication may mimic musculoskeletal symptoms.

Advanced Corner

We all may be faced with clinical scenarios that challenge us, and for these it is important not only to stick to first principles but also to have a degree of flexibility in order to adapt our examination routine to elicit clinical signs and come to logical conclusions.

Table 1.3 The characteristics of upper motor neuron and lower motor neuron lesions

	Upper motor neuron	Lower motor neuron
Site of lesion	Brain and spinal cord (above ant. horn cells)	Anterior horn cells, nerve root and peripheral nerve
Muscle wasting	Muscle mass maintained (some disuse atrophy)	Rapid muscle wasting
Tone	Increased	Decreased
Power	Decreased	Decreased
Tendon reflexes	Increased	Decreased
Pathological reflexes	Plantar response upgoing (Babinski's sign) Abdominal reflex absent (depending on spinal level)	Plantar response normal or absent Abdominal reflex present
Fasciculations/fibrillations	Absent	Could be present

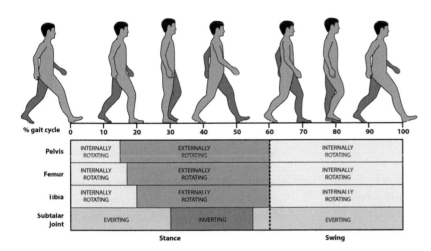

Figure 1.10 Illustration showing the position of the ankle, pelvis, femur, tibia and subtalar joints through the gait cycle.

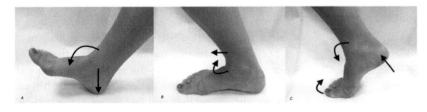

Figure 1.11 The three rockers. (A) Heel rocker with heel strike followed by ankle plantarflexion. (B) Ankle rocker with tibial advancement achieved by ankle dorsiflexion. (C) Forefoot rocker where heel raise is caused by forefoot dorsiflexion and ankle plantarflexion.

Clinical tips for these scenarios are invaluable, but in some cases the clinical presentation may be one that you have not encountered before, and these require you, the clinician, to think on your feet and formulate an appropriate examination sequence. It always helps if you have thought about these situations beforehand!

The following are a few examples of special scenarios where prior consideration would allow the candidate to feel more at ease with the clinical examination:

- A patient with significant abduction deformity of the hip will present with apparent lengthening of the affected side with compensatory pelvic tilt, tiptoeing, or shoe raise of the contralateral side, or with bending of the ipsilateral knee. There is a 2.5 cm of apparent lengthening for every 10 degrees of abduction deformity. The reverse is true

9

Table 1.4 The sensitivity and specificity of some of the common clinical tests and signs. Note that these values are very variable in the literature therefore studies showing the average values have been chosen.

Test	Sensitivity	Specificity
Neer's sign[7]	.76	.47
Hawkins–Kennedy test[7]	.75	.44
Speed's test[8]	.63	.58
Scarf (cross adduction) test[9]	.25	.80
O'Brien's test[10]	.63	.73
Kirk Watson test[11]	.69	.66
Tinel's sign (at wrist)[12]	.50	.77
Phalen's test[12]	.68	.73
Trendelenburg test[13]	.73	.77
Lachman's test[14]	.85	.94
Anterior draw test[14]	.55	.92
Pivot shift test[14]	.24	.98
McMurray's test[15]	.55	.77
Thessaly test[15]	.89	.97
Anterolateral ankle impingement test[16]	.95	.88
Straight leg raise (SLR)[17]	.52	.89
Allen's test[19]	.73	.91

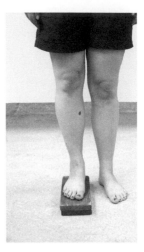

Figure 1.12 Blocks of varying thicknesses can be used to assess limb length discrepancy. These are most useful when the shortening is coming from below the medial malleolus (see text) and least useful if the patient has either a coronal or sagittal plane fixed deformity in either limb.

for adduction deformities, with patients presenting with apparent shortening to the same scale.

- Measuring limb length in a patient with varus or valgus deformities about the knee can be challenging and should be carried out in segments to prevent inaccurate results. Measure from the anterior superior iliac spine to the lateral or medial condyle (fixed bony point) of the femur and from the condyle to the medial malleolus.

- The use of a tape measure in leg length measurement is not helpful in patients with significant foot and ankle pathology where the shortening is coming from below the medial malleolus such as in subtalar arthritis or previous calcaneal fracture. In such cases, the use of standing blocks is advised. In turn, blocks are inaccurate for measuring leg length discrepancies in patients with flexed flexion deformities of the lower limb (Figure 1.12).

- Increased lumbar lordosis may be compensatory for a fixed flexion deformity of the hip joint. In a standing position, a patient wants to be upright so they will increase their lumbar curvature to compensate. Up to 30° of hip fixed flexion can be compensated for by this means.

- Thomas test can be carried out in a variety of conditions with slight modifications to the examination technique. In a patient with a fixed spine, such as ankylosing spondylitis, proceed as normal but bear in mind that complete elimination of the lumbar lordosis with progressive hip flexion, as described, will not be possible.

- If asked to perform Thomas test on a patient who has a contralateral arthrodesis of the hip how do you proceed? Answer: Lift that leg by the heel and allow the pelvis to tilt and reduce the lumbar lordosis.

- In a patient with a total hip replacement, when performing Thomas test, avoid flexing that hip beyond 90° to minimise the risk of dislocation. It can be safer to ask the patient to flex their hip to the point where they still feel secure (i.e. a patient-controlled Thomas test).

- When you are asked to examine a patient with a limb amputation, it is prudent in such cases to first perform a thorough inspection. Assess the residual limb length, the suture line, scar mobility, skin condition and sensation, bony/weight-bearing prominences and the soft tissue envelope. Look at orthoses or prostheses that may be present. Always remember to look for clues as to why the patient had an amputation. For example, in a lower limb amputation examining

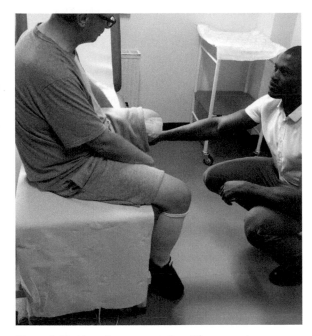

Figure 1.13 Above-knee amputation. When assessing a patient like this, remember to assess the residual limb length and shape. Also look at any prosthesis and assess the contralateral limb.

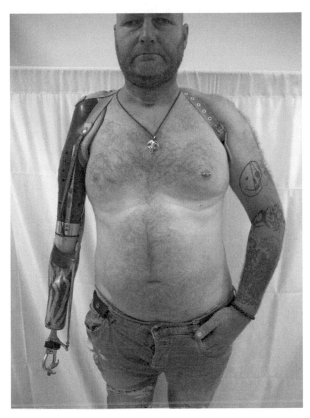

Figure 1.14 Right upper limb amputation with a prosthesis. Note that the clue for the reason for this amputation is in the face. This patient had a brachial plexus injury with Horner's syndrome (ptosis) and a flail upper limb that was subsequently amputated.

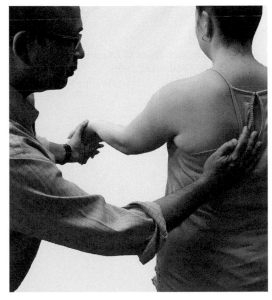

Figure 1.15 Testing serratus anterior without a wall. Note that the patient is forward flexing their shoulders at approximately 90° with the elbow extended. It will also help to demonstrate the winging by asking the patient to continue forward flexing against resistance.

the contralateral limb may reveal peripheral vascular disease or diabetic ulcers (Figures 1.13 and 1.14).

- What do you do if you are asked to demonstrate winging of the scapula in a patient with serratus anterior muscle weakness and there is no wall to push against? The technique is to stand by the side of the patient and ask them to push against your hand the same way they would against the wall. Observe the winging from the side (Figure 1.15).

Acknowledgement

We would like to acknowledge the help of Nicholas Adams and Sam Walters in the preparation of this chapter.

References

1. Apley AG, Solomon L. *Physical Examination in Orthopaedics*. Oxford: Butterworth–Heinemann, 1997.

2. Shaffer S, Harrison A, Brown K, Brennan K. Reliability and validity of Semmes-Weinstein monofilament testing in older community-dwelling adults. *J Geriatr Phys Ther* 2005;**28**(3):112–113.

3. Beighton PH, Horan F. Orthopaedic aspects of Ehlers–Danlos syndrome. *J Bone Joint Surg* 1969;**51**:444–453.

4. Miller MD, Thompson SR. *Miller's Review of Orthopaedics*, 7th ed. Philadelphia: Elsevier, 2016.

5. Banaszkiewicz PA, Kader, DF. *Postgraduate Orthopaedics: Guide to the FRCS (Tr & Ortho) Examination*, 3rd ed. Cambridge University Press, 2017.

6. McRae R. *Clinical Orthopaedic Examination*, 6th ed. Toronto: Churchill Livingstone, 2010.

7. MacDonald PB, Clark P, Sutherland K. An analysis of the diagnostic accuracy of the Hawkins and Neer subacromial impingement signs. *Shoulder Elbow Surg* 2000;**9**(4):299–301.

8. H-S Chen, S-H Lin, Y-H Hsu, S-C Chen, J-H Kang. A comparison of physical examinations with musculoskeletal ultrasound in the diagnosis of biceps long head tendinitis. *Ultrasound Med Biol* 2011;**37**(9);1392–1398.

9. Park HB, Yokota A, Gill HS, et al. Diagnostic accuracy of clinical tests for the different degrees of subacromial impingement syndrome. *J Bone Joint Surg Am* 2005;**87**:1446–1455.

10. Guanche CA, Jones DC. Clinical testing for tears of the glenoid labrum. *Arthroscopy* 2003;**19**:517–523.

11. LaStayo P, Howell J. Clinical provocative tests used in evaluating wrist pain: a descriptive study. *J Hand Ther* 1995;**8**:10–17.

12. MacDermid JC, Doherty T. Clinical and electrodiagnostic testing of carpal tunnel syndrome: a narrative review. *J Orthop Sports Phys Ther* 2004;**34**(10):565–588.

13. Bird PA, Oakley SP, Shnier R, Kirkham BW. Prospective evaluation of magnetic resonance imaging and physical examination findings in patients with greater trochanteric pain syndrome. *Arthritis Rheum* 2001;**44**:2138–2145.

14. Benjaminse A, Gokeler A van der Schans CP. Clinical diagnosis of an anterior cruciate ligament rupture: a meta-analysis. *J Orthop Sports Phys Ther* 2006;**36**:267–288.

15. Meserve BB, Cleland JA, Boucher TR. A meta-analysis examining clinical test utilities for assessing meniscal injury. *Clin Rehabil* 2008;**22**:143–161.

16. Molloy S, Solan MC, Bendall SP. Synovial impingement in the ankle. A new physical sign. *J Bone Joint Br* 2003;**85**:330–333.

17. Majlesi J, Togay H, Unalan H, Toprak S. The sensitivity and specificity of the Slump and the Straight Leg Raising test in patients with lumbar disc herniation. *J Clin Rheumatol* 2008;**14**:87–91.

18. van Kampen DA, van den Berg T, van der Woude HJ, et al. The diagnostic value of the combination of patient characteristics, history, and clinical shoulder tests for the diagnosis of rotator cuff tear. *J Orthop Surg Res* 2014;**9**:70.

19. Kohonen M, Teerenhovi O, Terho T, Laurikka J, Tarkka M. Is the Allen test reliable enough? *European J Cardiothoracic Surg* 2007:**32**(6):902–905.

Further Reading

Reider B. *The Orthopaedic Physical Examination*, 2nd ed. Philadelphia: Elsevier Saunders, 2005.

Examination of the Shoulder

Shantanu Shahane and David Limb

Steps in Shoulder Joint Assessment

A. History

B. Clinical Examination

Step 1

Stand the patient

Step 2

Look

Step 3

Feel

Step 4

Move (also assess scapulothoracic rhythm)

Step 5

Examine muscles

- Rotator cuff
- Consider other muscles (e.g. deltoid, pectoralis major, latissimus dorsi, rhomboids, trapezius and serratus anterior)

Step 6

Impingement tests

- Including acromioclavicular joint (ACJ) test, biceps tendon and superior labrum anterior and posterior (SLAP) lesion

Step 7

Instability (sit patient or lie)

- Anterior and posterior instability and laxity tests

Stand and Look

Have the patient undress appropriately. Stand the patient and look from the front. Ask to do a quick screen of neck movements and ask whether this reproduces the shoulder pain. Look from the side, look into the axilla and look from behind, describing any wasting, scars, etc.

It is good practice to keep some space behind the patient when examining, as the person examining can move around the patient and avoid having the patient turn around multiple times.

Feel

Feel the bony prominences, starting from the sternoclavicular (SC) joint and across the clavicle. Feel the acromioclavicular (AC) joint and feel the biceps tendon.

Move

Ask the patient to move. Start with cervical spine movements first, and then move on to the shoulder. Forward flexion, abduction, external rotation and internal rotation are all performed by demonstrating this to the patient. Active movement is followed by passive movement. Abduction must be done looking from the front and from behind, observing scapulothoracic movement.

Test Muscles

When testing the muscles, test them as a separate entity, i.e. test the four muscles of the rotator cuff together, then test the muscles of the shoulder girdle separately. Also, do not combine muscle testing with other tests, such as assessing infraspinatus, at the same time as assessing external rotation.

First, the four muscles of the rotator cuff are tested.

- Supraspinatus using Jobe's 'empty can' test
- Infraspinatus by external rotation plus the 'lag sign'
- Teres minor with the 'hornblower's sign'
- Subscapularis by performing the Gerber's 'lift-off' or 'belly-press' test

Tests for infraspinatus, teres minor and subscapularis can be performed in one sweeping motion.

Then, consider assessing other muscles of the shoulder girdle. It is not necessary in all cases to assess these muscles, but in some instances, especially if there is muscle wasting or weakness, it may be necessary to do so.

- From the front of the patient, assess deltoids, pectoralis major and latissimus dorsi.
- From the back, assess trapezius, rhomboids and serratus anterior.

Impingement

- Neer's sign and/or Hawkins' test for subacromial impingement
- Scarf test for ACJ pathology

Tests for subacromial impingement and ACJ tests can also be performed in one sweeping motion. Then:

- Speed's or Yergason's test for biceps tendonitis

Followed by:

- O'Brien's test for SLAP lesions

Instability

For this, it is wise to lie the patient down (if there is no couch, then sit the patient (with a backrest)). This is essential to stabilise the scapula.

Tests performed commonly for instability/laxity are:

- Sulcus sign
- Anterior and posterior drawer test (load and shift)
- Anterior apprehension/relocation
- Posterior apprehension/relocation

Note: if the patient has signs of multidirectional instability, then test for generalised laxity (Beighton's test).

History

Patients often present with shoulders that are painful, unstable and/or stiff. Age, handedness and occupation should be noted. Although an open mind should be kept at all times, instability tends to dominate in the younger age group, impingement symptoms and frozen shoulder in middle age and rotator cuff tears and arthritis in the older group.

Elements of the history are particularly useful in directing the subsequent clinical examination, and this merits further attention. In particular, the surgeon should consider the history of pain, weakness, stiffness and instability.

Pain

Patients with shoulder problems suffer night pain. It is a frequent complaint, often the main presenting symptom, that elsewhere would suggest tumour or infection. It is not a red flag symptom in this context, as it is so common in patients with shoulder pathology.

The patient may describe pain that is accurately localised or diffuse. Neck pain radiating to the scapula or tip of the shoulder should trigger an assessment of the cervical spine, whilst radiation into the forearm and hand, particularly with parasthesiae, suggests cervical root entrapment. Pain at the tip of the scapula may suggest abdominal pathology, though posterior pain in the upper, outer part of the shoulder blade is usually glenohumeral in origin.

Acromioclavicular joint pain is classically localised to the joint itself, the patient pointing with a single finger to the source of their problem.

The pain associated with impingement and rotator cuff disease is often diffusely felt over the deltoid region.

There are some conditions that can be associated with excruciating pain. Acute calcific tendonitis falls into this category. The early phases of frozen shoulder can also be extremely painful, and the above tests will be negative – this is particularly common in diabetic patients.

Parsonage–Turner syndrome or brachial neuritis can be normal on radiography and ultrasound, with neuralgic pain that is associated with weakness and wasting in the distribution of affected peripheral nerves, unlike the nerve root distribution of cervical disc disease.

Pain that occurs only through a particular range of movement is a painful arc. Rotator cuff disease, including subacromial impingement, often causes a midrange painful arc between about 60° and 120° of abduction and elevation. A high painful arc (e.g. the last 30° of elevation) is typical of ACJ disorders (Figure 2.1). A painful arc with pain felt posteriorly is less common, but can occur with subscapular disorders such as enchondromata, which typically produce ratchet-like crepitus as the lesion moves over the ribs.

Weakness

The commonest cause of perceived weakness of the shoulder is pain inhibition – if a movement hurts, the patient's brain will not let the muscles contract to produce the movement. Thus, subacromial impingement may present with weakness, but this may be

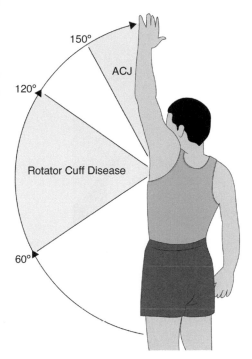

Figure 2.1 Painful arc of abduction. An arc of 60°–120° is usually due to subacromial impingement. High, painful arc of 150°–180° is usually due to acromioclavicular joint problems.

reversed by an injection of local anaesthetic into the subacromial space. Such diagnostic test injections are less commonly used now that diagnostic ultrasound is more freely available and can even be integrated into the clinical examination, observing deformation or bunching of the cuff as it moves under the acromion.

A history of inherited disorders or of generalised problems may alert the surgeon to rare neurological or myopathic conditions such as facioscapulohumeral dystrophy (FSHD).

However, the majority of patients presenting to shoulder clinic have a disorder either of the rotator cuff or of the nerves supplying the shoulder girdle muscles.

Other peripheral nerve problems that can manifest as shoulder pain and weakness include suprascapular nerve entrapment. This can occur in the suprascapular notch, in which case it is known as 'rucksack palsy' because prolonged downward traction on the shoulder has been implicated. Entrapment of the suprascapular nerve can also occur as it winds round the spinoglenoid notch, often a result of pressure from cysts or ganglia related to a degenerative posterior labrum. In this case, only infraspinatus is involved and the treatment relies on dealing with the labral tear and the cyst causing compression. Axillary nerve weakness, with deltoid wasting, may follow axillary nerve injury. Axillary and musculocutaneous nerve injury may follow anterior shoulder dislocation.

Common things being common, however, the most frequent cause of weakness in the shoulder clinic is rotator cuff disease and, in particular, rotator cuff tears.

Stiffness

If active movements are limited, then check passive movements. Frozen shoulder causes restriction of both active and passive movement in all planes (global restriction). Arthritic disorders can do the same, but the latter are often associated with crepitus and radiographs demonstrate the pathology, whilst radiographs are normal in cases of frozen shoulder. Arthritis is also seen in the slightly older population compared to frozen shoulder.

Frozen shoulder has been a loosely used term and should best be reserved for the specific condition that causes inflammation, myofibroblastic transformation and contracture associated with severe pain which, for reasons that we do not understand, eventually 'thaws out', even without treatment. So-called secondary frozen shoulder refers to stiffness associated with other pathology that is associated with fibrous scarring or contracture of the glenohumeral capsule and subacromial space and is often more resistant to complete reversal. This includes stiffness after even minimally displaced fractures or rotator cuff tears.

Instability

An assessment of generalised joint laxity is important in any patient in whom instability is suspected and can be documented using the Beighton score (Chapter 1). Instability refers to the symptomatic inability to maintain the humeral head centred in the glenoid. The patient will complain that they can feel the shoulder slipping out of the joint and back in, with or without a history of dislocation.

Silliman and Hawkins described a simple classification that broadly categorises patients into those likely to need surgical treatment and those who may not.[1] The acronyms TUBS (Traumatic, Unidirectional instability, Bankart lesion, Surgery) and AMBRI (Atraumatic, Multidirectional, Bilateral instability, Rehabilitation, Inferior capsular shift) are useful aide-memoires in this respect. However, this is an oversimplification, and the *Stanmore classification* considers three axes – traumatic structural, atraumatic structural and habitual non-structural (muscle patterning) – allowing any given patient to be plotted at a point recognising the contribution of all factors and allowing a more holistic treatment plan, and appreciating that more than one pathology can be present.[2] Thus, it is important to ask not only about previous dislocations and their treatment (including any previous surgery) but also about the evolution of symptoms and whether the patient can voluntarily produce subluxation or dislocation.

It should be noted that instability can present as pain in provocation positions of the arm. For example, anterosuperior instability can manifest as typical impingement symptoms.

Examination

Look

Inspection of the shoulder girdle should be systematic, and this requires the patient to be undressed to the waist. Garments worn for modesty should leave the scapulae visible and enquiry should be made as to any concealed scars. Observing preparation for examination may be an adjunct to the history, revealing functional difficulties in arm positioning.

The general appearance of the patient may help to identify underlying disease. The shoulder is inspected from the front, back and side. Inspection of the axilla (Figure 2.2) is also required but may more conveniently be carried out during 'move'.

Inspection is performed sequentially with the examiner moving from the front to the side and then inspecting from the back. From the front, bony contours may reveal prominence of the ACJ or sternoclavicular joint (SCJ) that could be degenerative or traumatic in origin. Deformity of the clavicle is most likely to be a consequence of past trauma (malunion). Look for a deltopectoral scar which is the commonest approach for open surgery of the shoulder joint. Deltoid wasting can give a 'squared-off' appearance to the shoulder. This can be a result of axillary nerve injury, but chronic shoulder pain and stiffness will also result in deltoid wasting (Figure 2.2a). Ruptured long head of biceps will make the biceps appear more prominent because of a dip appearing between the muscle and deltoid (the 'Popeye' sign – Figure 2.2b), whilst pectoralis major rupture will cause loss of the anterior axillary fold.

On moving from the side to the back of the patient, look for prominence of the shoulder blade

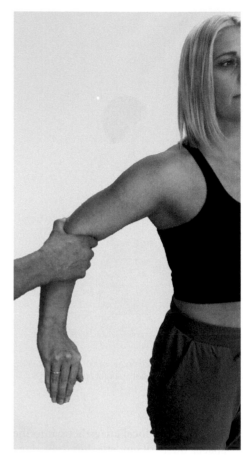

Figure 2.2 Inspect from the front, back and side. Remember to look into the axilla.

(scapular winging). Scapula positioning is checked from behind. This could be a result of structural problems, such as long thoracic nerve injury, malunion or osteochondroma, but is more often positional (static winging) and will be investigated further when movements are checked.

Evidence of muscle wasting is important, though it can be difficult if there is a substantial layer of subcutaneous fat. However, hollowing of the supraspinous and infraspinous fossae suggests tears of the supraspinatus and infraspinatus, respectively (Figure 2.2c). Often this gives as good an impression of the functional impact of a rotator cuff tear, as does detailed ultrasound examination of the cuff tendons. Look for arthroscopy scars all around the shoulder but these are mainly evident posteriorly. Also look for thoracic kyphosis. Exaggerated kyphosis can predispose to dynamic impingement syndrome (Figure 2.2d).

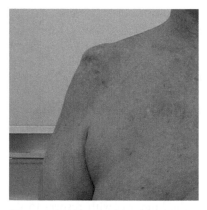

Figure 2.2a Wasting of the deltoid, in this case due to axillary nerve injury caused by a previous anterior dislocation of the shoulder.

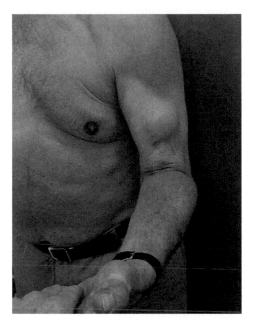

Figure 2.2b 'Popeye' sign – prominence of the belly of the long head of biceps due to rupture of its tendon in the intertubercular sulcus allowing distal retraction. Rupture of the distal biceps allows proximal retraction of the whole muscle belly, flattening the contour of the arm above the cubital fossa (reverse Popeye sign).

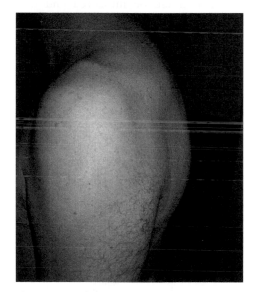

Figure 2.2c Infraspinatus and supraspinatus wasting caused by a massive rotator cuff tear.

Feel

Like inspection, palpation should proceed in a systematic manner (Figure 2.3). Start at the only synovial joint between the upper limb girdle and the trunk – the SCJ – and palpate from this, along the clavicle, to the ACJ. Pathology of the joints may cause local tenderness, but when the patient continues to flinch when the clavicle, acromion and scapular spine are palpated, one has to wonder about the significance of the finding and interpret tenderness with care!

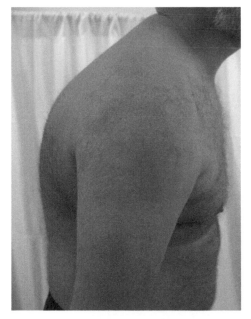

Figure 2.2d Significant thoracic kyphosis. This can predispose to dynamic impingement symptoms in the shoulder.

At the ACJ, gentle ballottement by downward pressure on the distal clavicle, followed by posteriorly directed pressure on the anterior margin of the distal clavicle, can help to identify symptomatic ACJ disease (degenerative change in the ACJ is almost universal with age, so imaging is often unhelpful in identifying whether the joint is culpable as a cause of symptoms).

Instability of the ACJ may be vertical (superior-inferior) or horizontal (anterior-posterior). Vertical instability signifies damage to the coracoclavicular ligaments and horizontal instability signifies damage to the acromioclavicular ligaments. Horizontal instability usually means that operative stabilisation procedures may be performed.

Tenderness along the subacromial margins can occur with impingement and cuff tears, particularly when there is bursitis, but this is a non-specific finding. Indeed, it is routine to document tenderness along the anterior and posterior joint lines and along the biceps groove about 5–7 cm distal to the tip of the acromion with the arm in neutral rotation, but diagnostic information is limited by low specificity.

Move

The 'shoulder' examination is really a composite examination of the glenohumeral (GH), scapulothoracic (ST), acromioclavicular and sternoclavicular joints. It is cervical spine pathology that is most easily confused with, and commonly coexists with, shoulder girdle pathology. Hence a *screening movement* of the cervical spine should be performed to see if it reproduces the shoulder pain (Figure 2.4).

Movements of the shoulder are documented as the sum of movements at the GHJ, STJ, ACJ and SCJ on the position of the humerus with respect to the axis of the torso. Be careful, therefore, to eliminate any trick movements such as leaning back to increase apparent elevation of the arm. As previously noted, active movements should be measured and then a check made to see if there is any additional passive range available. All movements can be measured

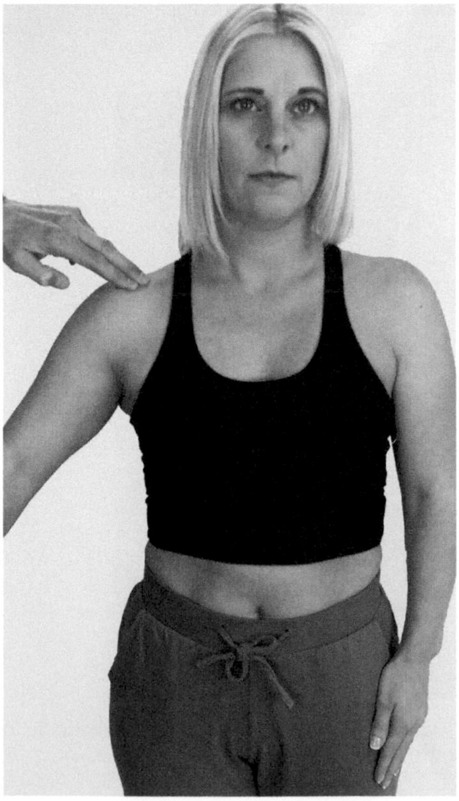

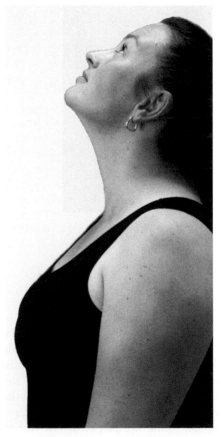

Figure 2.3 Palpate in a systematic manner starting at the sternoclavicular joint and progress laterally along the clavicle.

Figure 2.4 Screen the neck movements to see if the pain in the shoulder is reproduced.

with a goniometer – estimations are as poor in the shoulder as they are in any other joint, and this can be a huge source of interobserver discrepancy. Note also that, although the reference planes are sagittal and coronal, this does not correspond to the plane of the GHJ because the scapula faces forwards by approximately 30°.

Shoulder *flexion and extension* is conventionally measured in the sagittal plane. The humerus can be limited in flexion by the acromion (Figure 2.5).

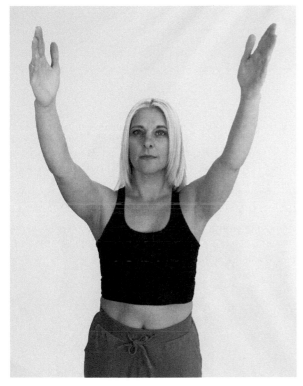

Figure 2.5 Forward flexion, limited by the acromion to 170°.

Extension is often not recorded but functionally can become very important (extension can be recorded later as part of assessment of functional internal rotation).

If the patient loses internal rotation, this can be compensated for by a combination of extension and adduction, another movement that is often not recorded as part of the routine shoulder examination.

Whilst *adduction* is not usually measured (as it can only be measured in positions of flexion and extension), *abduction* is recorded, and any painful arc is documented. Scapular rotation coupled with external rotation of the arm (proximal humerus) to take the greater tuberosity out of the subacromial space allows a full 180° of this movement in normal subjects (Figure 2.6).

External rotation during this stage of examination is usually measured passively. It is measured with the arms by the side and the elbows in 90° of flexion (to eliminate forearm rotations from interfering) (Figure 2.7). The neutral position is with the forearms pointing directly forwards in the sagittal plane. The 'normal' range of external rotation is very variable so should be carefully measured and recorded if any changes over time or with treatment are to be detected. Furthermore, any side-to-side difference may be significant. Reduced passive external rotation is indicative of either a frozen shoulder or an arthritic glenohumeral joint (differentiated by an X-ray).

Internal rotation cannot be measured in this position because the forearms become blocked by the abdomen long before the limit of internal rotation is reached.

Functional internal rotation (FIR) is more important to the patient in activities of daily living and so is more useful to assess than true internal rotation of the shoulder. FIR involves the patient internally rotating the shoulders to allow the thumb to reach the 'small' of their back. Functional internal rotation is a composite

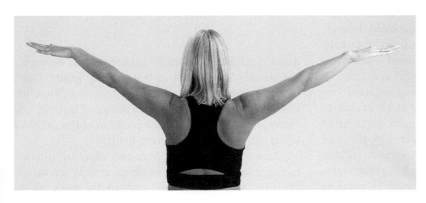

Figure 2.6 Abduction is possible to around 120 degrees if the shoulder is internally rotated, as shown, but can be increased to 180 degrees if the hand is turned palm-up.

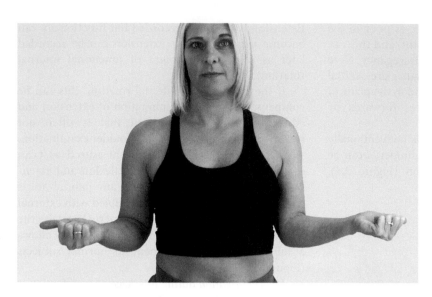

Figure 2.7 External rotation. Note that elbows are tucked into the side to isolate the movement.

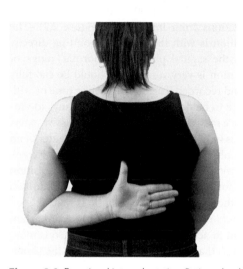

Figure 2.8 Functional internal rotation. Patient should be able to get their thumb to mid-thoracic level.

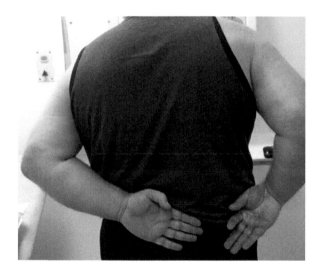

Figure 2.8a Patient attempting functional internal rotation (FIR) at the right shoulder. Note that because of the restricted internal rotation, he is tilting his trunk to the left as a compensatory manoeuvre.

movement, which involves extension, internal rotation and adduction of the shoulder, flexion of the elbow and abduction of the thumb. This can be quantified depending on how high the thumb reaches, i.e. from buttock, to the L5 level, T12 level and finally to T2 level. This can be compared to the opposite side (Figure 2.8 and 2.8a).

The range of internal and external rotation can also be documented with the shoulder at 90° of abduction, but note that the available range is different in this position when compared to the arms-by-the-side position. The anterosuperior capsule and rotator interval structures are under less tension at the starting position and the range of external rotation is

greater, whilst the inferior glenohumeral ligaments are already lengthened in the starting position and the range of internal rotation is less. It is therefore vital to document not only the range of internal and external rotation but also the position of the shoulder when the measurements were made.

Assess flexion, abduction and external rotation movement from the front of the patient. When assessing FIR, as the examiner goes to the back of the

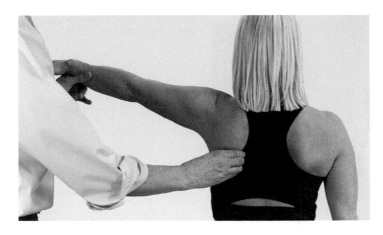

Figure 2.9 Stabilising the scapula in order to separate the glenohumeral and scapulothoracic components of abduction. This can be achieved by either manually fixing the tip of the scapula, as shown here, or more commonly fixing both the tip and the acromion.

patient, stay there and ask the patient to flex the shoulder again to observe the scapulae.

Scapular rhythm refers to the relative contributions of scapulothoracic and glenohumeral movement to the total range and is normally 1:2, delivered smoothly and simultaneously, with a slight predominance of glenohumeral movement in the lower range and scapulothoracic movement in the end range. An abnormal rhythm can arise with shoulder pathology. For example, an osteoarthritic glenohumeral joint may demonstrate little movement at the GHJ but full movement at the STJ. The contributions can be formally examined by stabilising the scapula. This is performed by manually fixing the tip of the scapula and the acromion (Figure 2.9). This will restrict abduction in the normal shoulder to about 80° with the arm in neutral rotation, or 120° if external rotation of the arm is allowed, bringing the greater tuberosity out from beneath the acromion.

Observing the rhythm of scapular movement is combined with observation for winging of the scapula. With paralysis of serratus anterior, there may be gross and obvious prominence of the medial border of the scapula, but many painful conditions (such as impingement syndrome) will cause pain inhibition of groups of muscles, resulting in dynamic winging that can be quite subtle, perhaps only occurring for part of the range of movement.

Muscle Testing

Rotator Cuff

The muscles of the rotator cuff are tested in sequence. This may be followed by testing the deltoid and other muscles around the shoulder girdle if indicated.

Supraspinatus

Supraspinatus is an abductor of the shoulder and, despite what is taught in undergraduate anatomy, most patients with a torn supraspinatus can still initiate abduction. Furthermore, the power of abduction can be good because deltoid is also a powerful abductor.

To test supraspinatus, the shoulder is elevated to 90°, in the plane of the scapula (which is 30° forwards from the coronal plane) and in line with the supraspinatus muscle. Downward pressure is then applied just above the elbow joint with the arm in internal rotation. The ability of the patient to maintain this position tests the strength of supraspinatus muscle and can be compared to the opposite side (Figure 2.10). This is also called the '**empty can test**' described by Jobe and Moynes.[3] The '**full can test**' uses the same position but uses a position of 45° external rotation rather than full internal rotation, which is less painful but has equal diagnostic accuracy.[4]

Anatomical explanation: In Jobe's test, while testing the supraspinatus, it is essential to reduce the contribution of deltoid in maintaining the arm position. By internally rotating the shoulder in 90° of scapular elevation, the deltoid attachment over the tuberosity moves internally, putting the deltoid at a maximal mechanical disadvantage. At the same time, it also puts the fibres of supraspinatus at a maximal mechanical advantage. This allows testing of supraspinatus in relative isolation. It is best to test the strength of supraspinatus by exerting pressure just above the elbow to reduce the contribution of triceps in reinforcing supraspinatus.

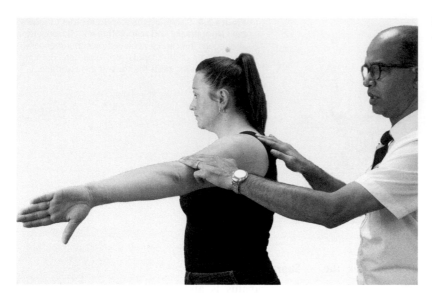

Figure 2.10 Testing supraspinatus. Jobe's 'empty can' test.

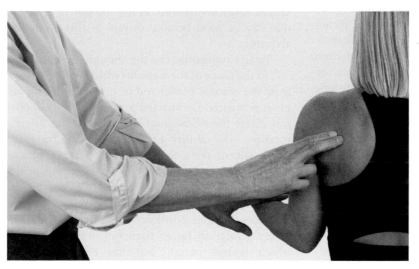

Figure 2.11 Testing infraspinatus and teres minor muscles by resisting external rotation.

Infraspinatus and Teres Minor

Infraspinatus is the most powerful external rotator of the shoulder when the arms are by the side. In this position, the patient's elbows are locked by the side of the trunk, flexed to 90°, and the power of external rotation is assessed (Figure 2.11). If the infraspinatus tendon is involved in a rotator cuff tear, this movement is very weak. With complete weakness, the patient cannot actively externally rotate the arm. Bigliani et al. described a **'drop/lag sign'** in which the arm is passively, maximally externally rotated and then released. If there is severe external rotator weakness, the arm will fall into internal rotation.[5]

Teres minor, the other external rotator, can also be tested similarly. Hertel et al.[6] described a sign in which the arm is supported at the elbow (bent at 90°) with the shoulder also elevated 90° in the scapular plane and almost fully externally rotated. Again, the patient is asked to maintain this position when the examiner releases the wrist. The sign is positive if the forearm moves forwards towards neutral rotation of the

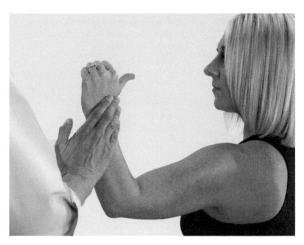

Figure 2.12 Hornblower's sign. The patient is unable to maintain a position of full external rotation, and the thumb falls towards the mouth.

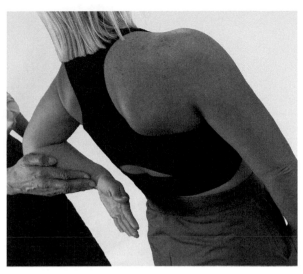

Figure 2.13 Testing subscapularis. Gerber's 'lift-off' test.

shoulder (hornblower's sign), similar to a position used to sound a hunting horn (Figure 2.12).

Subscapularis

Although subscapularis has the opposite action to infraspinatus, being a powerful internal rotator of the humerus when the arm is by the side, this cannot be used for testing because pectoralis major is equally strong in this respect. There are two strategies to use to get around this. If the patient has sufficient range of shoulder motion, then the hand is placed behind the back and from this position the strength of further internal rotation – pushing the examiner's hand away from the 'small' of the back – is tested (Figure 2.13). This **'lift-off' test**[7] is the most reliable test for subscapularis. A lag sign has also been described for the detection of subscapularis tears.[6] The hand is drawn away from the small of the back by the examiner and the patient is asked to hold their hand away from the back when it is released. The lag sign is positive if the patient cannot maintain the hand in this position and it falls back onto the lumbar region and suggests subscapularis rupture.

Not all patients with painful shoulders can reach behind their back. The patient is asked to keep the elbow forwards but to press their hand into their abdomen. The examiner can also exert gentle pressure on the elbow in a posterior direction. If pectoralis major is recruited, this pulls the humerus and brings the elbow back; therefore, to keep the elbow forwards requires that only subscapularis is used for this internal rotation movement (**Napoleon's test or belly-press test**) (Figure 2.14).

Anatomical explanation: Testing the subscapularis in 'lift-off test' and 'belly-press test' employs similar principles. Subscapularis is a powerful internal rotator of the shoulder. In both these tests, if the subscapularis is intact, the humerus remains in an internally rotated position while the wrist is lifted off the lumbar spine (in lift-off test) and the wrist presses the belly (in belly-press test). If the subscapularis is ruptured, the patient is unable to perform the above movement as the humerus falls into external rotation. The patient then tries to compensate this by flexion of the wrist.

Testing Other Muscles around the Shoulder Girdle

Sometimes on inspection, wasting of muscles is seen and the examiner is not sure that the wasting is that of the rotator cuff or other muscles. In these situations, it is necessary to progress by examining the other muscles around the shoulder girdle. For convenience, three muscles can be assessed whilst standing in front of the patient (deltoid, pectoralis major and latissimus dorsi) and three can be examined whilst standing behind the patient (rhomboids, trapezius and serratus anterior).

23

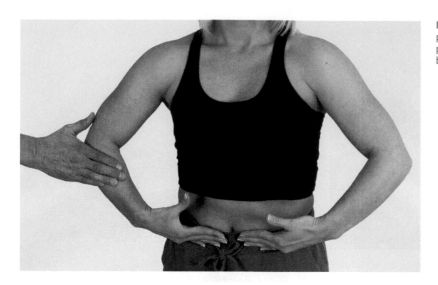

Figure 2.14 Napoleon's test or belly-press test for subscapularis. Useful for patients who cannot place their arm behind their back.

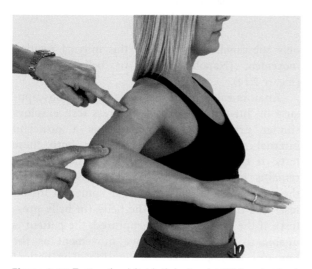

Figure 2.15 Testing the deltoid. Abduction (at 90°) is maintained against resistance and the deltoid palpated.

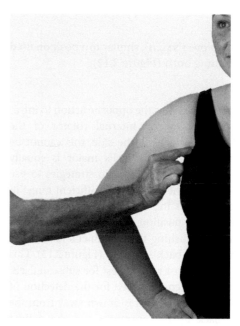

Figure 2.16 Testing pectoralis major. Patient is asked to squeeze into their waist. The muscle is palpated in the anterior axillary fold.

Test for deltoid: Deltoid can be tested either with the arm by the side or, if the patient allows, in 90° of abduction, which makes visualisation and palpation easier. From either of these positions, abduction, flexion and extension against resistance will lead to visible and palpable contraction of the lateral, anterior and posterior heads of deltoid, respectively (Figure 2.15).

Test for pectoralis major: The patient is asked to place their hands on their waist and squeeze inwards. Palpate the muscle, especially in the anterior axillary fold (Figure 2.16).

Test for latissimus dorsi: The patient is asked to perform downward/backward pressure of arm against resistance, as though climbing a ladder. Palpate muscle in the posterior axillary fold (Figure 2.17).

Test for rhomboids: The patient places their hands on their waist and then pushes their elbows back against resistance. Feel muscle (Figure 2.18). The muscles are felt at the medial border of the scapula.

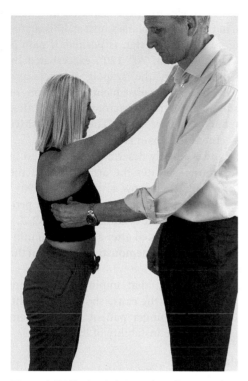

Figure 2.17 Testing latissimus dorsi. Downward pressure on the examiner's shoulder and palpate the muscle in the posterior axillary fold.

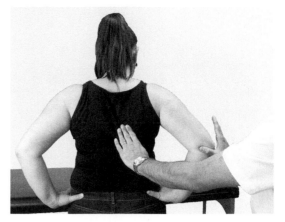

Figure 2.18 Testing the rhomboids. The patient pushes their elbows back against resistance. Feel the muscle between the scapulae.

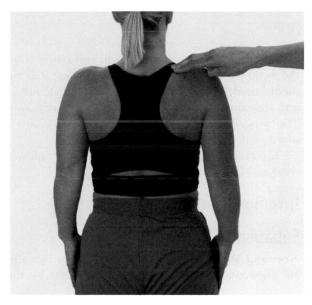

Figure 2.20 Testing trapezius by shrugging the shoulders against resistance.

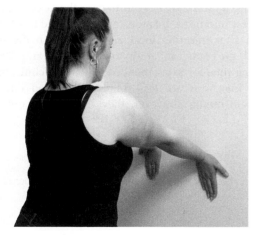

Figure 2.19 Testing serratus anterior. With the shoulders forward flexed to 90°, elbows extended and the fingers of the hands pointing downwards, pressure against the wall exaggerates the winging.

Test for serratus anterior: The patient pushes against the wall with both outstretched arms, the fingers and palm pointing downwards on the wall

(Figure 2.19). Scapular winging is observed with this manoeuvre if there is weakness.

Test for trapezius: The patient is asked to shrug shoulders against resistance (Figure 2.20).

The three muscles that are tested from the back of the patient can all manifest in *winging of the scapula*. Winging of the scapula can be medial or lateral. The type of winging is defined by the direction the superomedial border of the scapula moves due to the muscle weakness.

25

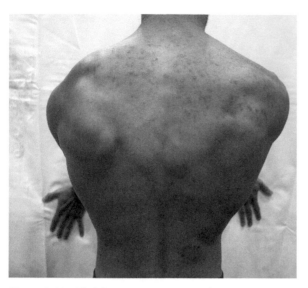

Figure 2.20a Medial winging in a patient with serratus anterior weakness.

Medial winging is more common and results from the weakness of one of the muscles that insert into the medial border – serratus anterior (long thoracic nerve) and rhomboids (dorsal scapular nerve) (Figure 2.20a). The winging seen with rhomboid weakness is much more subtle.

Lateral winging is usually caused by trapezius weakness (spinal accessory nerve).

Impingement Signs and Tests

Subacromial Space

Neer and Welsh described an *impingement sign* and an impingement test.[8] The sign is elicited by the examiner passively elevating the patient's internally rotated arm in the scapular plane whilst stabilising the scapula (Figure 2.21). The sign is positive if pain is felt, usually in the arc of 70°–120°, exacerbated by downward pressure on the scapula if necessary. *Neer's test* involves the subsequent instillation of local anaesthetic into the subacromial space, after which the manoeuvre is repeated. The test is positive if the impingement sign/pain is abolished.

Hawkins and Kennedy described a similar test in which the examiner elevates the arm to 90° in the scapular plane with the elbow also flexed to 90°.[9] From this position internal rotation of the arm provokes pain in impingement syndrome (Figure 2.22). Likewise, this can be repeated after subacromial infiltration of local anaesthetic, demonstrating relief of the provocation of pain.

It should be recalled that impingement is not a diagnosis in itself, and the cause should be sought. For instance, in the younger patient, impingement may be caused by subtle instability of the shoulder.

Acromioclavicular Joint

Acromioclavicular joint pathology may have been suggested by the localisation of symptoms, joint tenderness and a high painful arc. Pain is provoked by elevating the arm to shoulder height and then adducting across the chest (**scarf test/cross-arm adduction test**) (Figure 2.23). To continue the theme of diagnostic test injections, this too can be repeated 5–10 minutes after injecting local anaesthetic into the ACJ. With the ready availability of ultrasound and diminishing time for assessment of patients in clinic, these test injections are less frequently carried out but remain useful. However, they should be avoided if

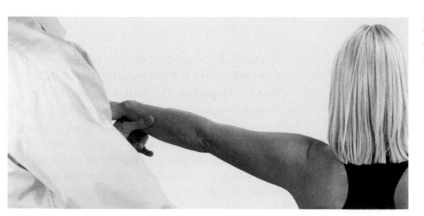

Figure 2.21 Neer's sign for impingement. This is performed in the scapular plane with the arm internally rotated. Pain occurs mainly in the 70°–120° arc.

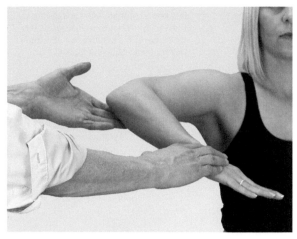

Figure 2.22 Hawkins' test for impingement. Internal rotation provokes the pain. This is classically done in the scapular plane, but in a modified technique internal rotation is carried out in a variety of positions.

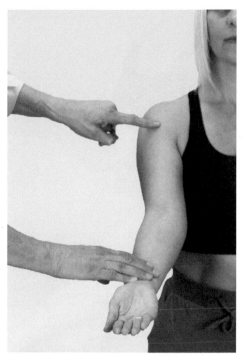

Figure 2.24 Speed's test for biceps tendonitis. The forearm is supinated. The examiner is to resist flexion of the patient's extended elbow. In a positive test, pain occurs over the proximal biceps tendon.

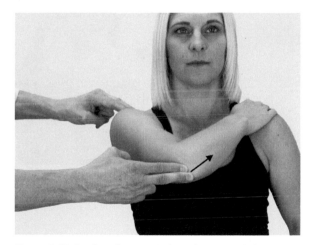

Figure 2.23 Scarf test for acromioclavicular joint pathology.

ultrasound is to be carried out within the next day or two, as the injection fluid itself can be misinterpreted to be a bursal or joint effusion.

Biceps Tendon Pathology and SLAP Lesion

The role of the long head of the biceps tendon is not fully understood, but inflammation of the tendon, structural damage to its insertion on the supraglenoid tubercle (SLAP tear) and structural injury to the biceps pulley, which supports the tendon as it turns from the intertubercular sulcus into the GHJ, have all been implicated as sources of pain. Several tests are available to detect biceps pathology, though all can be falsely positive in the presence of rotator cuff disease.

A rupture of the long head of biceps may have been identified by the 'Popeye' sign on inspection. In **Speed's test** the elbow is fully extended and the forearm supinated.[10] Anterior shoulder pain on flexion against resistance is indicative of biceps tendon pathology (Figure 2.24).

Yergason's test is performed by taking the patient's hand as if to perform a handshake. With the patient's elbow by their side, held at 90° flexion, the patient is asked to attempt to twist the examiner's hand by pronation and supination of their own forearm, and this is resisted.[11] Pain provoked by resisted supination of the patient's forearm but not pronation is indicative of biceps tendon pathology (Figure 2.25).

Injury to the biceps tendon attachment over the supra glenoid tubercle is also called a SLAP lesion. Numerous tests have been described to detect superior labral detachment. These tests have variable levels of accuracy.

In the **O'Brien's test**, the arm is elevated in flexion to 90°, adducted by 15° and fully internally rotated.

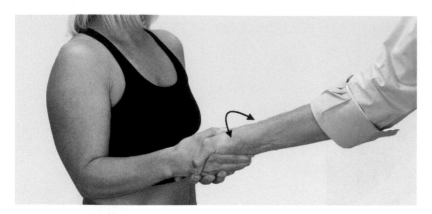

Figure 2.25 Yergason's test. The patient is asked to pronate and supinate their forearm while the examiner resists this movement. In a positive test, it is more painful on resisting supination.

(a)

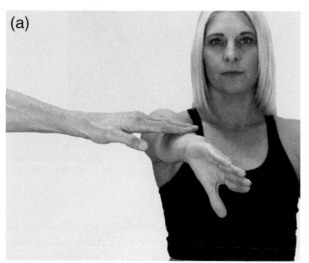

(b)

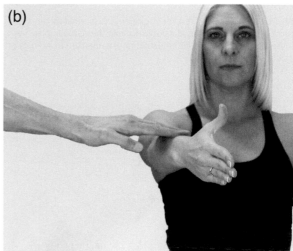

Figure 2.26a and b O'Brien's test can be used to detect SLAP lesions. The shoulder is elevated to 90° and the arm is adducted 15° and fully internally rotated. Downward pressure by the examiner causes more pain in this position compared to when the arm is fully externally rotated.

The patient is then asked to resist downward pressure exerted on the wrist. If the patient feels pain, the arm is then fully externally rotated and similar downward pressure exerted. If the pain now vanishes or reduces, it is indicative of a SLAP lesion (Figure 2.26a and b).[10]

Anatomical explanation: When the arm is elevated at 90°, 15° adducted and fully internally rotated, the biceps tendon has a tendency to slip out of the bicipital groove and become unstable in a medial direction due to lack of its superior attachment, also potentially damaging the medial pulley. If the patient has a SLAP lesion, this part of the test can cause pain. Once the arm is then externally rotated, the biceps tendon relocates back in the groove and is not dependent on its superior attachment, thereby eliminating pain.

Instability

It is important to realise that laxity is often physiological and asymptomatic, and not often associated with a major structural pathology (other than a capacious capsule). Instability, however, is pathological and mostly associated with a major structural lesion (labral lesion or bone loss).

It is useful in all cases to compare findings with the opposite shoulder. Evidence of generalised joint laxity may also be sought, expressed by the Beighton score. Anterior and posterior instability should be sought and either, or both, in combination with inferior laxity is termed multidirectional instability.

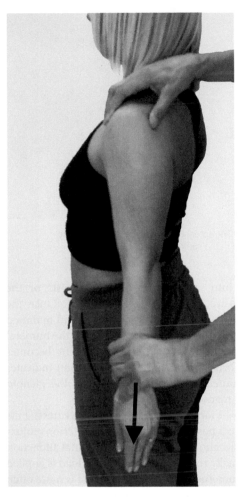

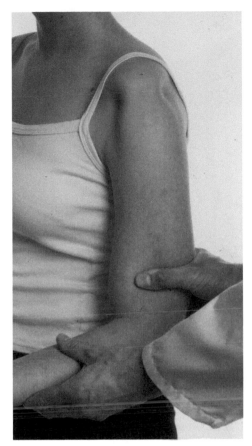

Figure 2.27a Sulcus sign in a patient with multidirectional instability.

Figure 2.27 The sulcus sign, elicited by downward traction on the humerus, causing inferior subluxation of the humeral head.

Inferior laxity can be identified by the presence of a **sulcus sign**, elicited by passive downward traction on the humerus in neutral rotation (Figures 2.27 and 2.27a). If this is also present in external rotation, it implies additional incompetence of the rotator interval structures (coracohumeral ligament and superior glenohumeral ligament).

The anterior and posterior capsulolabral structures can be tested in a similar manner using **load and shift tests** (Figure 2.28). The examiner stands behind the patient and stabilises the scapula by applying the thumb to the posterior acromion and the index finger on the coracoid process, using the examiner's left hand for testing the right shoulder and vice versa. The proximal humerus is grasped close to the humeral head between the thumb posteriorly and the index and middle fingers anteriorly. The humeral head is then translated backwards and forwards and the amount of passive movement between the humeral head and glenoid is estimated. The humeral head can be felt to glide up to the glenoid rim, moving laterally as it does, perch and then, with extreme laxity, pass beyond and begin to medialise and relocate again. The extent to which it translates is used to categorise the laxity. Pain or clicks during this test can be indicative of labral tears or damage to the glenoid rim.

Further evidence of anterior and posterior instability can be gained with the apprehension tests (though the posterior test may not be associated with much in the way of apprehension).

The **anterior apprehension test** can be performed with the patient seated or lying down, with the shoulder to be tested at the edge of the couch (Figure 2.29).

29

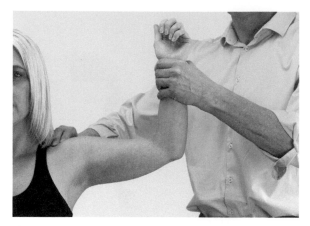

Figure 2.29 The anterior apprehension test. It is best demonstrated in the supine position.

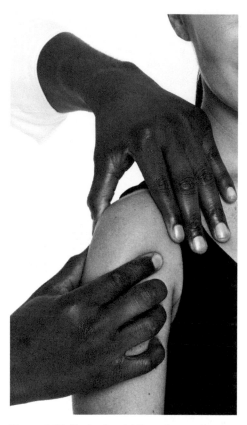

Figure 2.28 The load and shift test for anterior-posterior instability. This is essentially an anterior-posterior drawer test.

The important issue is to stabilise the scapula during this test (hence the reason that lying down or sitting on a chair with a backrest is best). The shoulder is abducted to 90° and the elbow flexed to 90°. Gentle passive external rotation from this position, with or without gentle anterior pressure applied to the back of the humeral head, can make the patient fearful that dislocation will occur if the apprehension test is positive. Indeed, they have good reason – this test can provoke dislocation if carried out too forcefully or in the presence of an engaging Hill–Sachs lesion.

To refine this test further in the seated position, gentle anterior pressure on the back of the humeral head can be maintained whilst external rotation is carried out to the point at which involuntary contraction of pectoralis major occurs or the patient stops the examination due to apprehension (augmentation). This can be repeated at various positions of abduction, e.g. 60°, 90° and 120°, to give more information on the likely extent of labral detachment (the more inferiorly the detachment extends, the greater degree of

abduction into which apprehension persists or the more extensive is the Hill–Sachs lesion). Once the patient experiences apprehension, apply and maintain gentle pressure over the anterior aspect of the humeral head (or proximal humerus). The patient becomes more comfortable, and end of apprehension indicates that the humeral head has relocated in the glenoid (relocation manoeuvre).

The **posterior apprehension test (Jerk test)** puts the arm into a position that provokes posterior subluxation or dislocation – achieved by horizontal adduction of the internally rotated arm whilst axial load is applied along the humerus (Figure 2.30). This test is more often associated with pain and sometimes apprehension. Even if apprehension does not occur or is equivocal, axial load should be maintained as the arm is brought out of internal rotation and adduction. Relocation of the subluxed humeral head may be felt, analogous to the Barlow/Ortolani combination in testing infant hips.

Conclusion

Clinical examination of the shoulder adds to diagnostic information gathered when taking a history and directs one to appropriate further investigations or treatments. However, the signs must be interpreted in context, as none of the tests described above has perfect sensitivity or specificity. None is truly diagnostic, and a meta-analysis suggested that no test for impingement or ACJ pathology demonstrated sufficient diagnostic accuracy.[10] A holistic view should be taken when examining a patient after listening to their description of the problems they are experiencing with their shoulder.

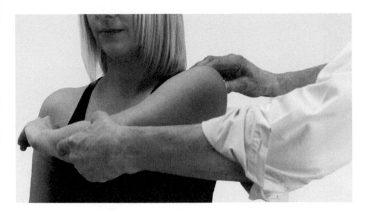

Figure 2.30 The posterior apprehension test (Jerk test). Shoulder at 90° and adducted. Then axial load along the humerus.

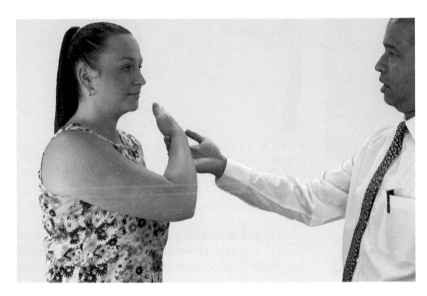

Figure 2.31 Bear-hug test for subscapularis tears. The patient puts the hand of their affected shoulder on top of the contralateral shoulder. Flex the shoulder to 90°. The examiner then tries to remove the hand from the shoulder (in an upward direction) while the patient tries to keep it there.

Advanced Corner

Bear-Hug Test

The bear-hug test is a good test that more accurately diagnoses *subscapularis tears* than the other described clinical tests. It was described by Barth, Burkhart and De Beer in 2006.[12]

The test is performed as follows:

Ask the patient to put the hand of the affected shoulder on top of the contralateral shoulder. Flex the shoulder to 90°. The examiner then tries to remove the hand from the shoulder (in an upward direction) while the patient is asked to continue to keep it there. Assess for strength and pain to confirm subscapularis integrity (Figure 2.31).

The bear-hug test was found to be the most sensitive test (60%) of all of those studied (belly-press test 40%; Napoleon's test 25%; and lift-off test 17.6%). In contrast, all four tests had a high specificity (lift-off test 100%; Napoleon's test 97.9%; belly-press test 97.9%; and bear-hug test 91.7%).

The bear-hug test optimises the chance of detecting a tear of the upper part of the subscapularis tendon. Moreover, because the bear-hug test represents the most sensitive test, it can be the most likely clinical test to alert the surgeon to a possible subscapularis tear. Performing all the subscapularis tests is useful in predicting the size of the tear.

31

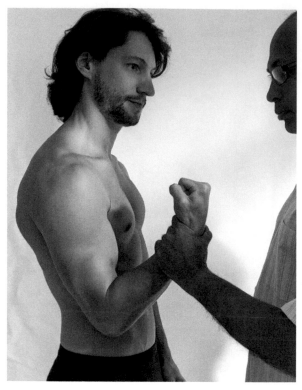

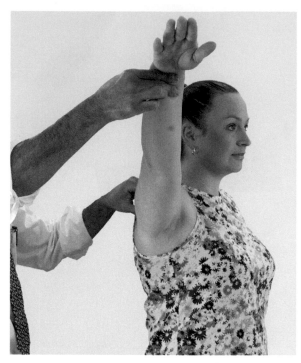

Figure 2.33 Drop arm test for a complete rotator cuff tear. There is poor ability to control the arm dropping to the side from a passively, fully abducted position. This lack of control starts at around 90° of abduction.

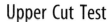

Figure 2.32 Upper cut test for biceps tendonitis. Pain occurs over the biceps tendon when the patient's attempt at an 'upper cut' (boxer's punch) is resisted.

Upper Cut Test

Biceps tendonitis is a difficult condition to diagnose. Numerous tests have been described in the literature to diagnose this pathology, but they lack adequate sensitivity and specificity. Recent studies have indicated that the upper cut test should be used as a screening test and that after a positive result; the Speed's and the Yergason's tests should be used as confirmatory tests to diagnose this condition.[13]

The upper cut test is performed as follows: The patient keeps the shoulder in neutral rotation with the elbow flexed to 90° in full supination. They are then told to make a grip and the examiner places their contralateral hand on the patient's wrist. The patient is then made to suddenly flex the elbow towards their chin (as in a boxer's punch). This manoeuvre can be repeated a few times. If this creates a pop or pain in the bicipital groove, then the test is deemed to be positive (Figure 2.32).

The test creates isometric contraction of the biceps tendon when the elbow is flexed and shoulder slightly internally rotated during this manoeuvre, creating stress on the biceps tendon in the groove.

Drop Arm Test

This is a test which can be used to diagnose a *complete rotator cuff tear*. When someone with an intact rotator cuff is asked to drop their arm to their side from a fully abducted position, they do so in a controlled manner. This control is lost from a position of around 90°–100° (when supraspinatus starts to act), down to the point where the arm is by the side, if there is a complete rotator cuff tear.[14]

It is performed as follows: The affected arm is passively abducted (with the elbow fully extended) to a point of near full abduction. The patient is then instructed to slowly drop their arm to the side. At about 90°–100° of abduction, their movement pattern becomes very jerky as they lose control of their arm (Figure 2.33).

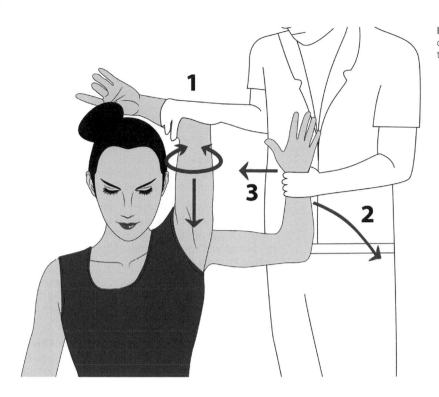

Figure 2.34 The three varieties of the crank test. The test for the SLAP lesion (1) is the most commonly performed.

This is a commonly performed test mainly by physiotherapists. The test has a very low sensitivity (about 24%) but a high specificity (90%).[15] It can also be seen with an axillary nerve palsy or deltoid tear. If on giving a subacromial joint injection, the test is repeated and the ability to drop the arm is more controlled, then some of the disability could be due to pain inhibition and therefore the rotator cuff may not necessarily be completely torn.

Crank Test

The term 'crank test' is confusing, as it is used to describe at least three different types of tests in the shoulder literature (Figure 2.34):

- **(1) Labral pathology** – SLAP lesions. This is the most common reference to a crank test. The arm is fully abducted and elbow flexed. Axial load is provided, followed by internal and external rotation of the humerus (similar to McMurray's in the knee). Pain is a positive result. Sensitivity is in the region of 46% and specificity 56%.[15]

- **(2) Anterior instability** – The anterior apprehension test is sometimes called the crank test. The shoulder is abducted 90° (and slightly extended). The elbow is flexed 90°. Passive external rotation of the humerus results in apprehension in the presence of anterior instability.[16]

- **(3) Biceps tendon pathology** – The shoulder is abducted to 90° and the elbow flexed to 90°. The patient is then asked to attempt to flex the elbow further against resistance, provoking pain with biceps tendon pathology.

Hyperabduction Test (Gagey)

This test assesses the laxity of the inferior glenohumeral complex. The examiner stands behind the seated patient with one hand firmly pressing downwards to stabilize the patient's scapula. With the other hand the examiner then abducts the patient's shoulder until the point where the scapula begins to rotate. The amount of glenohumeral abduction is assessed at this point. This is called the range of passive motion of the shoulder in abduction (RPA) by Gagey and Gagey.[17] The RPA should be less than 105°. If it is more than 105° then it is considered as positive for laxity of the inferior glenohumeral ligament.

33

References

1. Silliman JF, Hawkins RJ. Classification and physical diagnosis of instability of the shoulder. *Clin Orthop* 1993;**291**:7–19.

2. Lewis A, Kitamura T, Bayley JIL. The classification of shoulder instability: new light through old windows! *Curr Orthop* 2004;**18**(2):97–108.

3. Jobe FW, Moynes DR. Delineation of diagnostic criteria and a rehabilitation program for rotator cuff injuries. *Am J Sports Med* 1982;**10**:336–339.

4. Itoi E, Kido T, Sano A, Masakazu U, Sato K. Which is the more useful, the 'full can test' or the 'empty can test', in detecting the torn supraspinatus tendon? *Am J Sports Med* 1999;**27**(1):65–68.

5. Bigliani LU, Cordasco FA, McIlveen SJ, Musso ES. Operative treatment of massive rotator cuff tears: long term results. *J Shoulder Elbow Surg* 1992;**1**:120–130.

6. Hertel R, Ballmer FT, Lambert SM, Gerber C. Lag signs in the diagnosis of rotator cuff rupture. *J Shoulder Elbow Surg* 1996;**5**(4):307–313.

7. Kelly BT, Kadrmas WR, Speer KP. The manual muscle examination for rotator cuff strength: an electromyographic investigation. *Am J Sports Med* 1996;**24**:581–588.

8. Neer CS II, Welsh PR. The shoulder in sports. *Orthop Clin North Am* 1977;**8**:583–591.

9. Hawkins RJ, Kennedy JC. Impingement syndromes in athletes. *Am J Sports Med* 1980;**8**:151–157.

10. Hegedus EJ, Goode A, Campbell S, et al. Physical examination tests of the shoulder: a systematic review with meta-analysis of individual tests. *Br J Sports Med* 2008;**42**:80–92.

11. Yergason RM. Supination sign. *J Bone Joint Surg Br* 1931;**13**:160.

12. Barth JR, Burkhart SS, De Beer JF. The bear-hug test: a new and sensitive test for diagnosing a subscapularis tear. *Arthroscopy* 2006;**22**(10):1076–1084.

13. Cardoso A, Amaro P, Barbosa L, et al. Diagnostic accuracy of clinical tests directed to the long head of biceps tendon in a surgical population: a combination of old and new tests. *J Shoulder Elbow Surg* 2019;**28** (12):2272–2278.

14. Jain NB, Luz J, Higgins LD et al. The diagnostic accuracy of special tests for rotator cuff tear: the ROW Cohort Study. *Am J Phys Med Rehabil* 2017;**96** (3):176–183.

15. Stetson WB, Templin K. The crank test, the O'Brien test and routine magnetic resonance imaging scans in the diagnosis of labral tears. *Am J Sports Med* 2002;**30** (6):806–809.

16. Reider B. *The Orthopaedic Physical Examination*, 2nd ed. Philadelphia: Elsevier Saunders, 2005.

17. Gagey OJ, Gagey N. Assessment of the laxity of the inferior glenohumeral ligament. J Bone Joint Surg Br 2001;83-B:69–74.

Examination of the Elbow

Simon Booker, David Stanley and Amjid Ali

Steps in Assessment of the Elbow

A. History
B. Clinical Examination

Step 1
Stand the patient and look

Step 2
Move

Step 3
Feel

Step 4
Provocation tests (if indicated)

Step 5
Instability tests – medial, lateral and posterolateral

Stand and Look
Stand and look from the front, assessing the carrying angle. Look from the sides and then posteriorly; always look medially, especially for any scars.

Move
With the patient's shoulders abducted, ask them to extend both elbows and then to flex and compare the two. Ask them to put their elbows to the side and then test for pronation and supination. This pronation or supination can be quantified by either asking the patient to hold a pencil in the hand or to point the thumb upwards and compare each side.

Feel
Knowing the anatomy of the structures being palpated is essential, as the elbow is a superficial joint; therefore, tenderness over a specific structure indicates pathology in that structure.

Put one finger on the medial epicondyle, one finger on the lateral epicondyle and one on the tip of the olecranon. Feel for symmetry of the elbow by palpating these bony prominences. In extension, normally these three bony prominences form a horizontal line; in 90° of flexion, however, they form an isosceles triangle.

Feel for medial tenderness and then flex and extend the elbow and feel for a subluxing ulnar nerve. Palpate the lateral epicondyle and feel for lateral tenderness and then rotate the forearm and feel for the radial head.

Finally, palpate the anterior structures, especially for the biceps tendon insertion.

Provocation Tests
Provocation tests are then carried out, especially if the patient has medial or lateral tenderness. If the patient has medial tenderness, then the provocation test for golfer's elbow is performed. If the patient has lateral tenderness, then the provocation test for tennis elbow is performed.

The provocation test for the medial side is performed first by extending the elbow and then by asking the patient to flex the wrist and prevent the examiner from straightening it. This results in increased pain in the region of the medial epicondyle. A similar test is done for tennis elbow. Try to straighten an extended wrist against resistance. If this results in pain in the region of the lateral epicondyle, then this is a positive provocation test for lateral epicondylitis.

Instability Tests
Instability tests are for the medial collateral (valgus) and the lateral collateral (varus) ligaments.

Medial (Ulnar) Collateral
Stability is assessed by externally rotating the shoulder to lock it and by slightly flexing the elbow to unlock it from the olecranon fossa and then providing a valgus force to the elbow.

Lateral Collateral
The test for the lateral collateral ligament is performed by internally rotating the shoulder to lock

35

it, slightly flexing the elbow to unlock it and providing a varus force.

Posterolateral Rotatory Instability

Posterolateral rotatory instability (PLRI) is assessed by the pivot shift test. This is a painful test and is usually not required in the clinical examination. It is usually performed on an anaesthetised patient in the supine position. The shoulder and elbow are both flexed to 90°. An axial force is applied to the supinated forearm. At the same time, a valgus force is applied to the elbow and the elbow is slowly extended. In the presence of PLRI, the radial head will subluxate/dislocate as the elbow is taken into extension and will reduce when the elbow is flexed.

It is important that, as the patient describes the symptoms, the clinician interprets the information in the light of the local anatomy, most of which, because the elbow is a superficial joint, can be palpated and assessed during the examination.

History

It is always essential when taking a history to record the patient's age, sex and hand dominance. Age will give an immediate clue as to the likelihood of certain conditions being responsible for the patient's complaints. For example, osteochondritis dissecans may be the underlying cause of elbow locking in a young patient, whereas the same symptom in an older patient is more likely to be caused by loose body formation associated with degenerative disease.

The elbow may be the first presenting site of rheumatoid arthritis and, since this occurs more commonly in women, the sex of the patient should alert one to the possibility of this diagnosis if the initial symptoms are pain and slight swelling. Conversely, osteoarthritis is far more common in males, especially manual workers.[1]

Hand dominance is of importance because a disorder of the dominant elbow may result in the patient's inability to work, participate in sporting activity or undertake activities of daily living.

In addition to the current symptoms, it is important to enquire about the patient's previous medical health, particularly regarding whether there is any history of previous similar problems. Enquiry should also be made about trauma, occupation and current sporting activity.[2]

Presenting Symptoms

Most patients with elbow disorders present with pain, often associated with tenderness, or reduced elbow movement. Intermittent swelling and locking may also occur. More unusually, recurrent instability of the elbow is a significant problem. Combinations of these symptoms are not infrequent.

The nature of the patient's pain, together with its location and frequency, should be noted. It is important to record whether the pain is associated with movement and whether there is a history of pain radiation. For example, patients with ulnar nerve entrapment may experience local pain and tenderness at the elbow together with pain radiation down into the hand affecting the little and ring fingers, often with intermittent pins and needles or numbness.

Reduced elbow movement can be the result of a variety of conditions but is perhaps more commonly seen after elbow trauma or as a result of degenerative and inflammatory arthropathies. Loose bodies within the elbow joint may be another cause of reduced elbow movement, and this pathology is also often associated with intermittent elbow locking.

Although rare, recurrent instability of the elbow does occur following elbow trauma, particularly if the coronoid process has been damaged or the collateral ligaments torn. Recurrent dislocation is easily recognised, but posterolateral rotatory instability is much more subtle. Patients present with vague elbow discomfort, complaining of painful clicking, snapping, locking or giving way, which is frequently worse in supination.[3] Instability may also be a feature of inflammatory arthropathy, especially when the disease has resulted in significant bony destruction.

Symptoms of crepitus are not often reported by the patient and should be specifically asked about, because this may indicate mechanical derangement of the elbow or an inflammatory arthropathy.

As with all upper limb disorders it is essential to ask the patient specifically about neck symptoms since, at times, cervical spine pathology may result in symptoms referable to the elbow.

It is of relevance to enquire about the patient's general health since this may indicate a generalised musculoskeletal disorder. In addition, enquiry as to the patient's family history may reveal problems such as haemophilia or osteochondromatosis.

The patient's occupation is of relevance since there is some evidence to suggest that heavy manual work may be associated with degenerative change within the elbow joint.[1] Similarly, an enquiry regarding sporting activity is of importance. Throwing athletes may develop symptoms of ulnar collateral ligament insufficiency, occurring primarily during the late cocking and early acceleration phases of the throwing movement. Other athletes who undertake recurrent flexion and extension movements of the elbow, i.e. boxers, may develop posterior elbow impingement resulting from recurrent impact of the tip of the olecranon into the olecranon fossa.

Examination

Inspection (Look)

It is important to note the posture in which the patient holds the elbow. A painful elbow will often be protected with the arm being held adjacent to the patient's body, whilst patients who are unable to extend the elbow fully often find it most comfortable resting the arm by placing the hand in a trouser pocket.

Inspection should also include a close assessment of the elbow for evidence of previous scars, either traumatic or surgical, or the presence of elbow swelling such as will occur with an acute injury, inflammatory arthritis or a neoplastic lesion (Figure 3.1).

Rheumatoid nodules may be noted on the extensor aspect of the elbow. Always remember to inspect the medial aspect of the elbow. After an acute injury, bruising here is a sign of instability. Lateral bruising suggests an even higher-grade injury.[4]

The carrying angle of the elbow should be assessed with the elbow in full extension and supination. If this is not possible because of elbow pathology, then the assessment of the carrying angle is compromised (Figure 3.2).

Although the carrying angle varies, the average valgus angulation is 10° in males and 15° in females. An increase in valgus angulation may result from a previous bony injury to the lateral distal humerus (Figures 3.2a and 3.2b).

Varus deformity is always abnormal and most commonly occurs as the result of a supracondylar fracture in childhood or a growth arrest on the medial side of the distal humerus (Figure 3.2c). Be aware that patients with cubitus varus malunion may have an abnormal lateral thrust which can result in chronic attenuation of the lateral ulnar collateral ligament (LUCL) leading to posterolateral rotatory instability.

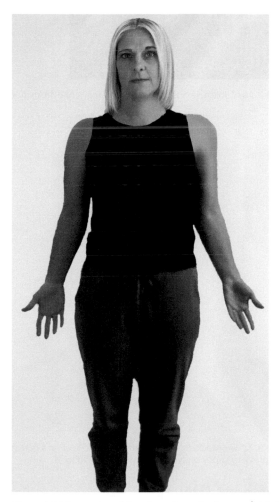

Figure 3.2 Inspection of the elbow from the front and side is followed by inspection from behind and medially. From the front, the carrying angle is noted.

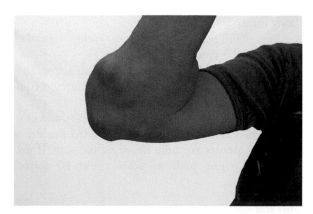

Figure 3.1 Large rheumatoid nodules seen on the extensor side of the arm, but most prominent when the patient is asked to flex the elbows.

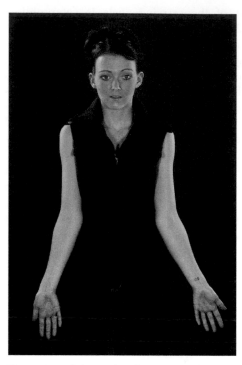

Figure 3.2a Cubitus valgus from previous lateral condyle fracture of humerus.

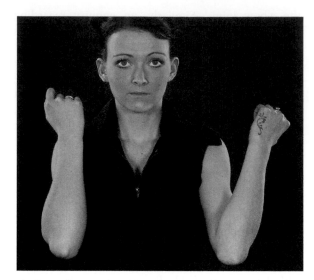

Figure 3.2b Note that the valgus is maintained even with flexion of the elbow.

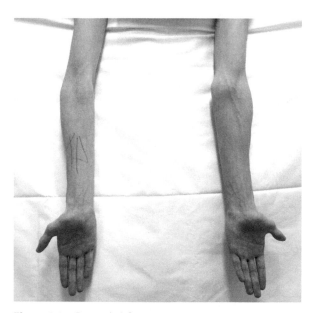

Figure 3.2c Gunstock deformity in the right arm seen in a patient with a previous supracondylar fracture during childhood.

Movement (Move)

Movement of the elbow can only adequately be assessed in a patient whose top clothes have been removed. It is important to compare both upper limbs to identify subtle changes in elbow movement clearly.

It should be noted that when the elbow is flexed from the fully extended position, the carrying angle changes from being valgus to varus.[5]

Flexion/Extension

With the forearms supinated and extended, the arms are forward flexed at the shoulders, then abducted to 90° at the sides (Figure 3.3a). The normal range of movement is from 0° to 140° of flexion (Figure 3.3b). Up to 10° of hyperextension (recorded as a negative integer) is not abnormal, but hyperextension beyond that level is suggestive of hypermobility or previous bony injury.

Loss of full extension is often the earliest sign of an intra-articular elbow abnormality.

A discrepancy between the passive and active range of movement is suggestive of either a musculotendinous or neurological abnormality.

It is important to look at the posterior aspect of the elbow either at the point of forward flexion or when the elbows are fully flexed by the side. If not, important signs such as scars could be missed (Figure 3.3c).

Forearm Rotation

Forearm rotation is assessed with both elbows flexed to 90° and with the arms adducted to the body

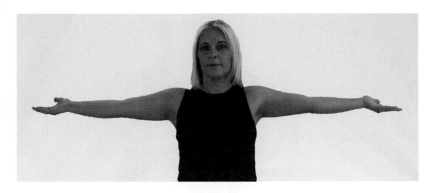

Figure 3.3a Extension of the elbows can be easily compared when the shoulders are abducted.

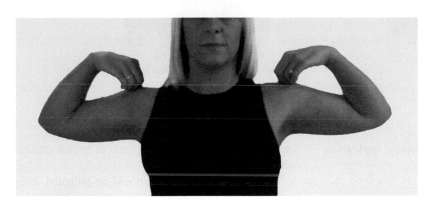

Figure 3.3b Flexion of the elbows can be compared when the shoulders are abducted.

(Figure 3.4a,b). This prevents compensatory shoulder movement.

Variation in supination and pronation movement occurs in normal patients, although the average range of supination is 85°, whilst pronation is normally a few degrees less. Rotation can be assessed by holding a pen in the hand or with 'thumbs up'.

Strength

Although detailed assessment of muscle strength is not possible in the setting of the consulting room, it is possible to obtain a gross assessment of muscle strength by comparing both arms. Flexion is tested with the elbow flexed to 90° and the forearm in neutral rotation. Resistance to the flexion movement is applied and the two arms compared. Extension is tested with the arm in a similar position, but on this occasion resistance to extension movement is provided. Pronation and supination strength is assessed with the elbows flexed to 90° and in neutral rotation. The

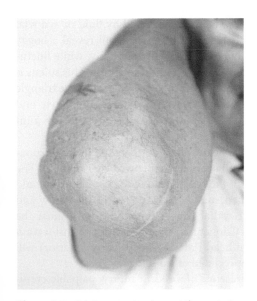

Figure 3.3c It is important to inspect the posterior aspect of the elbow when the elbow is flexed, as this could reveal important signs such as scars.

39

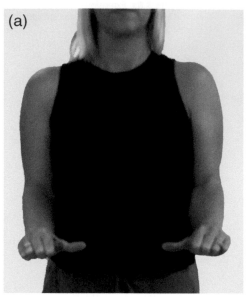
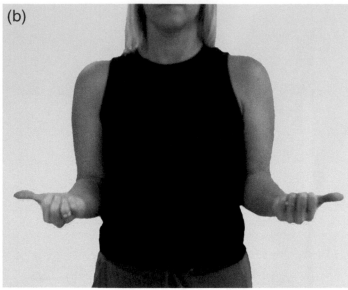

Figure 3.4a,b The range of pronation (a) and supination (b) is best assessed with the elbows held against the sides in order to minimise compensation from the shoulders.

movement under test is resisted. Normally, supination is slightly stronger than pronation.

Palpation (Feel)

A systematic approach to examination of the elbow must be developed. Much of the elbow is subcutaneous and, therefore, by careful examination most of the structures likely to be causing the patient's symptoms can be individually examined and assessed.

The lateral and anterior aspects of the elbow can be palpated with the examiner standing in front of the patient, whilst the medial and posterior aspects of the elbow are best examined from behind with the shoulder slightly abducted and extended.

Lateral

Examination of the lateral aspect of the elbow joint begins at the lateral supracondylar ridge (Figures 3.5a and 3.5b). This is easily palpable. Examination should extend down the ridge to the lateral epicondyle, common extensor origin and lateral collateral ligament.

The extensor carpi radialis brevis and extensor carpi radialis longus muscles can be assessed by resisted wrist extension in neutral and radial deviation, respectively. Tenderness, particularly at the site of the extensor carpi radialis brevis, should alert

the clinician to a possible diagnosis of lateral epicondylitis or tennis elbow.[6]

The capitellar joint line should be palpated since tenderness and discomfort at this site may indicate an articular injury or the presence of osteochondritis dissecans.

Inspection of the infracondylar recess between the lateral condyle and radial head will normally reveal a small sulcus. This is obliterated by fluid or synovial distension. Palpation of the area will reveal a boggy swelling if due to synovial hypertrophy, while fluctuation is noted if fluid is within the joint. This sulcus is formed within the anconeus triangle, with the triangle points being the radial head, lateral epicondyle and the tip of the olecranon. This is the site for joint aspiration in a flexed and pronated elbow.

The radial head is best appreciated during pronation and supination movement of the forearm. The orientation of the radial head to the capitellum should be determined, and in all positions of the elbow and forearm the radial head should line up against the capitellum. Congenital or post-traumatic dislocation of the radial head (lateral, posterior or anterior) will be easily appreciated at this stage.[7]

In the presence of a recent injury, palpable crepitus over the radial head, together with pain on rotation movements of the forearm, is usually indicative of a radial head fracture, although at times there may

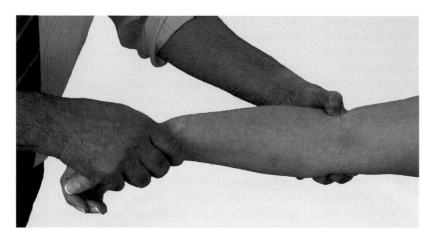

Figure 3.5a Palpation of the lateral aspect of the elbow.

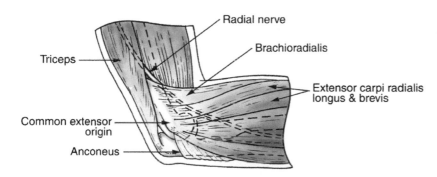

Radial nerve

Brachioradialis

Triceps

Extensor carpi radialis longus & brevis

Common extensor origin

Anconeus

Figure 3.5b The anatomy of the lateral aspect of the elbow.

also be an associated capitellar injury. In the absence of a recent injury, pain and crepitus at the radiocapitellar joint are usually indicative of degenerative change. The symptoms may be exacerbated by asking the patient to grip the examiner's fingers during forearm rotation.

Anterior

Anteriorly, the brachioradialis muscle and the biceps tendon, together with the lacertus fibrosus, the brachial artery and the median nerve, can be palpated from lateral to medial. It is therefore important to know the anatomical relationship of these structures (Figure 3.6a).

Although uncommon, myositis ossificans may occur after elbow dislocation and may be palpated as an abnormal hard swelling during examination of the anterior aspect of the elbow joint.[8]

Another reasonably common condition that may be appreciated on anterior elbow palpation is rupture of the insertion of the biceps tendon (Figure 3.6b).[9] The patient will normally present with a history of

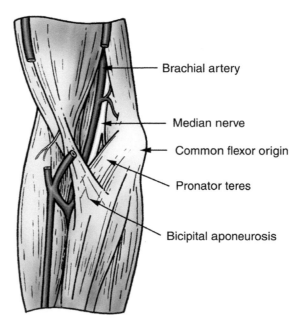

Brachial artery

Median nerve

Common flexor origin

Pronator teres

Bicipital aponeurosis

Figure 3.6a The anatomy of the anterior aspect of the elbow.

41

recent injury, most frequently caused by an eccentric load on the supinated forearm. Examination of the arm reveals a retracted biceps with the muscle bulge appearing more proximally in the arm as opposed to the more common long head of biceps rupture where the muscle bulge is distal. Assessment of power usually reveals moderate loss of flexion strength at the elbow but more marked weakness of supination in 90° of elbow flexion.

The **'hook' test** will demonstrate the presence or absence of the distal biceps tendon at the anterior aspect of the elbow (Figure 3.7a).[10] It is performed as follows: The patient actively fully supinates the forearm with their elbow in 90° flexion. The examiner then uses their finger from the *lateral* side to feel the cord-like structure and 'hook' their finger around it if

the distal biceps tendon is intact. If it is not intact, then this structure will not be felt.

If the distal biceps is attempted to be felt from the medial side, a false result may be obtained. This is because the bicipital aponeurosis (lacertus fibrosus), which is medial to the biceps tendon, can obstruct the examiner's finger (Figure 3.7b).

Medial

Tenderness on palpation of the medial epicondyle and origin of the common flexors will indicate medial epicondylitis, whilst tenderness over the belly of pronator teres should suggest the diagnosis of pronator syndrome.[11] Clinical features of this syndrome are often rather vague. They consist primarily of diffuse

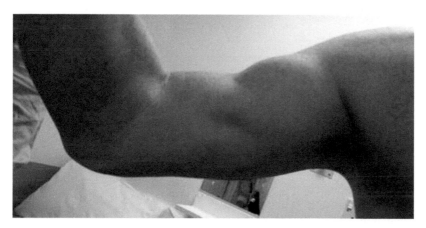

Figure 3.6b Rupture of the insertion of the biceps. Note the proximal position of the biceps muscle (reverse Popeye sign).

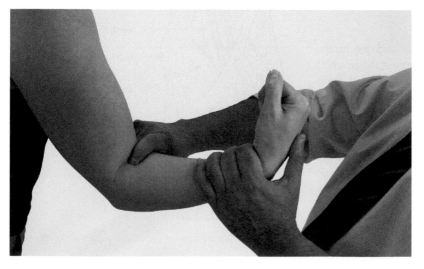

Figure 3.7a Demonstration of the 'hook' test. Note that the finger is hooked from the lateral side of the biceps tendon. The patient is actively supinating a flexed elbow.

proximal forearm discomfort and weakness that, in addition, may be associated with distal sensory changes in the distribution of the median nerve. Phalen's test and Tinel's sign are negative at the

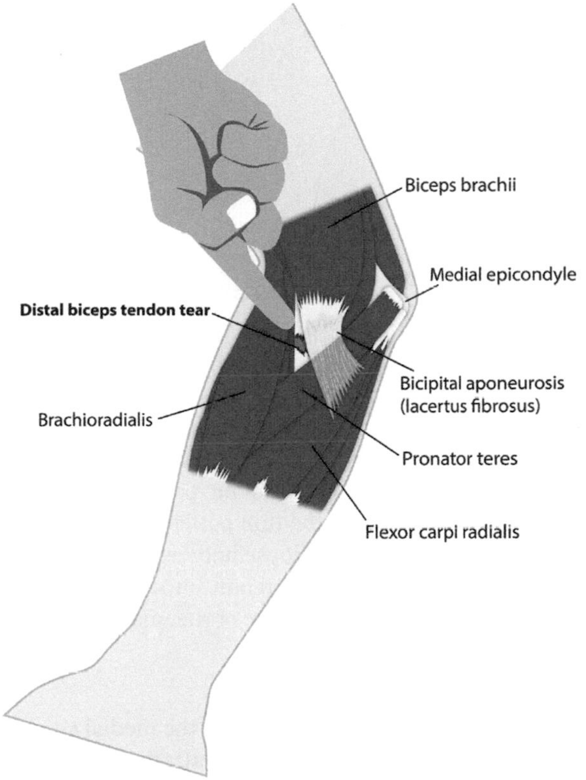

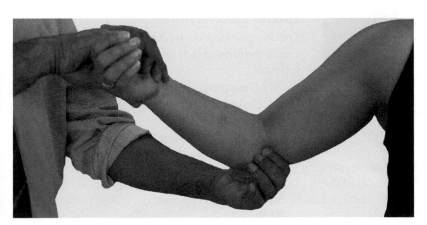

Figure 3.7b This illustration of the 'hook' test shows how a ruptured biceps tendon may be missed if it is performed from the medial side. This is because the bicipital aponeurosis is in the way.

wrist, whilst percussion over the median nerve at the elbow results in tingling distally.

Provocation tests, when positive, are helpful in confirming the diagnosis. These include resisted pronation for 60 seconds, resisted elbow flexion and forearm supination and resisted middle finger flexion at the proximal interphalangeal joint.

The ulnar nerve should be palpated and can be easily felt behind the medial epicondyle (Figures 3.8a and 3.8b). It should be remembered that in up to 10% of patients the ulnar nerve may sublux anteriorly, and it is important to identify the position of the ulnar nerve during flexion and extension movements of the elbow. A subluxing ulnar nerve may give rise to medial elbow pain.

More commonly, compression of the ulnar nerve gives rise to sensory and/or motor symptoms.[12] These may occur secondary to degenerative or inflammatory arthritis, medial epicondylitis, elbow instability and fracture dislocations. The nerve is most commonly compressed at the cubital tunnel and between the two heads of flexor carpi ulnaris. Tinel's sign is usually positive at the point of maximal nerve tenderness.

Posterior

With the elbow extended, the tip of the olecranon process and the medial and lateral epicondyles form a straight line. On flexion of the elbow to 90°, these landmarks form an isosceles triangle (Figures 3.9a and 3.9b). Any abnormality of this normal arrangement is suggestive of previous bony injury. For example, in an old supracondylar fracture these landmarks would be maintained, but if there was a chronic dislocation of the elbow, then they would not.

Figure 3.8a Palpating the medial side of the elbow. Subluxation of the ulnar nerve may be picked up on flexion and extension of the elbow.

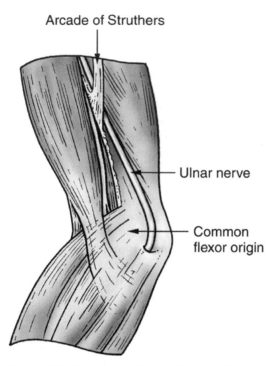

Arcade of Struthers

Ulnar nerve

Common flexor origin

Figure 3.8b The anatomy of the medial aspect of the elbow.

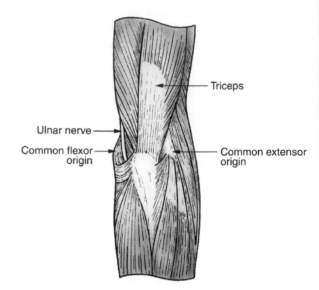

Triceps

Ulnar nerve

Common flexor origin

Common extensor origin

Figure 3.9b The anatomy of the posterior aspect of the elbow.

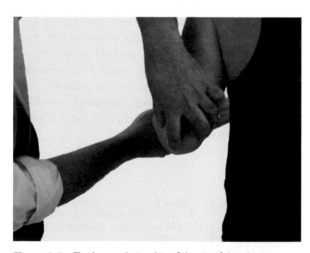

Figure 3.9a The bony relationship of the tip of the olecranon process to the medial and lateral epicondyles with the elbow flexed to 90°. Here an isosceles triangle is formed. When the elbow is extended, the triangle becomes a straight line.

With the arm extended, the triceps insertion onto the olecranon can be palpated and the integrity of the triceps tested by resisted extension. Tenderness on this manoeuvre may represent a partial tear of the triceps, whilst an inability to extend against gravity is indicative of a complete triceps avulsion.[13]

The olecranon fossa can be palpated with the elbow flexed to 30°. In the thin patient, it is occasionally possible to palpate a loose body within the fossa.

Examination of the olecranon bursa may reveal a bursitis or indicate the presence of rheumatoid nodules.

Provocation Tests

Both the long flexors that attach to the medial epicondyle and the long extensors which attach to the lateral epicondyle are inserted distally in the hand. Hence, the position of the wrist affects the length of these muscles, and therefore this concept can be utilised to perform the provocation tests.

Lateral Epicondylitis

Specific provocation tests of the wrist extensors that can be performed to help confirm the diagnosis are as follows:

- With the elbow extended, resisted wrist extension results in localised pain over the lateral epicondyle (Figure 3.10a).[14]
- Pain may also occur if the test is undertaken with the elbow flexed, the forearm pronated and the wrist in extension and radial deviation. Resisted extension of the wrist in this position causes pain over the lateral epicondyle; Cozen's test (Figure 3.10b).

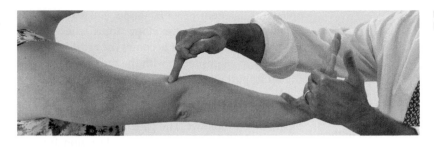

Figure 3.10a Provocation testing for lateral epicondylitis.

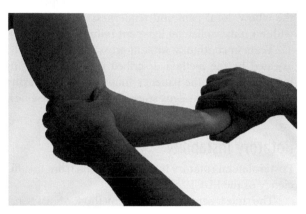

Figure 3.10b Cozen's test. The elbow is flexed, the forearm pronated, and the wrist is placed in extension and radial deviation.

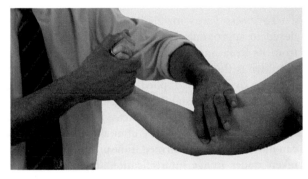

Figure 3.11 Provocation testing for medial epicondylitis.

Medial Epicondylitis

This is characterised by tenderness of the common flexor origin at the medial epicondyle. Provocation tests include the following:

- Resisted wrist flexion causes pain at the medial epicondyle (Figure 3.11).
- Passive extension of the wrist and elbow results in pain at the medial epicondyle.
- Clenching of the fist may also cause pain at the medial epicondyle.

Impingement

Elbow impingement most commonly occurs in the posterior compartment of the elbow joint but can also occur anteriorly.

In the posterior compartment, the symptoms are normally associated with osteophytic changes at the tip of the olecranon, which impinge on the olecranon fossa during extension. Loose bodies within the olecranon fossa may produce similar symptoms in the absence of osteophytic change. Clinically, there is often a history of repetitive hyperextension movements of the elbow.

The condition can be clinically demonstrated as follows: With the patient's elbow just short of full extension, applying a gentle, rapid passive extension force reproduces the posterior pain.

Anterior impingement occurs most commonly due to osteophytes on the coronoid process impinging into the coronoid fossa. Occasionally, anterior impingement is the result of osteophytic change within the radial fossa such that on full flexion the radial head impinges with the osteophytes.

The condition can be clinically demonstrated as follows: With the patient's elbow just short of full flexion, applying a gentle, rapid passive flexion force reproduces the anterior pain.

Instability of the Elbow

The elbow depends on bony (ulnohumeral, radiocapitellar and proximal radioulnar), capsular, ligamentous and musculotendinous structures for stability. The bony articulations are the main stabilisers at the extremes of motion (less than 20° and greater than 120° flexion).

Varus Instability

The lateral ligament complex is Y-shaped and is composed of four ligaments: the lateral collateral ligament (LCL), lateral ulnar collateral ligament (LUCL), accessory ligament and annular ligament. The LUCL is a thickening of the capsule that extends from its origin deep to the common extensors on the lateral humeral epicondyle to its tubercle on the supinator crest of the ulna. The LUCL is a restraint to varus stress and also acts to stabilise the radial head from posterior subluxation or dislocation.

To assess varus instability, the elbow should be flexed to approximately 30° (to unlock the olecranon from its fossa and to relax the anterior capsule). The shoulder is then locked in full internal rotation and a varus stress then applied to the elbow.[15] In the presence of varus instability, the gap between the capitellum and radial head will increase (Figure 3.12). This can often be appreciated by clinical examination but can more easily be confirmed if the procedure is undertaken under image intensification. The elbow under examination should be compared with the normal side.

Valgus Instability

With the elbow in full extension, the ulnohumeral articulation, anterior capsule and ulnar (medial) collateral ligament provide almost equal restraint to valgus translation. As the elbow approaches 90°, the ulnar collateral ligament becomes the most important stabiliser to valgus force, with the radial head becoming an important secondary stabiliser.

Valgus instability is most commonly seen in throwing athletes. Assessment of the ulnar collateral ligament is as follows: The patient's elbow is flexed to approximately 30° (to unlock the olecranon from its fossa), the shoulder locked in full external rotation and then a valgus stress is applied to the elbow. Opening of the elbow, local pain and tenderness are compatible with an ulnar collateral ligament injury (Figure 3.13).

Tears in continuity without gross instability can be assessed by the method described by O'Brien.[16] This involves holding the patient's thumb and fully flexing the elbow whilst a valgus stress is applied to the elbow joint.

Rotatory Instability

Posterolateral rotatory instability results from insufficiency of the LUCL.

The most sensitive clinical method of assessing insufficiency of the LUCL is the **lateral pivot shift test** (O'Driscoll), which is most commonly performed under general anaesthesia with image intensifier screening.

Although the originally described technique starts in full extension, the technique has been modified over the years (and is the authors' preference) where the patient is positioned supine with the shoulder and elbow flexed to 90°. The patient's forearm is fully supinated, and the examiner holds the patient's wrist and forearm and slowly extends the elbow whilst applying a valgus and axial compression force. As the elbow is extended, subluxation/dislocation of the radius and ulna from the humerus causes a prominence posterolaterally over the radial head and a dimple between the radial head and the capitellum. This subluxation/dislocation reduces when the elbow is again flexed. This may be accompanied by a palpable and visible clunk (Figure 3.14).[17]

Apprehension Signs

These are representative of posterolateral rotatory instability and the principles are similar to the pivot shift test.

Asking a patient to rise from a chair (**chair push-up test**) using their arms to push them into the standing position may reproduce symptoms of instability.

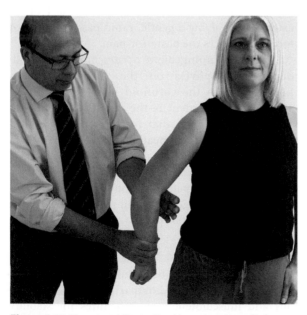

Figure 3.12 Varus instability testing. Varus stress is applied across the elbow with the humerus in full internal rotation. If instability is present, the gap between the capitellum and radial head increases.

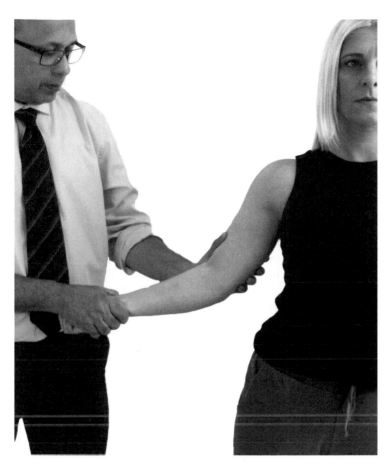

Figure 3.13 Valgus instability testing. Valgus stress is applied across the elbow with the humerus in full external rotation.

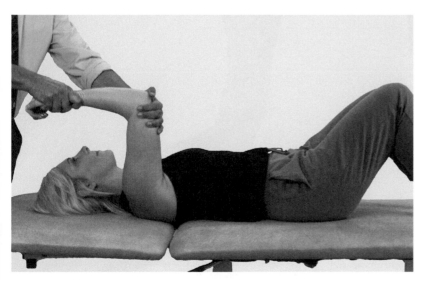

Figure 3.14 The lateral pivot shift test. With the patient lying supine, elbow flexed to 90°, and the arm above the head and forearm supinated, a valgus force with axial compression is applied to the elbow. With extension of the elbow, there is subluxation of the radial head, which produces a prominence and a dimple in the skin behind it. Subsequent flexion causes a reduction to occur with a palpable, audible clunk.

In such a situation, the patient is reluctant to extend the elbow fully since the manoeuvre involves an axial load, valgus and supination of the forearm (Figure 3.15).

A similar situation occurs if the patient is asked to perform a press-up (**floor push-up test**). The same forces are applied to the elbow and once more result in apprehension.[18] The patient is reluctant to extend the elbow fully.

Another test using the same concept is the **table top relocation test**. In this test, the patient experiences apprehension at around 40° of elbow flexion when lifting off with one arm from a table top with a supinated forearm. This pain is improved if the procedure is repeated with the examiner pressing on the radial head to prevent subluxation.[19]

Advanced Corner

Rotational Deformity

Rotational deformity is often not appreciated and results from an abnormality of either the shoulder or humerus. If both shoulders are normal, an asymmetrical range of rotation is indicative of a humeral rotational deformity. This may result from previous humeral fractures.

The deformity is best demonstrated by the technique described by Yamamoto et al.[20]

The examiner stands behind the patient with the elbow flexed to 90° and the forearm behind the back. With the patient bent forwards and the shoulder in full extension, the forearm is lifted maximally, resulting in maximal internal rotation. The angular difference above a horizontal line is the internal rotation deformity (Figure 3.16).

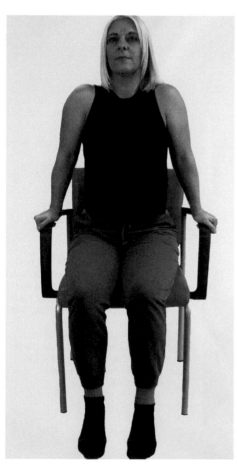

Figure 3.15 The chair push-up test. Note that the arms are slightly abducted, the elbows are initially flexed to 90° and the forearms are supinated. The patient is reluctant (because of pain) to fully extend the elbow when rising from a chair and pushing up with their arms.

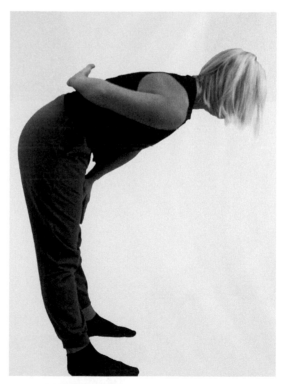

Figure 3.16 The assessment of rotational deformity. The patient is bent forwards, the shoulder fully extended and the elbow flexed to 90°. If there is no rotational deformity, the forearm is parallel to the ground. If there is increased internal rotation in the humerus, then the acute angle between the line of the forearm and the horizontal gives a measure of the internal rotation deformity.

Posterolateral Rotatory Instability

O'Driscoll first described the concept of PLRI in 1991.[17] In the presence of an LUCL injury, the combined valgus, supination and compression forces across the elbow produce a rotatory subluxation of the ulnohumeral joint. Anatomically, the semilunar notch of the ulna is displaced from the trochlea of the humerus. This rotation dislocates the radiohumeral joint posterolaterally by a coupled motion. The LUCL is the structure that prevents the ulna from rotating on its long axis away from the trochlea, ultimately allowing the radiohumeral joint to sublux or dislocate.[21]

The posterolateral rotatory displacement is at a maximum at approximately 40° of flexion. Additional flexion results in a sudden reduction of the radiohumeral and ulnohumeral joints. Flexion and extension through the very small arc in the identified range will cause the radiohumeral joint to be alternately dislocated and reduced.

Varus Posteromedial Rotatory Instability

Varus posteromedial rotatory instability (VPMRI) of the elbow is a recently recognised concept. It is seen after trauma with the shoulder in an abducted and flexed position, with the elbow in varus alignment, causing pronation and internal rotation.

It is usually associated with a coronoid anteromedial facet fracture and disruption of the lateral ligamentous complex.

To test: It can be identified under anaesthesia with the **hyperpronation test** where passive pronation of the elbow at 90° flexion produces palpable ulnohumeral subluxation.

Gravity-assisted varus stress with shoulder abducted and elbow moved from flexion to extension in neutral rotation causing instability/pain/crepitus can be performed in clinic.[22]

References

1. Stanley D. Prevalence and aetiology of symptomatic elbow osteoarthritis. *J Shoulder Elbow Surg* 1994;**3**:386–389.

2. Andrews JR, Whiteside JA. Common elbow problems in the athlete. *J Orthop Sports Physiother* 1993;**6**:289–295.

3. Lee ML, Rosenwasser MP. Chronic elbow instability. *Orthop Clin North Am* 1999;**30**(1):81–89.

4. Robinson PM, Griffiths E, Watts AC. Simple elbow dislocation. *Shoulder Elbow* 2017;**9**(3):195–204.

5. Morrey BF, Chow EY. Passive motion of the elbow joint. *J Bone Joint Surg Am* 1976;**58A**:501–508.

6. Major HP. Lawn tennis elbow. *BMJ* 1883;**ii**:557.

7. Mardam-Bey T, Ger E. Congenital radial head dislocation. *J Hand Surg* 1979;4:316–320.

8. Thompson H, Garcia A. Myositis ossificans: aftermath of elbow injuries. *Clin Orthop* 1967;**50**:129–134.

9. Baker BE, Bierwagen D. Rupture of the distal tendon of biceps brachii. *J Bone Joint Surg Am* 1985;**67A**:414–417.

10. O'Driscoll SW, Goncalves LB, Dietz P. The hook test for distal biceps avulsion. *Am J Sports Med* **35** 2007;**35** (11):1865–1869.

11. Hartz CR, Linscheid RL, Gramse RR, Daube JR. The pronator teres syndrome: compressive neuropathy of the median nerve. *J Bone Joint Surg Am* 1981;**63A**:885–890.

12. Spinner M, Kaplan EP. The relationship of the ulnar nerve to the medial intermuscular septum in the arm and its clinical significance. *Hand* 1976;**8**:239–242.

13. Bennett BS. Triceps tendon rupture. *J Bone Joint Surg Am* 1962; **44A**:741–744.

14. Nirschl RP. Elbow tendinosis/ tennis elbow. *Clin Sports Med* 1992;**4**:851–870.

15. Regan WD, Korinek SL, Morrey BF, An KN. Biomechanical study of ligaments about the elbow joint. *Clin Orthop* 1991;**271**:271.

16. Jobe F, Flattrache N. Reconstruction of the MCL. In Morrey BF (ed), *Master Techniques: The Elbow*. Philadelphia: Raven Press, 1994.

17. O'Driscoll SW, Bell DF, Morrey BF. Postero-lateral rotatory instability of the elbow. *J Bone Joint Surg Am* 1991;**73A**:440–446.

18. Regan WD, Morrey BF. Physical examination of the elbow. In Morrey BF (ed), *The Elbow and Its Disorders*, 3rd ed. Philadelphia: WB Saunders, 2000.

19. Arvind CH, Hargreaves DG. Tabletop relocation test: a new clinical test for posterolateral rotatory instability of the elbow. *J Shoulder Elbow Surg* 2006;**15**:707–708.

20. Yamamoto I, Ishii S, Usui M, Ogino T, Kaneda K. Cubitus varus deformity following supracondylar fracture of the humerus: a method for measuring rotational deformity. *Clin Orthop* 1985;**201**:179–185.

21. McAdams TR, Masters GW, Srivastava S. The effect of arthroscopic sectioning of the lateral ligament complex of the elbow on posterolateral rotatory stability. *J Shoulder Elbow Surg.* 2005;**14**(3):298–301.

22. Chan K, Athwal GS. Varus posteromedial rotatory instability. In Tashjian RZ (ed), *The Unstable Elbow*. Cham: Springer, 2017.

Examination of the Wrist

Stephen Bostock and Meg Birks

Assessment of the Wrist

A. History

B. Clinical Examination

Step 1

Look

Step 2

Move

Step 3

Feel

Step 4

Provocation tests (if indicated)

Step 5

Instability tests (if indicated)

As with the elbow, the sequence *look, move, feel* (followed by provocation then instability tests) appears to flow better than the traditional *look, feel, move*.

Look

Sit the patient. Look at both palmar and dorsal aspects of the wrist.

Move

Dorsiflexion – Hands together and lift both elbows up comparing sides.

Palmarflexion – Dorsum of hands together and move both elbows downwards.

Radial and ulnar deviation.

Pronation and supination – With elbows tucked into side.

Feel

For tender areas (remember Lister's tubercle just proximal to scapholunate ligament.

Then depending on tender area this will direct you to perform the relevant special test.

Special Tests

The following are the more commonly performed provocation or instability tests:

- Snuffbox tenderness – palpate scaphoid tubercle and perform first metacarpal axial compression.
- Radial tenderness – perform Finklestein's test.
- Tenderness over the scapholunate ligament – perform Kirk Watson test.
- Tenderness over lunotriquetral ligament – perform lunotriquetral ballottement test.
- Tenderness over triangular fibrocartilage complex (TFCC) – perform TFCC compression test.
- Prominence of the ulna head – perform piano key test.

History

Patients with wrist problems often have a paucity of clinical signs. Specific provocation tests can be both difficult to perform and equivocal in their interpretation. A thorough history is therefore essential.

This should start by recording the age, occupation and handedness of the patient. Affected recreational activities should also be recorded, including sports and hobbies. Different sport will typically result in a characteristic problem related to that sport. For example, rowers, weightlifters and tennis players can get intersection syndrome. Golfers may get De Quervain's disease and, if so, it is usually on the dominant side.

The basic complaint must be established. Is it pain, weakness, a swelling, stiffness or a combination of these? Are there other symptoms? How long has there been a problem? Was there an injury, or has the onset been insidious? What was the nature of the injury? Was it a single event or repetitive trauma and, if so, did it receive treatment at the time?

The site and nature of **pain** should be established (Figure 4.1). The patient should be asked to try to localise it as accurately as possible (e.g. by

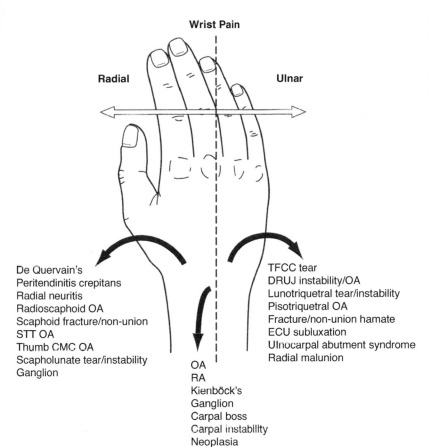

Wrist Pain

Radial ⟷ Ulnar

Figure 4.1 Sites of commonly occurring pathologies about the wrist.

CMC, carpometacarpal; DRUJ, distal radio-ulnar joint; ECU, extensor carpi ulnaris; OA, osteoarthritis; RA, rheumatoid arthritis; STT, scaphotrapeziotrapezoid; TFCC, triangular fibrocartilage complex

De Quervain's
Peritendinitis crepitans
Radial neuritis
Radioscaphoid OA
Scaphoid fracture/non-union
STT OA
Thumb CMC OA
Scapholunate tear/instability
Ganglion

TFCC tear
DRUJ instability/OA
Lunotriquetral tear/instability
Pisotriquetral OA
Fracture/non-union hamate
ECU subluxation
Ulnocarpal abutment syndrome
Radial malunion

OA
RA
Kienböck's
Ganglion
Carpal boss
Carpal instability
Neoplasia

pointing). What is its nature; is it constant or intermittent, sharp, dull or 'burning'? Is it worse with use and eased by rest? Are there particular movements that aggravate the pain such as turning taps, opening jars?

Stiffness may be a part of the presenting problem. If so, determine and record which movements are restricted. Is there associated discomfort; if so, how does this interfere with the use of the arm in functional terms?

Swelling may be present. If so, is this the main problem? Is it painless? Is the swelling growing or does its size vary?

Other symptoms may also be present, e.g. a 'click' or a 'clunk'. If so, is it painful? Has there been an injury? Is the wrist weak? Does the weakness appear to be secondary to pain?

The history also needs to document the impact that the patient's wrist problem has had on activities of daily living, work, sports and other hobbies.

Examination

Inspection (Look)

The patient should be sat comfortably in a chair directly facing the examiner. Patients will usually offer their wrist forward in pronation (Figure 4.2). Observe this and then place the opposite side in a corresponding position with the elbows to the sides. Look carefully and systematically at the wrists. Look at the overall alignment and shape of the forearm wrist and hand. Is there obvious deformity? What is the likely nature of this deformity (e.g. Madelung's deformity, rheumatoid arthritis, radial malunion)? Is there an obvious swelling in the wrist (dorsal wrist ganglion, carpal boss)?

Be aware of the particular clinical signs of each of the possible pathologies, as this will help with the description of the correct pathology. These are described in the following sections.

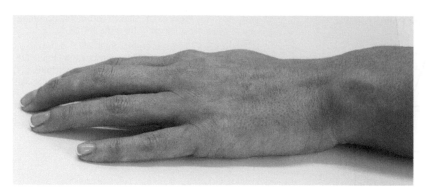

Figure 4.2 Inspection usually starts on the dorsum of the wrist.

Rheumatoid Arthritis

Features of rheumatoid arthritis are usually prominent around the wrist.[1] These include:

- Extensor synovitis
- Extensor tendon rupture
- Dorsal subluxation of the distal radioulnar joint (DRUJ)
- Volar subluxation and supination of the carpus
- Ulnar translocation of the carpus with radial metacarpal drift and ulnar drift of the fingers
- Flexor synovitis
- Flexor tendon rupture
- Finger deformities
- Bilaterality
- Other joint involvement.

Radial Malunion

Deformity most commonly follows the pattern of the original fracture, e.g. most commonly radial shortening and prominence of the distal ulna.

Madelung's Deformity

This condition arises in childhood. There is volar bowing of the distal radius, with dorsal prominence of the distal ulna. Look for hypoplastic radius, family history, absence of trauma, bilaterality.[2] (Dorsal bowing may occur and is described as 'reverse Madelung's deformity'.)

Dorsal Wrist Ganglion

This usually arise from and overlie the scapholunate ligament[3] (just distal to Lister's tubercle). They will transilluminate if large. Pain without swelling in this area may represent an 'occult' ganglion[4] (a small ganglion that is not large enough to see or palpate). Diagnosis is by ultrasound or magnetic resonance imaging (MRI).

Carpal Boss

Bony hard swelling at the level of the second and third CMC joints dorsally. More distal than most simple ganglia. To confuse matters however, a carpal boss may have an associated small overlying bursa.[5]

Extensor Digitorum Brevis Manus

This is an extra (vestigial) muscle whose presence distal to the extensor retinaculum may confuse it with a ganglion or extensor synovitis. This muscle will move with finger extension.

Once the dorsum has been inspected, ask the patient to supinate. Determine whether this movement is pain free or restricted.

Then carefully inspect this volar surface from its ulnar aspect back to the radial side, thus completing the circumference of the wrist. Look for scars and swelling, comparing right with left.

Volar Ganglion

A volar ganglion on the radial side must be examined with the underlying radial artery in mind using Allen's test (Chapter 5). This is because it may increase in size and cause compression; alternatively, surgery may be contemplated, and the surgeon therefore needs to ensure that the ulnar artery is adequately supplying the hand in case the radial artery is damaged during surgery.

On the volar side of the wrist look for swelling which can contribute to a carpal tunnel syndrome or compression in Guyon's canal. If present, this should prompt the examiner to look for signs of median or ulnar nerve compression, respectively.

Finally, fully flex the elbows and inspect the ulnar aspect of the wrists looking at the profile

(a) 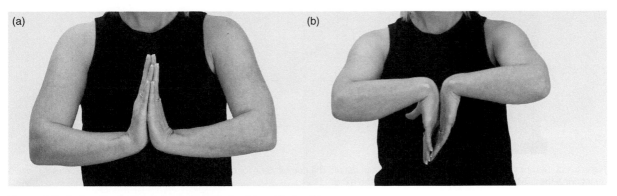 (b)

Figure 4.3a,b A method of assessing wrist extension (a) and flexion (b).

(c) 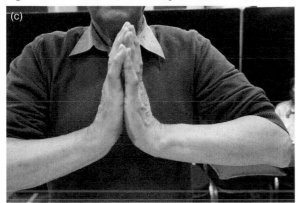 (d)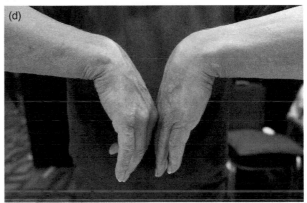

Figure 4.3c,d Patient with restricted extension (dorsiflexion) (c) and flexion (palmar flexion) (d) of right wrist.

of the distal ulna in relation to the radius. Asymmetry suggests possible DRUJ subluxation (dorsal or volar).

Range of Motion (Move)

Flexion/Extension (Palmar Flexion/Dorsiflexion)

Both palmar and dorsiflexion measure about 75°.

Extension can be assessed by placing the palms of the hands together and lifting up the elbows (this allows for direct comparison of the right and left sides).

Flexion can be measured in a similar way with the dorsum of both hands in apposition (Figures 4.3a,b and 4.3c,d).

A goniometer may be used to quantify the range more accurately. Each wrist is measured in turn. For wrist extension, the goniometer is placed on the volar aspect in line with the radius and third metacarpal. For flexion, the goniometer is placed dorsally in the same line.

Radial and ulnar deviation are assessed with the wrists in pronation and the elbows to the sides (Figure 4.4). The range can also be assessed with a goniometer by alignment with the radius and the

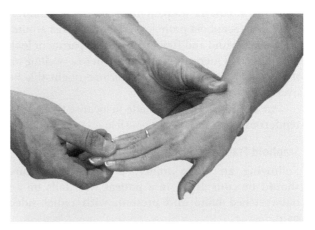

Figure 4.4 Demonstration of ulnar deviation (perform active followed by passive).

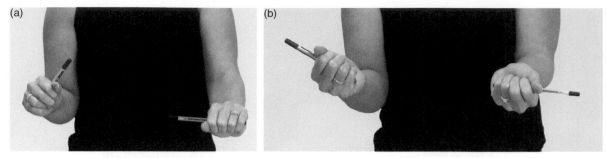

Figure 4.5 Demonstrations of (a) pronation and (b) supination. The normal value for both movements is approximately 80°. A useful way of quantifying this is asking the patient to hold a pen in the hand.

third metacarpal on the dorsum of the wrist. Typically, radial deviation is slightly less than ulnar deviation (20° and 35°, respectively).

Pronation and supination are measured with the elbows to the sides (Figure 4.5a,b), again with a comparison of right and left (about 80°for both pronation and supination). Note that it is difficult to separate the contributions to pronation and supination from the wrist and the elbow (see 'Advanced Corner').

For all movements, it may be appropriate to assess 'active' range of motion in addition to the passive measurements.

Palpation (Feel)

Palpation should also follow a system. Work across the wrist initially on its dorsal aspect and then volarly (Figure 4.6). Palpation should be aimed at specific anatomical landmarks (Figures 4.7).

Start on the dorsal aspect and work across from radial to ulnar. Is there fullness in the anatomical snuffbox? (Scaphoid pathology.) Does the area around the radial styloid and first extensor compartment look swollen? (De Quervain's disease.) Is there a swelling on the dorsum and, if so, what structure might this be overlying?

An attempt should be made to localise the area of tenderness as accurately as possible

Scaphoid Fracture

Following an acute injury, a scaphoid fracture should be considered in a patient who falls on an outstretched hand and presents with radial sided pain.

There is no single reliable test to diagnose a scaphoid fracture. The three most common ones are snuffbox tenderness, scaphoid tubercle tenderness and axial pressure along the first metacarpal (Figure 4.8a,b,c). These tests each have a sensitivity of around 100%. However, their specificity is 9%, 30% and 48%, respectively. If all three of these tests are combined, then the specificity improves to 74%.[6] Therefore, to make a diagnosis of scaphoid fracture, it is recommended that the three clinical tests be used in combination. Three other additional signs have also been used to help with the clinical diagnosis: wrist swelling, reduced thumb movement and reduced grip strength.[7]

De Quervain's Disease

Swelling and pain are localised to the first extensor compartment (overlying the radial styloid). Crepitus may be present ('wet leather sign') on active and passive movements of the thumb. There may be an associated ganglion.

Radial Neuritis (Wartenberg's Neuralgia)

Radial neuritis presents as pain and tenderness over the terminal cutaneous branches of the radial nerve. Look for a history of trauma.

Intersection Syndrome (Peritendinitis Crepitans)

This is a bursitis between abductor pollicis longus (APL) and extensor pollicis brevis (EPB) and the wrist extensors extensor carpi radialis longus (ECRL) and extensor carpi radialis brevis (ECRB). Crepitus is often palpable together with tenderness. This area of discomfort is more proximal (about

5 cm proximal to Lister's tubercle) and central than that in De Quervain's disease.[8]

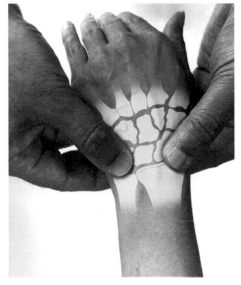

Figure 4.6 Palpating in sequence dorsal (usually first), volar, radial and ulnar aspects of wrist.

Kienböck's Disease

There is very specific tenderness over the lunate. This is usually associated with some wrist swelling, reduced range of movement and reduced grip strength.

Hamate Fracture/Non-union

Tenderness over the hook of the hamate (distal and radial to the pisiform) may indicate an underlying fracture or non-union. In these conditions, the pain may be made worse by resisted flexion of the little and ring fingers with the wrist in ulnar deviation.

Provocation and Instability Tests

Several provocation tests for various conditions about the wrist have been described (Table 4.1). Clearly, it would be inappropriate to perform all the available tests in every patient. A strategy is needed based on the history and examination. In particular, the location of the tenderness, and therefore presumed diagnosis, will dictate the best tests to perform.

Carpal instability is a term that is used to describe a wide variety of pathological conditions, all of which

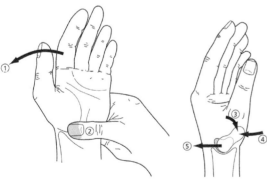

1. The wrist is moved from ulnar into radial deviation
2. Pressure is applied by the examiner's thumb to resist scaphoid flexion
3. Scaphoid rotates (flexes) with radial deviation of the wrist
4. Applied force (examiner's thumb)
5. Subluxation (may be felt by examiner's index/middle finger)

Figure 4.7 Demonstration of the anatomical structures around the wrist. A point of tenderness will indicate the underlying pathology and prompt the examiner as to which special test to perform.

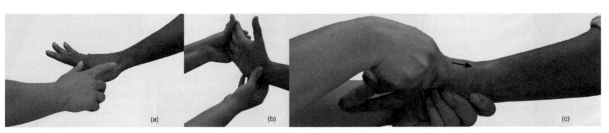

Figure 4.8a,b,c (a) Tenderness in the anatomical snuffbox may signify a scaphoid fracture. Similarly, tenderness over the scaphoid tubercle (b) or with axial pressure down the first metacarpal (c) may also signify a scaphoid fracture.

Table 4.1 Provocation and instability tests

Condition	Main site	Test
De Quervain's disease	Radial	Finkelstein's test
Intersection syndrome	Radial	Resisted wrist extension and thumb extension
Scapholunate instability	Radial	Scaphoid shift (Kirk Watson) test Also 'scaphoid thrust' and 'scaphoid lift'
Midcarpal instability	Central	Midcarpal shift test Pivot shift test
Ulnar-sided pathology – general	Ulnar	Ulnocarpal stress test
Lunotriquetral instability	Ulnar	Ballottement test (Reagan) Shear test
Pisotriquetral arthritis	Ulnar	Grind test
DRUJ instability	Ulnar	Piano key test Compression test Radioulnar drawer test Dimple sign
TFCC tear	Ulnar	Compression test

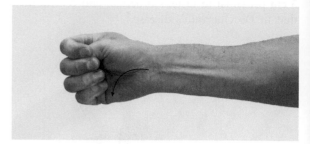

Figure 4.9 Finkelstein's test, which stresses the first extensor compartment, is a provocative test for De Quervain's tenosynovitis. The thumb is flexed, followed by ulnar deviation of the wrist.

over the inflamed area in the region of the radial styloid (i.e. within the first extensor compartment).[9] This can be a painful test, and sometimes rather than passively ulnar deviating the wrist the examiner can perform an active 'patient-controlled' Finkelstein's test.

Intersection Syndrome: Provocative Test

Palpable crepitus over the area of tenderness is key to diagnosis. However, pain is increased with resisted wrist extension and thumb extension.[10]

Scapholunate Instability

Rupture of the scapholunate ligament permits abnormal movement between the scaphoid and the lunate. Kirk Watson described a provocative test to reproduce and clinically detect this abnormal movement. This test is known variously as the 'Kirk Watson test', the 'Watson test', the 'scaphoid test' or the 'scaphoid shift'.[9] Two other tests for scapholunate instability are the 'scaphoid thrust' and the 'scaphoid lift' tests.[11,12,13] These are described later in the chapter.

Scaphoid Shift Test (Kirk Watson)

The examiner uses one hand to grasp the wrist, placing the fingers dorsally (index or middle fingertips to lie over the area of the scapholunate ligament). The thumb is placed over the scaphoid tubercle volarly. With the examiner's other hand, the patient's wrist is moved from **ulnar into radial** deviation whilst maintaining pressure on the scaphoid tubercle (Figure 4.10a,b). With radial deviation, the scaphoid will usually flex. The thumb pressure resists this, and in the presence of a scapholunate tear the scaphoid subluxes over the dorsal lip of the radius. A positive test occurs when this abnormal movement is felt by the examiner, often as a 'click'. Pain may also be

stem from disruption of the complex ligament system that controls the relative motion of the bones that form the carpus. A considerable number of instability patterns have been described. The common tests are for scapholunate, lunotriquetral and midcarpal instability.

Although there is overlap, broadly speaking, wrist symptoms and signs can be divided into those that are predominantly radial, central or ulnar.

Radial Pain/Tenderness

The main conditions to think of are De Quervain's disease, intersection syndrome and scapholunate instability.

De Quervain's Disease: Finkelstein's Test

The examiner supports the forearm with one hand. With the other hand, the thumb is adducted and the wrist ulnarly deviated to put tension on the APL and EPB tendons (Figure 4.9). A positive test will elicit pain

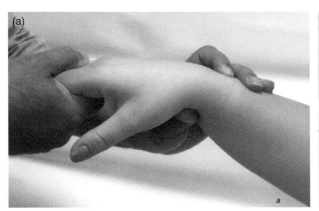

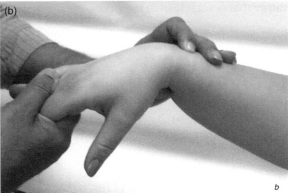

Figure 4.10a,b The scaphoid shift test (Kirk Watson). Pressure over the scaphoid tubercle with the examiner's thumb whilst radially deviating the wrist causes a click or pain in scapholunate instability.

a significant finding but is less specific for scapholunate instability. The 'scaphoid shift' is positive in up to 36% of 'normal' individuals (and especially those with hyperlaxity).[14]

Central Pain/Tenderness

The possible diagnoses are radiocarpal arthritis, Kienböck's disease and midcarpal instability. There are no specific tests for arthritis or Kienböck's.

Midcarpal Instability

The 'drawer tests' may be positive in patients with midcarpal instability, although they are more commonly an assessment of general ligamentous laxity. More specific tests for midcarpal instability are the 'midcarpal shift test' and the 'pivot shift'

Radiocarpal and Midcarpal Drawer Tests

The examiner firmly grasps the patient's forearm with one hand. With the other hand, the examiner holds the patient's hand at metacarpal level and a distracting force is applied. A dorsal and volar translating force is then applied, and the amount of movement assessed (comparing sides). This tests the radiocarpal joint.

If the examiner then repeats the manoeuvre but moves the proximal hand distally to the level of the proximal carpal row, it has been suggested that it is possible to assess laxity across the midcarpal joint (Figure 4.11).

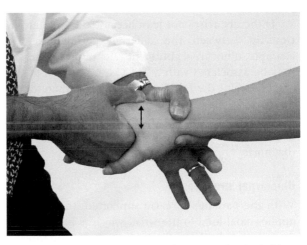

Figure 4.11 Midcarpal drawer test. The patient's hand is held at the level of the proximal carpal bones and a distracting force is applied. At the same time, the examiner exerts a translating force in both dorsal and volar directions.

Midcarpal Shift Test

The examiner stabilises the forearm with one hand. With the other hand, the examiner places their thumb over the capitate dorsally. A volarly directed force is applied as the wrist is ulnarly deviated. If there is a palpable 'clunk' as the wrist approaches full ulnar deviation, then this is a positive test. The degree of laxity and clunking has been graded (I–V). It is thought that in patients with midcarpal instability, the proximal carpal row is slow to dorsiflex as the wrist ulnarly deviates and that the clunk represents a catch-up movement.[15,16]

57

A slight variation on this test applies an axial rather than a volar load as the wrist is ulnarly deviated.

Pivot Shift Test

The elbow is placed on a firm surface and the hand is fully supinated. The forearm is held firmly. The hand is radially deviated, and pressure applied to the dorsoulnar aspect of the carpus. The hand is then ulnarly deviated. A normal wrist 'notches' into a less supinated position as the capitate engages the lunate.[15,17]

Ulnar Sided Wrist Pain/Tenderness

The diagnosis of ulnar sided wrist pain is difficult. The ulnocarpal stress test is a general screening test for ulnar-sided pathology. More specific tests have been described to try and separate out the underlying pathology.

Difficulty arises not least because of the interrelationship between the different pathologies. For example, ulnocarpal abutment (also ulnar impaction) may be associated with a TFCC tear.[18] The TFCC is a stabiliser of the DRUJ and a tear may therefore be associated with painful instability of the DRUJ. Thus, in the context of clinical examination it may be impossible and inaccurate to try to establish a single diagnosis.[17]

Ulnocarpal Stress Test

With the patient's forearm supported, the examiner applies axial load to the wrist, which is held in ulnar deviation and neutral flexion/extension. The forearm is then rotated. A positive test elicits pain on the ulnar side of the wrist.[19]

A variation of this test is to hold the forearm with the wrist in neutral pronation and supination but ulnar deviation. The wrist is then flexed and extended. A positive test elicits pain.

Lunotriquetral Ligament Injuries

Carpal instability associated with predominantly ulnar sided symptoms may be secondary to a lunotriquetral ligament tear. Reagan et al. have described a ballottement test.[20] There is also the shear test.

Ballottement Test (Reagan)

The lunate is fixed between the thumb and index finger of one hand. With the other thumb and index

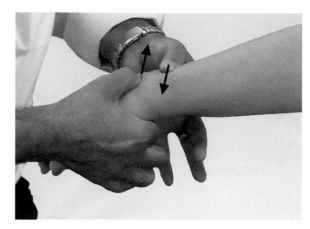

Figure 4.12 Ballottement test. Fixing the lunate between the finger and thumb of one hand and displacing the triquetrum dorsally and volarly with the other causes pain or demonstrates laxity in patients with lunotriquetral instability.

finger, the triquetrum (and pisiform) is displaced dorsally and volarly (Figure 4.12). Laxity, pain or crepitus indicates a positive result.

Shear Test

The lunate is stabilised with the thumb over the dorsal aspect of the wrist. A force is the applied to the pisiform volarly, thus indirectly applying a shear force across the lunotriquetral joint.

Pisotriquetral Arthritis

Pisotriquetral arthritis is a cause of ulnar-sided wrist pain. Many of the tests described for lunotriquetral tears apply compression across the pisotriquetral joint, and these tests are likely to be positive for pain where there is arthritis. A grind test has also been described that is a bit more specific for pisotriquetral arthritis.

Grind Test

In this test, the pisiform is held between the thumb and index finger. Compression is applied and the pisiform displaced back and forth in a radial and ulnar direction.

Distal Radioulnar Joint

Problems with the DRUJ may be isolated or part of a complex of injuries. Pain on pronation and supination may be exacerbated by compression. The (radioulnar) drawer test, 'piano key' test and 'dimple sign' may indicate joint subluxation.

Compression Test

Pain on pronation and supination of the forearm may not be specific to the distal radioulnar joint. The compression test applies a force across the joint by squeezing the forearm, which is then pronated and supinated. A positive test occurs where this increases pain in the region of the DRUJ.

Piano Key Test

The examiner stabilises the forearm distally with their fingers over the volar aspect. The thumb then presses over the distal ulna. Increased excursion suggests dorsal subluxation (this test can be used to demonstrate caput ulnae seen in conditions such as rheumatoid arthritis) (Figure 4.13).

Radioulnar Drawer Test

The flexed elbow is rested on a firm surface. The radius is stabilised with one hand. The ulna is grasped between the fingers and thumb of the other hand and moved dorsally and volarly. This can be repeated with the forearm in different positions of pronation and supination and should be compared with the opposite side. Laxity of the DRUJ can be assessed, and if excessive may be a sign of instability, especially if this is associated with discomfort.

Dimple Sign

Longitudinal traction is applied across the wrist. A force is applied to the dorsal aspect of the ulna shaft. If a 'dimple' appears at the level of the DRUJ, then this suggests volar subluxation.

TFCC Compression Test

The diagnosis of TFCC tears may be suspected from tenderness in the hollow just distal to the ulna head. This can be confirmed by the TFCC compression test. Here, the patient's forearm is pronated and the elbow flexed. The examiner grasps the forearm with one hand and grasps the fingers with the other hand. The wrist is then loaded by compressing the hand proximally against the forearm. It is then moved in radial and ulnar directions. A painful click may indicate a TFCC tear (Figure 4.14).[21]

Extensor Carpi Ulnaris Subluxation

Subluxation of the extensor carpi ulnaris (ECU) tendon may be provoked by placing the forearm in supination and ulnar deviation. With dorsiflexion, the tendon may be painful and can sometimes be felt to sublux volarly.

Measurement of Grip Strength

Grip strength can be measured using a Jamar dynamometer. This provides an objective measurement of one aspect of hand function.

With the shoulder adducted and the elbow flexed to 90°, the patient is asked to squeeze the dynamometer with maximum strength. The test can be repeated three times for each wrist to provide an average reading.

Maximum grip strength occurs at 35 degrees wrist extension. It is useful to note that wrist arthrodesis is performed at 20 degrees extension because at 35 degrees activities of daily living are difficult to perform.

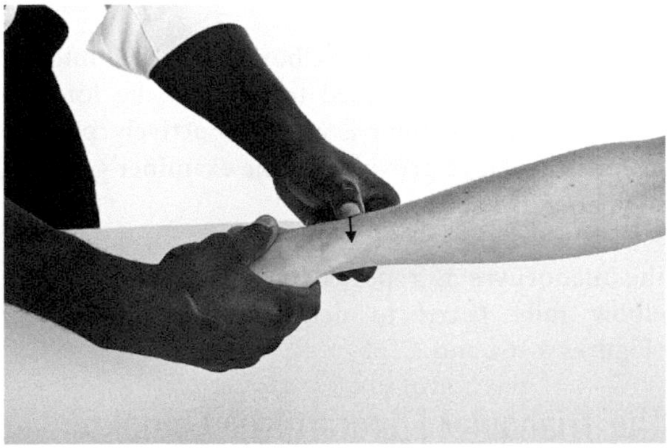

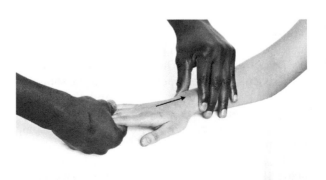

Figure 4.13 Demonstration of the piano key test. Pressure over the ulnar styloid by the examiner's thumb in a dorsal-to-volar direction will demonstrate increased excursion in patients with dorsal subluxation.

Figure 4.14 The TFCC compression test. Axial load across the wrist followed by radial and ulnar deviation will result in a painful click.

Advanced Corner

Scapholunate Instability

The most common test for assessing scapholunate instability is the Kirk Watson scaphoid shift test. No test is conclusive, and it is helpful to know other tests to aid in the diagnosis. Scaphoid thrust and scaphoid lift tests are described here.

Scaphoid Thrust Test

Lane has described a modification of the Kirk Watson test, which he originally, rather confusingly, named the scaphoid shift test, but which has been renamed the scaphoid thrust test.[12] The patient's hand is held in the same way as for the scaphoid shift with the examiner's thumb over the scaphoid tubercle. The wrist is rocked backwards and forwards from radial to ulnar deviation and back again until the patient is relaxed and guarding has been eliminated. The scaphoid tubercle is then quickly pressed by the examiners thumb with the wrist in slight radial deviation and neutral flexion/extension. For a positive test, the scaphoid should be felt to move dorsally.

Scaphoid Lift Test

A third test has been described in which the lunate is stabilised with the thumb and index finger of one hand whilst the scaphoid is translocated volarly and dorsally using the other thumb and index finger.[11]

Pronation and Supination

Full pronation and supination of the forearm depends on the distal radioulnar joint as well as the proximal radioulnar joint. The final positioning of the hand also involves a contribution from the carpal joints. The main muscles that provide pronation are pronator teres and pronator quadratus. The main muscles of supination are biceps brachii and supinator. Supination is approximately 15% stronger than pronation.

To test supination: The elbows are tucked into the side to remove any compensation from the shoulder. The elbow is then flexed to 90° and the forearm pronated. The patient is asked to actively supinate against resistance provided by the examiner grasping the patient's hand.

To assess the contribution of supinator, the manoeuvre is repeated but this time with the elbow fully *extended* to minimise the effect of biceps brachii (Figures 4.15a and 4.15b).

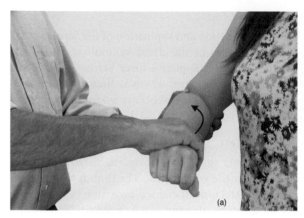

Figure 4.15a Supination strength is tested with the forearm fully pronated the elbow flexed to 90°. The patient's hand is grasped and then the patient is asked to actively supinate.

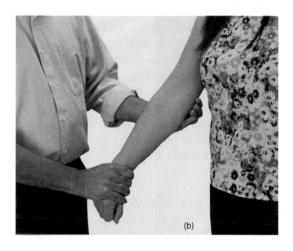

Figure 4.15b To isolate the supinator muscle, the same procedure is repeated but this time with the elbow fully extended.

To test pronation: The elbows are tucked into the side. They are then flexed to 90° and the forearm supinated. The patient is asked to actively pronate against resistance provided by the examiner grasping the patient's hand.

To assess the contribution of pronator quadratus, the manoeuvre is repeated but this time with the elbow fully *flexed* to defunction pronator teres (Figures 4.16a and 4.16b).

The Triangular Fibrocartilage Complex

The TFCC is attached along the relatively broad ulnar margin of the radius (Figure 4.17). From here it overlies the ulna head and inserts into the ulna.

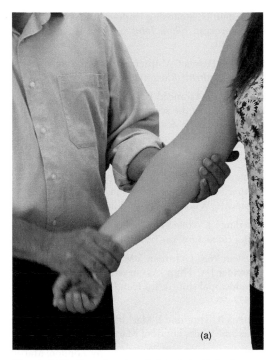

Figure 4.16a Pronation strength is tested with the forearm fully supinated and the elbow flexed to 60°–90°. The patient's hand is grasped and then the patient is asked to actively pronate.

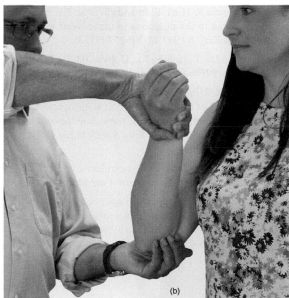

Figure 4.16b To isolate the pronator quadratus muscle, the same procedure is repeated but this time with the elbow fully flexed.

A superficial limb attaches to the ulna styloid (1) and a deep limb to the ulna fovea (2). In the axial plane,

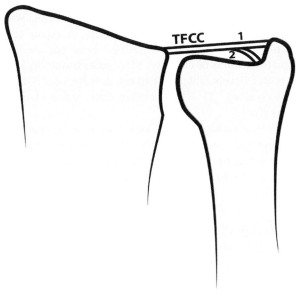

Figure 4.17 Anatomy of the TFCC.

this structure is triangular in shape, with the strongest parts along the volar and dorsal margins (the radioulnar ligaments).

The TFCC is the principal soft tissue stabiliser of the DRUJ. Damage to this structure can give rise to pain and can underlie DRUJ instability. Tears are classified according to the system described by Palmer.[22]

Class 1 tears are traumatic, and the most common of these is a peripheral avulsion at the ulna attachment, with or without an associated ulna styloid fracture (Class 1B)

Class 2 tears are degenerative, almost invariably a central perforation and part of 'ulna abutment syndrome'.

Clinical Considerations

Where DRUJ instability exists, check for a history of bony injury and assess very specifically for a potential malunion of the radius. If this is present, then an osteotomy may be required to restore stability.

Although ulna styloid fractures are commonly associated with distal radius fractures, they are rarely the cause of significant ongoing DRUJ instability. However, styloid fractures closer to the base have a greater chance of disrupting the foveal attachment with an increased potential for instability.

Isolated traumatic TFCC tears can produce ulnar-sided wrist pain, and this may not be associated with clinically detectable DRUJ instability. A repair (e.g. a peripheral reattachment using a bone anchor into the fovea) may be effective. More gross instability with greater (irreparable) soft tissue damage occasionally necessitates TFCC reconstruction using tendon transfer.[23]

Degenerative tears (Class 2) cannot be repaired. Symptoms associated with these usually require a levelling procedure to shorten the ulna or a 'wafer procedure' to excise the impacted surface of the ulna head.

References

1. Wolfe SW (ed). *Green's Operative Hand Surgery*, 6th ed. London: Churchill Livingstone, 2010.

2. Schmidt-Rohlting B, Schwöbel B, Pauschert R, Niethard FU. Madelung deformity: clinical features, therapy and results. *J Pediatr Orthop B* 2001 Oct; **10** (4):344–348.

3. Angelides AC, Wallace PF. The dorsal ganglion of the wrist: its pathogenesis, gross and microscopic anatomy, and surgical treatment. *J Hand Surg Am* 1976;**1**(3):228–235.

4. Sanders WE. The occult dorsal carpal ganglion. *J Hand Surg B* 1985;**10-B**(2):257–260.

5. Park MJ, Namdari S, Weiss A-P. The carpal boss: review of diagnosis and treatment. *J Hand Surg Am* 2008 Mar;**33**(3):446–449.

6. Parvizi J, Wayman J, Kelly P, Moran CG. Combining the clinical signs improves the diagnosis of scaphoid fractures. A prospective study with follow up. *J Hand Surg B* 1998;**23**(3):324–327.

7. Clementson M, Bjorkman A, Thomsen N. Acute scaphoid fractures: guideline for diagnosis and treatment. *EFFORT Open Rev* 2020 Feb;**5**(2):96–103. Published online.

8. Grundberg AB, Reagan DS. Pathological anatomy of the forearm: intersection syndrome. *J Hand Surg Am* 1985 Mar;**10**(2):299–302.

9. Finklestein H. Stenosing tendovaginitis of the radial styloid process. *J Bone Joint Surg Am* 1930;**12-A**:509–540.

10. Browne J, Helms CA. Intersection syndrome of the forearm. *Arthritis Rheum* 2006 Jun;54(6):2038.

11. Watson HK, Ashmead D, Makhlouf MV. Examination of the scaphoid. *J Hand Surg Am* 1988;**13-A**(5):657–660.

12. Lane LB. The scaphoid shift test. *J Hand Surg Am* 1993 **18-A**:366–368.

13. Cooney W (ed). *The Wrist: Diagnosis and Operative Treatment*, 2nd ed. Philadelphia: Wolters Kluwer / Lippincott, Williams and Wilkins, 2010.

14. Easterling KJ, Wolfe SW. Scaphoid shift in the uninjured wrist. *J Hand Surg Am* 1994;**19-A**(4): 604–606.

15. Feinstein WK, Lichtman DM, Noble PC, Alexander JW, Hipp JA. Quantitative assessment of the midcarpal shift test. *J Hand Surg Am* 1999;**24-A** (5):977–983.

16. Tubiana R, Thomine J, Mackin E. *Examination of the Hand and Wrist*. London: Martin Dunitz, 1998.

17. Stanley J, Saffar P. *Wrist Arthroscopy*. London: Martin Dunitz, 1994.

18. Sammer DM, Rizzo M. Ulnar impaction. *Hand Clin* 2010 Nov;**26**(4):549–557.

19. Nakamura R, Horii E, Imaeda T, et al. The ulnocarpal stress test in the diagnosis of ulnar-sided wrist pain. *J Hand Surg B* 1997;**22-B**(6):719–723.

20. Reagan DS, Linscheid RL, Dobyns JH. Lunotriquetral sprains. *J Hand Surg Am* 1984;**9-A**(4):502–514.

21. Sachar K. Ulnar sided wrist pain: evaluation and treatment of triangular fibrocartilage complex tears, ulnocarpal impaction syndrome, and lunotriquetral ligament tears. *J Hand Surg Am* 2008 Nov;**33** (9):1669–1679.

22. Palmer AK. Triangular fibrocartilage complex lesions: a classification. *J Hand Surg Am* 1989;**14**;594–606.

23. Adams BD, Berger RA. An anatomic reconstruction of the distal radioulnar ligaments for posttraumatic distal radioulnar joint instability. *J Hand Surg Am* 2002;**27**;243–251.

Chapter

Examination of the Hand

Michael Gale and Joe Garcia

General Assessment of the Hand

A. History
B. Clinical Examination

Step 1
Perform the screen test

Step 2
The subsequent path taken depends on what is found on screening. In virtually all cases a provisional diagnosis can be made, e.g. Dupuytren's disease, rheumatoid arthritis, lumps, nerve lesions.

There are so many varied pathologies in the hand, and each necessitates a different pattern of examination. The easiest way to approach clinical examination of the hand is to have a screening test that will help to determine the pathology, and then tailor the subsequent examination based on the observed findings. For example, a nerve lesion would be examined differently to a patient with Dupuytren's disease or a swelling in the hand.

Screening

The screening test for picking up hand pathology is as follows:

- Expose the patient adequately, to above the elbows.
- Ask them to show you their palms, make a fist and then spread the fingers wide.
- Ask them to show the backs of the hands, make a fist and then spread the fingers.
- Ask the patient to lift their hands up to show you their forearms and elbows. Look at the profile, look for scars, including around the elbow and axilla, and for rheumatoid nodules or psoriasis.

Function

It is important to be able to assess the functions of the hand, as many surgical decisions are based on function, such as in rheumatoid arthritis.

Hand function is 45% grasp, 45% pinch, 5% hook and 5% paperweight.

- Grasp – 'Grip my forearm.'
- Hook – 'Pull my fingertips with yours.'
Types of pinch:
- Chuck – 'Pick this coin up from my hand.'
- End – 'Hold this pen.'
- Side – 'Hold this key.'

Tips for Assessing Patients with a Swelling in the Hand

The diagnosis of a swelling in the hand depends to a large degree on the location of the swelling.

Volar
Lumps on the volar side of the hand are:

- Inclusion dermoid cysts
- Ganglion of A1 pulley (pearl ganglion)
- Giant cell tumour of the flexor sheath usually located in relation to the proximal phalanx

A swelling in relation to the radial artery at the wrist may be the volar ganglion which comes from the scaphotrapeziotrapezoidal (STT) joint. If considering surgery, remember to perform Allen's test to check for the contribution of circulation from the radial and ulnar arteries.

Dorsal
On the dorsum of the hand, the possible swellings are:

- Dorsal ganglion over the wrist
- Rheumatoid nodules on the extensor surface
- Gouty tophi
- Subungual exostosis under the nail
- Heberden's nodes over the distal interphalangeal (DIP) joint
- Mucous cyst in relation to the DIP joint
- Bouchard's nodes in relation to the proximal interphalangeal (PIP) joint
- Carpometacarpal boss

63

Examination of the Rheumatoid Hand

It is important to know all the possible abnormalities that can occur in rheumatoid disease affecting the hand. With this knowledge, description becomes easier.

Step 1

Ask the patient to lift their arms, if possible, above their head to gain a general impression of neck, shoulder and elbow function. At the same time, look for rheumatoid nodules on the extensor side of the arms.

Step 2

Describe from proximal to distal, first on the extensor side and then from proximal to distal on the flexor side. Knowledge of what to look for will aid description.

Step 3

Perform functional tests of the hand.

On the extensor side some common abnormalities are:

- Rheumatoid nodules
- Distal radioulnar joint (DRUJ) instability with caput ulnae (piano key sign)
- Extensor tendon rupture (Vaughan-Jackson syndrome)
- Metacarpophalangeal (MCP) joint subluxation and ulnar deviation
- Finger deformities such as mallet finger, Boutonnière deformity, swan neck deformity
- Z-deformity of the thumb

On the flexor side some common abnormalities are:

- Thickening of the carpal tunnel resulting in carpal tunnel syndrome
- Thenar wasting
- Tendon ruptures such as flexor pollicis longus (FPL) (Mannerfelt lesion)
- Trigger finger

Most of the above findings are obviously visible. There are two findings that have to be specifically looked for by asking the patient to demonstrate movements. On the dorsal side the extensor tendon rupture (Vaughan-Jackson) as it may be very subtle, and on the volar side a Mannerfelt lesion.

Examination of Dupuytren's disease

Step 1

Palpate the cords and the rest of the palm

Step 2

Look for Garrod's pads

Step 3

Perform Hueston's table top test (failure to put the hand flat on the table indicates either a PIP joint flexion contracture or an MCP joint flexion contracture)

Step 4

Measure fixed flexion deformities at MCP joint and the PIP joint (with a goniometer)

Step 5

Ask the patient about family history, age of onset and any other parts of body affected

Step 6

If previous surgery to the hand, perform neurovascular assessment including digital Allen's test

If this system of examination is carried out, the examiner is then able to answer the following two important questions: Are there signs of aggressive disease? Is there any indication for surgery?

Signs of aggressive disease:

- Early age of onset
- Garrod's pads
- Involvement of other sites such as feet, penis and other hand
- Radial-sided disease

Indications for surgery:

- Positive Hueston's table top test
- MCP joint flexion contracture (>30°)
- PIP joint flexion contracture (>0°)

Introduction

The hand is anatomically and functionally complex, and there are numerous pathologies that affect the hand. This complexity makes having a standard approach helpful. **A simple history, screening test and careful observation will usually identify the location and basic nature of the pathology. We can**

then move on to a more focused examination. It is simply impossible to do a detailed examination of every part of the hand within the timescale of a clinic appointment or an examination station. Special tests for individual pathologies may then complete the examination.

History

Examination of a patient's hand should always follow a comprehensive history. The history will usually point to a limited differential diagnosis, give crucial information about how the hand affects the patient's quality of life and guide potential treatments. Other medical problems have a bearing on hand pathology, especially diabetes, smoking and thyroid problems. Always remember to ask for hand dominance, occupation and recreational activities.

A patient will likely complain of one or more of the following: pain, stiffness, loss of function, sensory disturbance or abnormal appearance

Pain

Pain is often the presenting symptom in a hand clinic. Degenerate joints will become painful before any stiffness or deformity develops. Even peripheral neurological problems are often described as pain by patients. A standard pain history should be taken:

- Location. This will identify a shortlist of anatomical structures involved. For example, pain at the base of the thumb is likely arising from the base of thumb joints or the thumb tendons.
- Distribution. Pain in the distribution of a peripheral nerve could indicate entrapment. Pain along the course of a tendon suggests a problem here. Cramp in the muscles that move a joint could mean arthritis in that joint (a consequence of *Hilton's law*: the nerve supplying a muscle that crosses a joint also supplies the joint and the skin overlying it).
- Character
- Duration
- Exacerbating factors
- Effect on function

Stiffness

Loss of movement in the hand is particularly troublesome. It is important to determine what is causing the loss of movement. Ask the patient which parts of the hand have lost movement and whether this affects any particular tasks. Is there a loss of active movement, passive movement or both? Is there loss of flexion or extension?

Loss of Function

Loss of function or loss of strength causing an inability to perform a task may be another presenting symptom. Inability to perform activities of daily living or simple tasks such as holding a spoon or a key may be an indication for surgery.

Sensory Disturbance

Patients usually describe altered sensation in the fingertips. Try to determine whether this is in the distribution of a peripheral nerve or could be attributed to a cervical or brachial plexus lesion. Commonly, patients describe loss of dexterity. Buttons on clothes are a particular problem; the loss of sensation means the patient cannot feel where the button is relative to the hole.

Abnormal Appearance

This is particularly the case with ganglia and other hand swellings. Remember that deformity occurs in degenerative, and especially inflammatory, joint disease. Osteoarthritis in the DIP joints is often relatively painless and the patient will first notice deformity. Ask when the swelling was first noticed, and whether it has changed over time.

Examination

The complexity of the hand means that the examination first will have to focus on broadly identifying the pathology. Then, more specific examination tests are performed relevant to the identified pathology.

To accomplish this, first a **screening manoeuvre** must be performed, which will help narrow down the possibilities.

Screening

Both upper limbs should be exposed to above the elbows. Jewellery is ideally removed. Both hands should be screened together; this gives a useful comparison if the other hand is normal and allows identification of bilateral/symmetrical pathologies.

First, inspect the hands with the palm facing upwards then ask then to spread their fingers apart

(Figure 5.1a). Then ask the patient to close the hands to make a fist (Figure 5.1b).

Ask them to turn the hands over to face the floor and inspect the dorsum (Figure 5.1c). Again, ask them to make a fist (Figure 5.1d).

Last, ask the patient to flex the elbow and lift their arms above their head. By doing this, the examiner can view the elbows, forearm and hands in profile (Figure 5.1e).

Look

It is helpful to look for, and comment on, the following when inspecting (Figure 5.2a,b):

- **Attitude** – The relaxed hand has a normal attitude, with a gradual cascade from one finger to another. Any deviation from this normal attitude is quite obvious to the eye and will point to joint problems and/or musculotendinous imbalance.
- **Deformity** – Commonly a result of joint damage, arthritis, subluxations or trauma.
- **Swelling** – For example, synovitis, ganglia or osteophytes.

- **Wasting** – Look at intrinsic muscle bulk. Can occur through disuse or because of neurological compromise.
- **Discolouration** – Bruising, effects of steroid injections, circulatory phenomena. Comment on nail problems.
- **Scars** – Surgical or traumatic. Beware, the hand heals very well so look carefully.

After careful inspection, it should be possible to determine the pathology and focus the rest of the examination specific to the presumed diagnosis.

Feel

Knowing the surface landmarks of the underlying anatomical structures is important when palpating areas of pathology. Focal points of tenderness will often point to an abnormality in the anatomical structure that the examiner is palpating (Figure 5.3).

Feel each joint briefly in turn. Start proximally or distally; it doesn't matter. Just be systematic. Feel for tenderness, swelling, synovitis, deformity or bony abnormalities, e.g. osteophytes.

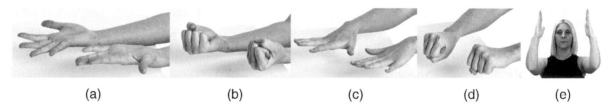

(a)	(b)	(c)	(d)	(e)

Figure 5.1 Screening for hand pathology: (a) Hands open and palms up. Spread fingers apart. (b) Make a fist. (c) Look at the hand, palms down. (d) Make a fist. (e) Flex elbows and observe profile (hands open).

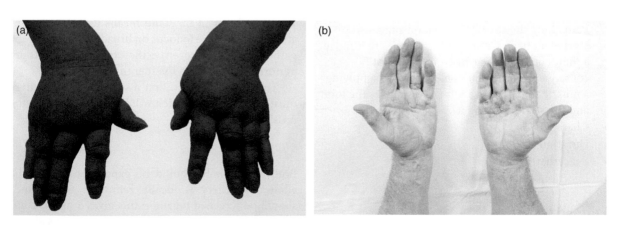

Figure 5.2a,b (a) Arthritis mutilans affecting the hands. There is underlying severe joint destruction. Remember to assess hand function and also to look for the underlying cause especially psoriasis.
(b) Dupuytren's disease. On the right side, the patient was operated on so remember to do a digital Allen's test. On the left hand, remember to remove the ring for a full assessment.

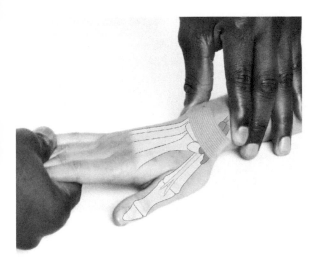

Figure 5.3 Palpation is only usually necessary at this point if the diagnosis is not immediately obvious. The hand is a superficial joint; therefore, tenderness at a point signifies pathology in the underlying structure. As such, knowing the surface anatomy is crucial.

Feel any swelling or lump according to an established system (site, size, shape etc.).

Feel for the cords of Dupuytren's disease. A simple screen is to passively extend the fingers and run an index fingertip across the palm. The tension of finger extension should make early cords palpable.

A rapid neurological screen can be performed if required using the 'autonomous sensory areas' of the three nerves.

Move

Assess first active and then passive range of movement in the joints of interest.

The *composite movements* of the finger joints allow the fingers to go fully straight in extension and for the fingertips to touch the palm in full flexion (Figure 5.4a,b). An inability to do this with one or more fingers suggests a restriction in movement secondary to an underlying problem. You can document the distance of the fingertip to the palm as a quick measure of movement loss, e.g. 'pulp to palm is 1 cm'.

The MCP joints also allow ad/abduction by the action of the interossei. A simple comparison of the two hands will show up an obvious deficit.

If abnormalities are picked up during screening, proceed to assess the individual joints. Range of movement can be quantified by use of a goniometer (Figure 5.4c,d).

The normal range of movements for the individual joints of fingers are:

- Distal interphalangeal joint (DIP): 0°–80°
- Proximal interphalangeal (PIP) joint: 0°–100°
- Metacarpal phalangeal (MCP) joint: 0°–40° of hyperextension to 90° flexion

Remember, anatomically speaking, the thumb is pronated 90° out of the plane of the hand. Therefore, the normal range of movements for the individual joints of the thumb are:

- Carpometacarpal joint: Metacarpal in line with palm on adduction to 45° of abduction. Metacarpal in line with palm on flexion to 60° of extension.
- Metacarpophalangeal joint: 10° of hyperextension to 55° of flexion.
- Interphalangeal joint: 15° of hyperextension to 80° of flexion.

Figure 5.4e,f summarises the movements of the thumb.

Functional Assessment

An assessment of hand function should be performed (Figure 5.5a,b,c,d).

Treatment discussions often revolve around which particular functions the patient needs or has lost. Particularly in the rheumatoid hand, surgery is aimed at retaining and improving those functions. The functions of the hand can be divided into:

- Power grip/grasp (45% of function), e.g. holding a larger object like a bottle
- Pinch (45%), three types

    ○ End pinch (hold a pen)
    ○ Side pinch (turn a key)
    ○ Chuck or tripod pinch (pick up a coin)

- Hook (5%), e.g. carrying a shopping bag
- Paperweight (5%), e.g. holding paper still while writing

The **tenodesis effect at the wrist** is a passive 'grasp and release' mechanism that is caused by wrist extension and flexion, respectively. It results from the fact that the tendons that cross multiple joints of the hand maintain the same length and tension whatever the position of the wrist. Hence, if the wrist extends, then the fingers will flex, and if the wrist is flexed, then the fingers will extend (Figure 5.6). This concept can be used to help diagnose tendon rupture and nerve

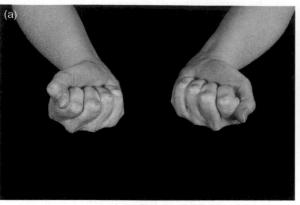 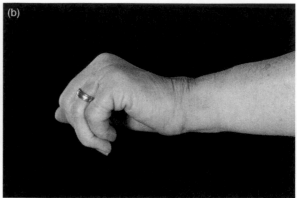

Figure 5.4a,b (a) Composite movements of small joints of fingers allow fingertips to touch palm. (b) Reduced composite movements of the hand because of arthritis.

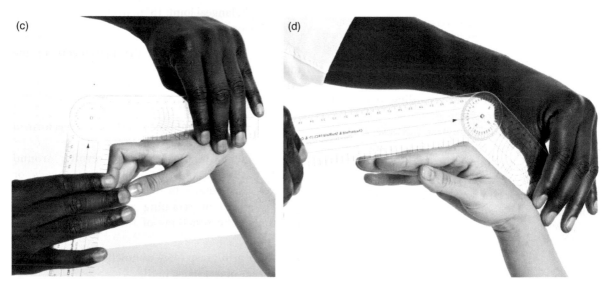

Figure 5.4c,d Measure the range of movements with a goniometer.
(c) Proximal interphalangeal joint (PIP joint).
(d) Metacarpophalangeal joint (MCP joint).

injuries. It is also use in occupational therapy and rehabilitation.

The concept of wrist tenodesis can also be applied to the digits, e.g. the thumb.

Specific Pathologies

Osteoarthritis

Almost any joint can be affected, but common sites for osteoarthritis in the hand are the base of the thumb, the metacarpophalangeal joints and the interphalangeal joints. Typical symptoms are pain, swelling and stiffness. Typical signs are swelling, tenderness and restricted range of motion.

First Carpometacarpal (CMC) Joint Arthritis

Arthritis at the base of the thumb is one of the commonest arthritic conditions in the hand. The thumb is involved in almost all of the functions of the hand and in pinch grip the joint reaction force through the carpometacarpal (CMC) joint can be up to 8 times the pinch force. The CMC joint is saddle shaped, which allows excellent range of movement but means that the actual joint surface area in contact at any given time is very small. This leads to very high pressures on the articular cartilage and consequent risk of wear.

This condition presents with pain at the base of the thumb, extending into the thumb and sometimes proximally along the radial aspect of the wrist. Patients often

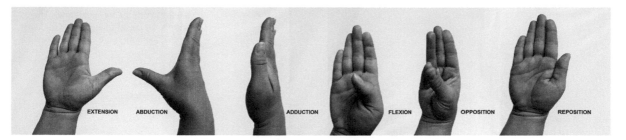

Figure 5.4e Movements of the thumb: extension, abduction, adduction, flexion, opposition, reposition.

Figure 5.4f Retropulsion of the thumb.

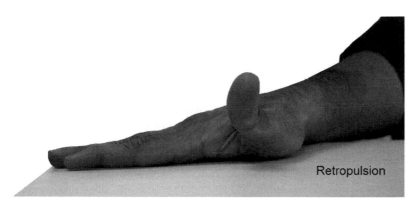

Retropulsion

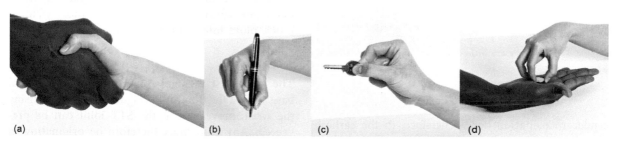

(a) (b) (c) (d)

Figure 5.5a,b,c,d Functions of the hand.
(a) Grasp. (b) End pinch. (c) Side pinch. (d) Chuck pinch.

describe an ache in the thenar eminence (Hilton's law). Associated symptoms include a reduction in the range of movement and weakness in many functions of daily activity. Any movement involving grasping and gripping is painful and feels weak. The patient may also notice and complain of a deformity involving the thumb.

Look

Initial inspection may reveal a characteristic deformity of the thumb (Figure 5.7).

- A prominent base of thumb caused by subluxation of the CMC joint after attrition of the beak ligament. This may be described as '**squaring**'.

- An adduction deformity of the metacarpal, caused by the now abnormal pull of adductor pollicis brevis (and the other thenar muscles). This gives the '**thumb in palm**' appearance.
- A secondary **hyperextension of the MCP** joint as the patient stretches out the volar plate to try to maintain hand span.

Feel

Palpation of the affected area may be commenced away from the problematic area. Palpation from distal to proximal along the thumb may reassure the patient. Arthritis in this joint frequently starts on the palmar aspect, and the inflamed adjacent joint capsule is

69

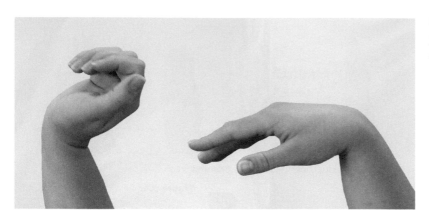

Figure 5.6 Tenodesis effect 'grasp and release'. With the wrist extended, the fingers are flexed (grasp). With the wrist flexed, the fingers are extended (release).

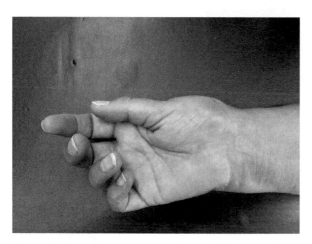

Figure 5.7 Typical deformities found in first CMC joint arthritis.

tender to palpation here. Therefore, in the earliest stages tenderness may be most pronounced on the palmar aspect of the joint, palpating at the base of the thenar eminence. In established arthritis, tenderness is present all around the joint and can be elicited directly over the dorsum of the joint.

The CMC joint is best identified dorsally by palpating proximally along radial border of the index metacarpal; the first joint you come to is the CMC joint. Palpating along the inner border of the thumb metacarpal also meets at the first CMC joint. The STT joint is identified on the volar side by identifying the scaphoid tubercle and moving distally.

Move

The thumb CMC joint can be assessed further by asking the patient to actively move the thumb into extension, flexion, adduction and abduction. Note and measure any restriction in active movement and whether this reproduces pain. Measurement may be a simple comparison to the uninvolved side. It is especially useful to comment on any loss of hand span. Composite adduction/flexion/opposition can be measured using the Kapandji score[1] (Table 5.1). Passive movement of the thumb CMC joint may again demonstrate these restrictions in movement and reproduce pain, although in this scenario passive movement is likely to cause discomfort while not yielding much more information.

Special Tests

The **grind test** involves rotation of the metacarpal base against the trapezium (Figure 5.8). By stabilising the wrist, movement at the STT joint can be prevented. Any pain must therefore be originating in the first CMC joint.

Next, stabilising the thumb to reduce CMC movement, the STT joint can be moved by deviating the wrist ulnar-radially (this causes the scaphoid to flex and extend against the trapezium). Increased pain at that point will suggest pain from the STT joint (arthritis) or even more proximally from a scaphoid pathology (fracture or non-union) or radioscaphoid arthritis.

DIP Joint Arthritis

Arthritis in these small joints is very common but fortunately not always symptomatic. Patients will present with pain, stiffness and deformities.

Examination will identify the deformities and bony and soft tissue swellings. There may be a fixed flexion

Table 5.1 The Kapandji score describes the degree of thumb opposition possible on a scale of 0–10 depending on where the thumb is able to touch the hand

Kapandji score[1]	Extent of thumb opposition
1	Index finger proximal phalanx
2	Index finger middle phalanx
3	Index finger distal phalanx
4	Middle fingertip
5	Ring fingertip
6	Little fingertip
7	Little finger DIP joint
8	Little finger PIP joint
9	Little finger MCP Joint
10	Distal palmar crease

DIP, distal interphalangeal; MCP, metacarpophalangeal; PIP, proximal interphalangeal

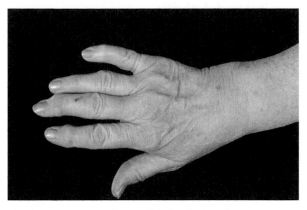

Figure 5.9 DIP joint arthritis with Heberden's nodes.

side of the midline (Figure 5.9). Soft tissue swelling may be diffuse because of an inflamed joint or more localised as a result of a mucoid cyst.

A mucoid cyst is a ganglion cyst arising from the joint and lying dorsally, often distal to the joint. They appear away from the midline because the presence of the extensor tendon prevents direct dorsal emergence. It may affect the nail bed and/or deform the germinal matrix, leading to ridging of the nail plate. The cysts can sometimes burst and leak typical ganglion fluid. Rarely infection can ensue. Mucoid cysts may be present without other obvious signs of an arthritic joint. Closer scrutiny will reveal a tender joint and movements may be significantly restricted.

PIP/MCP Joint Arthritis

Arthritis in these joints is common and often symptomatic. Patients will present with pain, stiffness and deformities. Examination will identify the deformities and bony and soft tissue swellings.

There may be a fixed flexion deformity of the joint because of the articular degeneration. More typically, there will be a loss of flexion causing difficulty with grip. Osteophyte formation gives the typical bony swellings, described as Bouchard's nodes in the PIP joint, on either side of the midline. Soft tissue swelling may be diffuse because of an inflamed joint. Range of movement may be restricted, and this will be more severe with chronic problems as the volar plate and accessory collaterals fibrose.

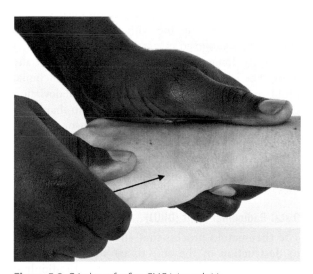

Figure 5.8 Grind test for first CMC joint arthritis.

deformity of the joint because of the articular degeneration. There is often a coronal plane deformity, more in an ulnar direction, because the forces applied to the fingertips usually come from the thumb on the radial side. Osteophyte formation gives the typical bony swellings described as Heberden's nodes on either

71

Rheumatoid Arthritis

Improvements in medical management of inflammatory arthritis means that the classic, severe, rheumatoid hand is becoming rare. When seen, inflammatory arthritis presents most commonly as a polyarticular, symmetrical and potentially destructive disease. Classically rheumatoid spares the DIP joints.

Inflammatory arthritis causes problems by soft tissue and cartilage inflammation and subsequent destruction and periarticular bony erosion. Normally, the hand works because the opposing forces (e.g. flexors/extensors) are in balance and act across stable joints. Joint and soft tissue damage causes loss of joint stability and can cause subluxation and even rupture of tendons. Several classic deformities tend to result, and these are described below (Figure 5.10).

Inspection is vital in the inflammatory hand. Often one can identify the classic features of inflammatory arthritis purely by looking carefully.

Arguably the most important information you can get in the inflammatory hand is an *assessment of function*. Often a patient will complain about a specific function loss and may have some ideas of their own about what they want to use the hand for. Surgical treatment for the inflammatory hand is almost always an attempt to maintain or restore a specific set of functions. Carry out an assessment of hand function as detailed above (Figure 5.11).

Wrist

The wrist itself can be the site of considerable pain, leading to functional problems. But even when there is minimal pain, significant deformities of the wrist can have an impact on the other joints of the hand.

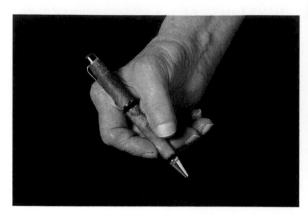

Figure 5.11 End (pen) pinch in a rheumatoid hand.

Assessing the condition of the rheumatoid wrist is therefore particularly important when there are other hand deformities.

The typical wrist deformity is radial deviation with volar subluxation and ulnar translation. As the rheumatoid process weakens and eventually destroys the intrinsic and extrinsic ligaments (particularly the radioscaphocapitate), the carpus slides ulnarwards and subluxes volarly. Radial deviation ensues to try to keep the hand in line with the forearm, partly allowed by a subluxed extensor carpi ulnaris (ECU) tendon no longer stabilising the ulnar side of the wrist. The loss of a stable base results in functional problems and progressive deformity. Radial deviation of the carpal and metacarpal bones leads to changes in direction of pull of the flexor and extensor tendons, contributing to abnormal lines of pull at the MCP joints. Any surgery to the MCP joints requires a careful assessment and treatment of wrist abnormalities to obtain a stable, well-oriented base for the hand.

Distal Radioulnar Joint (DRUJ)

The rheumatoid process that affects this joint leads to destruction of the soft tissue stabilisers of the joint, namely the volar and dorsal distal radioulnar ligaments and the triangular fibrocartilage complex (TFCC), resulting in dorsal subluxation of the distal ulna (although, strictly speaking, it is the radius which subluxes volar). The ECU tendon also subluxes ulnar and volar, allowing further DRUJ instability. The subsequent prominence is called a *caput ulna*. Being able to push down on the ulna head and return it to its original position is a positive **'piano key' sign.**

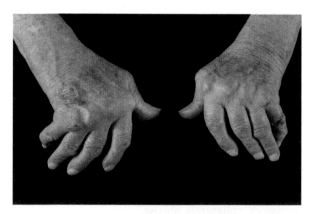

Figure 5.10 Overview of the rheumatoid hand.

The presence of a caput ulnae should be noted as it may predispose to attritional damage to the extensor tendons. This, in combination with dorsal tenosynovitis, is a typical clinical sign found in a Vaughan-Jackson syndrome (see below).

Metacarpophalangeal Joint (MCP)

The typical deformity is volar subluxation with ulnar drift. MCP joint deformities in the hand are caused by a combination of pathologies:

- Radial deviation of the wrist and metacarpals causing abnormal tendon forces
- Articular destruction
- Synovitis damaging the collateral ligaments and palmar plates
- Stretching of, and damage to, the sagittal bands on the radial side and subsequent ulnar subluxation of the extensor tendons
- Intrinsic tightness

On examination it may be possible to identify the presence of some of these problems with simple inspection (Figure 5.12). It can then be determined whether the MCP joints are reducible, i.e. can they be straightened out? Chronic subluxed joints often cannot be reduced because of secondary changes. If they can be reduced, assess whether this reduction can be held temporarily. This gives an idea about the integrity of the extensor tendons. The relocation of the extensor tendon onto the dorsum of the metacarpal head may maintain the joint in a more normal position for a small period of time. Subsequent re-subluxation of the extensor tendon may also be seen, with the finger dropping back into flexion. If this is absent, question whether the tendon has been ruptured.

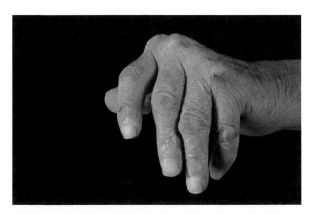

Figure 5.12 MCP joint deformities of the hand.

Fingers: Boutonnière Deformity

If the dorsal extensor tendon structures, particularly the central slip, are destroyed by rheumatoid disease, the PIP joint subluxes dorsally, resulting in PIP joint flexion. The lateral bands may secondarily collapse volarly, leading to an increased flexion force to the PIP joint and hyperextension of the DIP joint.

Nalebuff and Millender Staging[2] is according to severity:

- Stage 1 – mild extensor lag of 10°–15° and the PIP joint is passively correctable. On passive PIP joint extension, DIP joint flexion becomes limited.
- Stage 2 – more severe extensor lag of 30°–40°, but it is still passively correctable. There is no DIP joint flexion with correction.
- Stage 3 – there is a fixed deformity of the PIP joint.

Fingers: Swan Neck Deformity

If the volar plate and associated structures are damaged and attenuated by rheumatoid disease, then the PIP joint may hyperextend. Subsequently, a secondary DIP joint flexion occurs from muscle imbalance.

The Nalebuff classification[3] is based around the mobility of the PIP joint:

- Type I – PIP joint flexible in all positions.
- Type II – PIP joint flexibility is affected by the presence of intrinsic tightness. Bunnell's test will demonstrate decreased flexibility with MCP joint extended compared to increased flexibility with MCP joint flexed.
- Type III – PIP joint has limited flexibility in all positions, and X-rays show a well-preserved joint.
- Type IV – PIP joint has limited flexibility in all positions, but X-rays show joint destruction.

Thumb Deformities

Deformities may be present at the first CMC joint, MCP joint and IP joint (Figure 5.13).

The typical patterns of deformity in rheumatoid arthritis were described by Nalebuff:[4]

- Type I – Boutonnière deformity. Damage to the extensor tendon mechanism leads to dorsal subluxation of the MCP joint with secondary hyperextension of the IP joint (most common).
- Type II – type I deformity with additional subluxation of the first CMC joint.
- Type III – swan neck deformity. Subluxation of the first CMC joint with adduction of the

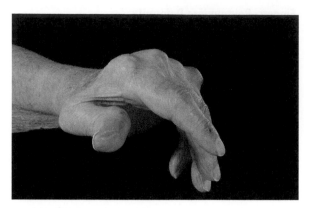

Figure 5.13 Thumb deformity in rheumatoid disease. Z-deformity consists of hyperextension at the IP joint and fixed flexion/subluxation at the MCP joint.

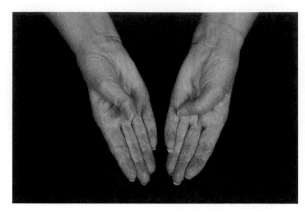

Figure 5.14 FPL rupture of the right thumb. Evident with the patient being asked to flex the thumb across the palm.

metacarpal leading to secondary hyperextension of the MCP joint and flexion of the IP joint.

- Type IV – gamekeeper's thumb. Instability from laxity of the ulnar collateral ligament of the MCP joint.
- Type V – volar plate damage leads to hyperextension of the MCP joint with secondary flexion of the IP joint, but differs from type III as there is no adduction of the metacarpal from first CMC joint dislocation.

Type I (and Type 2) deformities are sometimes referred to as Z-deformities because of the flexion at the MCP joint and the hyperextension of the IP joint.

Tendons

Tenosynovitis can occur in extensor and flexor tendon sheaths. This will lead to swelling around the tendons, hampering their movements, and inflammatory soft tissue changes. This causes damage to the tendons and can potentially lead to complete ruptures. Two classic tendon rupture patterns are described below.

Mannerfelt Lesion

Flexor pollicis longus (FPL) rupture[5] occurs as a result of attritional damage to the FPL around the distal pole of the scaphoid. Irregularities here are caused by wrist capsule synovitis and joint destruction (Figure 5.14).

If the rheumatoid process has not destroyed the thumb IP joint, then active movement is lost but the IP joint will flex passively. A destroyed joint will have both passive and active loss of movement and will be more difficult to assess.

The differential diagnosis for an FPL rupture is:

- A triggering thumb locked in extension – the thumb is unable to flex because the FPL is scarred down within the flexor sheath.
- An anterior interosseous nerve (AIN) injury – an AIN palsy can be differentially assessed with index finger flexor digitorum profundus (FDP) function. Absence of active index finger DIP joint flexion in combination with loss of thumb IP joint flexion may suggest an AIN palsy (OK sign).

The tenodesis effect may also be used to assess whether an FPL tendon is intact and therefore useful in differentiating an FPL rupture from an AIN palsy. If the tendon is in continuity and attached to the distal phalanx, extending the wrist and thumb proximal to the IP joint should result in IP joint flexion. In a ruptured FPL, the joint will not flex. Remember to compare one side to the other.

Extensor Tendon Rupture

As described previously, tenosynovitis around the extensor tendons and a caput ulna resulting from rheumatoid disease can ultimately lead to rupture of the extensor tendons. The little finger is the first and most commonly involved. Sequential ruptures of the ring and middle fingers can then occur; this is Vaughan-Jackson,[6] or caput ulnae, syndrome (Figure 5.15).

The clinical features include an extensor lag of one or more fingers in the presence of dorsal tenosynovitis and a caput ulna.

Extensor tendon rupture needs to be differentiated from:

1. *MCP joint dislocation or subluxation.* Passive extension may reduce the joint, at which point the extensor tendons can function and retain extension until the joint subluxes once again. If there is a fixed deformity, with no passive correction, then one can assume that it is an intrinsic joint problem.

2. *Subluxation of the extensor tendon* caused by sagittal band rupture or stretching. If the joint is not subluxed and the extensor lag is corrected passively, the extensor tendon may reduce onto the apex of the metacarpal head. While there, it will maintain extension, but if it subluxes ulnarly because of a deficient sagittal band, the extensor lag will return. This subluxation may be seen or felt.

3. *Posterior interosseous nerve palsy.* All the fingers will be affected, as well as the thumb. There may also be weakness in wrist extension. Tenodesis effect will show tendons are intact. Look carefully at the elbow in this case; there may be signs of elbow joint destruction and/or previous surgery here.

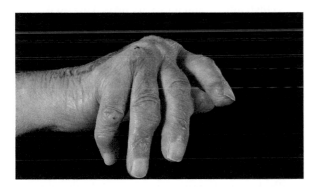

Figure 5.15 Extensor tendon rupture of right little and ring fingers (Vaughan-Jackson syndrome). Note the synovitis on the dorsal region of wrist.

If you have determined the presence of an extensor tendon rupture, check for the presence of extensor indicis proprius (EIP), as this is a popular choice of donor for tendon transfer. (See extensor pollicis longus (EPL) rupture).

Rheumatoid Nodules

Rheumatoid nodules occur usually on the extensor surface of the arm, including the olecranon, ulnar border of the forearm and over the IP joint of the fingers. They are the most common extra-articular manifestation of rheumatoid arthritis and are usually associated with aggressive disease (Figure 5.16).

Psoriatic Arthritis

Psoriatic arthritis is a chronic inflammatory arthritis that develops in up to approximately 20% of patients with psoriasis.[7] The differentiating features include distal joint involvement and arthritis mutilans (mutilans may less commonly be seen in rheumatoid arthritis). Although DIP joint involvement is considered a classic and unique symptom of psoriatic arthritis, it occurs in only 5–10% of patients.

On initial inspection psoriatic nail pitting may be seen. Psoriatic arthritis may be present with or without obvious skin lesions. Minimal skin involvement may be hidden (e.g. scalp, umbilicus, intergluteal cleft).

By looking at the arm in profile, psoriatic plaques on the back of the elbow may be identified. Simply asking the patient whether they have any dry skin problems is often enough to confirm your suspicions.

Mutilans is a rare form of psoriatic arthritis, being found in 1–5% of patients[8] (Figure 5.17). In this severe arthritis, there are radiographic changes of bone resorption, with dissolution of the joint. This gives rise to the typical 'pencil-in-cup' appearance on X-ray.

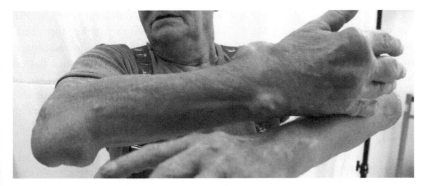

Figure 5.16 Large rheumatoid nodules on the extensor surface of the arm.

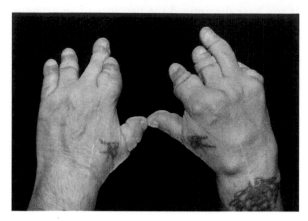

Figure 5.17 Collapsed skeleton of arthritis mutilans.

Severe deformities of the joints occur. Overlying skin may be redundant, and a telescoping motion of the joint is possible.

Psoriatic dactylitis with sausage digits is seen in as many as 35% of patients. It is very easy to confuse this with the signs of a flexor sheath infection, and sometimes the diagnosis is made on biopsy.

Flexion Contractures

Flexion contractures of the small joints of the hand are a frequent problem. Their cause is multiple, but the common outcome is poor hand function. Patients may have problems with work or sporting activities, but even simple day-to-day actions like putting hands in pockets or gloves may prove frustratingly difficult. The cosmetic appearance may also be a concern to the patient.

The patient's history may provide valuable information with regard to the aetiology. A history of injury to the hand or to the specific joint may be present. A history of multiple joint pathology may be consistent with an inflammatory arthropathy. Specific co-morbidities or a family history may be present in Dupuytren's disease.

On examination, it is important to decide if the contracture is fixed. In other words, can it be passively straightened? If there is a fixed flexion contracture, it is still necessary to know how much further flexion the patient has. If contractures are not fixed, the range of passive extension can be measured.

It is important to isolate each joint in turn when assessing contractures; overall deformity may be cumulative across more than one joint. *When assessing the PIP joint, hold the MCP joint in flexion. When*

assessing the MCP joint, hold the wrist in flexion using the tenodesis effect (these manoeuvres exclude any 'tenodesis' affect by the underlying pathology, e.g. a Dupuytren's cord extending across two joints). An extensor lag will highlight the active functional loss of the extensor mechanism, such as can occur with mallet injuries and flexible Boutonnière.

Specific Pathologies Causing a Flexion Deformity

Dupuytren's Contracture

Dupuytren's is thickening of the palmar fascia. Palmar fascia is normally concentrated in definable bands (pre-tendinous, commissural, natatory, spiral and lateral digital sheet). When these bands become thickened, they are termed 'cords'. Contraction of these thickened cords causes the recognisable deformities.

In Dupuytren's disease, the extent of the disease should be determined:

- Does it involve both hands?
- Which fingers and joints are involved, and by how much?
- Are there any extrapalmar manifestations?

The little finger is by far the most commonly affected, at either the MCP or PIP joints, followed by ring and middle fingers, and thumb (Figure 5.18a,b).

History

Dupuytren's is sometimes associated with diabetes mellitus, chronic liver disease and epilepsy (probably via prolonged use of anticonvulsants) but family history is most prevalent. Ask about functional limitations, and about any extrapalmar manifestations.

Screen

A simple test to demonstrate contractures of the PIP and MCP joints is **Hueston's table top test**[9] (Figure 5.19). It may also be used as a guide for surgery. Ask the patient to place the palm of the hand flat on a table top. If there is a significant contracture of any of the PIP or MCP joints, then the patient would be unable to perform this manoeuvre and the hand will not lie flat.

Look

When looking at obvious contractures, the slightly less obvious problems may be missed. Pay attention to see

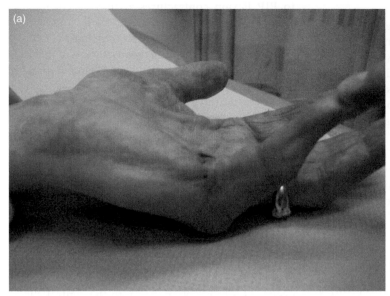

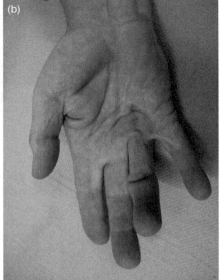

Figure 5.18a,b (a) Dupuytren's disease involving the abductor digiti minimi and the lateral sheet of finger. Note profile of the finger shows the deformity most clearly. (b) Dupuytren's disease leading to a pretendinous cord affecting the ring finger.

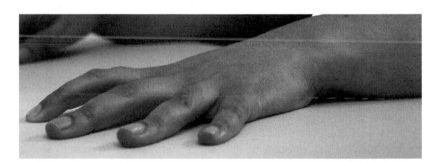

Figure 5.19 Hueston's table top test. Inability to put hand flat on the table signifies contractures of the MCP or PIP joints.

whether the thumb is involved, as cords in the first web space may lead to an adduction contracture. This leads to a loss of the smooth 'sail' of skin in the first web space on attempting full span. The fingers may also be adducted because of natatory cord involvement.

Assessing the condition of the skin is important. Look for and describe pitting and nodular formations. Severe contractures may lead to maceration of the skin. Any scars from previous surgery may affect your surgical decisions. Also look at the forearm for any skin graft donor site scars.

Dupuytren's fibromatosis may be associated with other fibromatosis. Therefore, do not forget to check for the presence of these, including *Garrod's pads* on the dorsal aspect of the PIP joint and nodules on the plantar aspect of feet (Ledderhose disease, 5%

association). The patient may provide a history of penile involvement (Peyronie's disease, 3% association).

Multiple site fibromatosis, multiple finger involvement, bilateral or radial-sided disease, young age of onset and a family history may suggest the presence of a Dupuytren's diathesis and may result in less rewarding surgical intervention with a higher risk of recurrence.

Feel

Assess and describe the palpable cords. As previously stated, gentle passive finger extension can make early pitting or cords easier to feel.

The skin condition (previous scarring, loss of elasticity or volume) may determine the need for dermofasciectomy and skin grafting.

Move

Measure the degree of fixed flexion with a goniometer, being careful to isolate each joint in turn.

An assessment of the subsequent loss of function is important. As in the rheumatoid hand, simple tests for hand function can be performed. Loss of ability to extend fingers and thumb so as to grasp may be very limiting. Patients often describe problems with grip, pockets and gloves.

Special Tests

If previous surgery has been performed, then a *digital Allen's test* is important to assess the competence of both digital arteries (Figure 5.20) (see below).

Flexion Contractures of PIP Joints Secondary to a Previous Ligamentous Injury

The PIP joint is stabilised by the collateral ligaments, accessory collateral ligaments and the volar plate. Injuries, and subsequent scarring, to the accessory collateral ligaments or to the volar plate may lead to contractures. This is fairly common after finger dislocations, particularly where these injuries are neglected or treated inappropriately. Even when treatment is appropriate, a gradual and progressive flexion contracture can still occur.

It is also possible for hand injuries not directly involving the PIP joint to have similar consequences. Traumatic swelling or oedema of the hand can lead

to PIP flexion contractures as fibrosis ensues. For this reason, it is important for these joints to be protected in a position of safety intrinsic (POSI) or 'Edinburgh' splint.[10] POSI means flexion of the MCP joints to nearly 90° and full extension of the PIP joints.

These flexion contractures are characteristically fixed and isolated to the PIP joint only. The degree of contracture can vary from mild to severe. There are no nodules or scarring to be seen or palpated. Some tenderness may be found on the palmar aspect over the volar plate and along the collateral ligaments, particularly if it is soon after the injury.

Boutonnière Deformity

This is a flexion deformity of a finger PIP joint with a secondary hyperextension of the DIP joint. It occurs as a result of an injury to the central slip of the extensor mechanism. Damage to the central slip can occur as a result of a direct injury from sharp or blunt trauma (especially a volar PIP joint dislocation). This results in a laceration or avulsion of the central slip. Attenuation and rupture of the central slip may also occur following synovial proliferation in the dorsal aspect of the PIP joint in inflammatory arthropathies.

As a result, the head of the proximal phalanx buttonholes (Boutonnière) through these damaged tissues, leading to the PIP flexion deformity. The typical deformity includes extension of the DIP joint because as the central slip tears or stretches the two

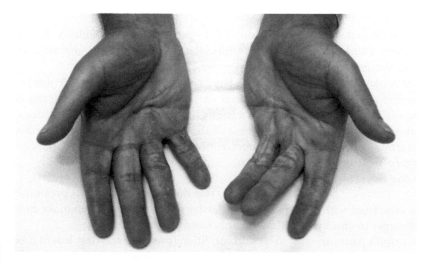

Figure 5.20 Patient with Dupuytren's disease who had previous surgery including an amputation of a digit on the left hand. Hence it is very important to perform a digital Allen's test here.

lateral bands are allowed to retract, increasing extension force at the DIP joint. The lateral bands also separate and begin to sublux around the PIP joint. Eventually they slip palmar to the axis of the PIP joint and become PIP flexors, producing further flexion of the PIP joint and secondary hyperextension of the DIP joint (Figure 5.21).

Elson's test[11] (Figure 5.22) may be used to assess the presence of a competent central slip. Place the hand flat on a table with the PIP joints at the edge of

the table. Flex the PIP joint over the edge of the table. Ask the patient to actively extend the finger against resistance. An intact central slip will try to extend the PIP joint and the lateral bands will remain slack (the extensor mechanism is tethered by the intact central slip); the DIP will remain relaxed. A ruptured central slip will cause weakness of extension at the PIP joint while allowing tensioning of the lateral bands and thus hyperextension and stiffness of the DIP joint.

Mallet Finger

This is a flexion deformity of the DIP joint. It occurs following a distal injury to the lateral slips of the extensor. The tendon can be lacerated proximal to its insertion, or may be avulsed from the distal phalanx by a sudden flexion force. This may be an intra-substance avulsion or may involve an avulsed fragment of bone (Figure 5.23).

Doyle[12] classified these injuries into closed, open and bony injuries. Bony injuries are further classified into:

- Those that are physeal (in children).
- Those involving less than 50% of the joint surface (which tend to be stable).
- Those >50% of the joint surface (which tend to be unstable).

The resulting consequence is an inability to extend the DIP joint. Inspection following the injury will identify an extensor lag. However much a patient

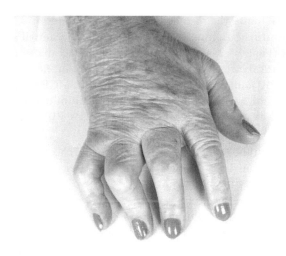

Figure 5.21 Boutonnière deformity with synovial proliferation on the dorsal aspect of the PIP joint.

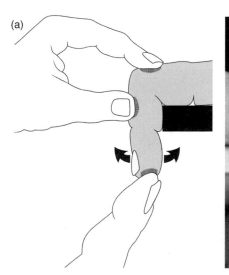
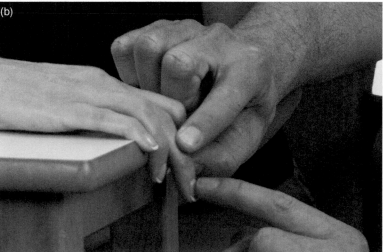

Figure 5.22 Elson's test for Boutonnière deformity.

tries, he or she is unable to extend the joint actively. The joint may be passively correctable by the clinician, but the corrected position will not be maintained when the pressure is released. If the injury is chronic, it is possible for the deformity to become fixed, at which point it is no longer passively correctable. Determining these facts will guide what treatment options are available to the patient. Mallet injuries are one cause of a swan neck deformity (see explanation below).

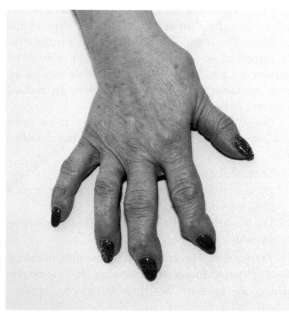

Figure 5.23 Mallet finger. Flexion deformities of the DIP joint. In this patient the deformity was fixed indicating it is chronic.

Intrinsic Tightness Leading to Flexion Contracture of the MCP Joint

The intrinsic muscles include the dorsal and palmar interossei and the lumbrical muscles. The lumbrical muscles work through the extensor mechanism and by their direct attachment to the base of the proximal phalanx. Their actions through these insertions are to flex the MCP joint and extend the PIP and DIP joints. As a result of scarring following injury or increased tone from a neurological problem, shortening of these structures leads to a fixed flexion deformity of the MCP joint and extension, or decreased flexion, of the IP joints: the so-called **intrinsic plus hand.**

Intrinsic tightness can be assessed by **Bunnell's test** (Figure 5.24a,b).[13] This relies on the fact that the lumbricals are at least tension with MCP joint flexion and PIP joint extension, most tension with MCP joint extension and PIP joint flexion, and medium tension in other positions. Bunnell's test assesses PIP joint flexion in two positions:

- With the MCP joint flexed – this will relax the tight intrinsic muscles and allow greater passive flexion of the PIP joint.
- With the MCP joint extended – this will tighten the already tight intrinsic muscle and will reduce the passive flexion of the PIP joint.

In the normal hand passive flexion will be the same in all positions of the MCP joint.

Ulnar Claw Hand

In this situation, the ulnar two digits will assume a position of extension at the MCP joint and flexion

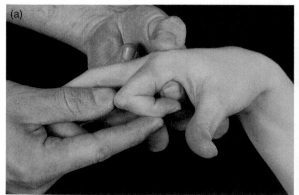
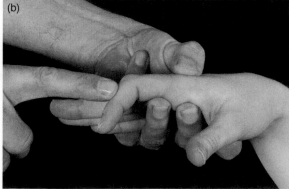

Figure 5.24a,b Bunnell's test. (a) Assess PIP joint flexion with the MCP joint flexed. (b) Then compare the PIP joint flexion with the MCP joint extended.

of the PIP and DIP joints (**'intrinsic minus'**). Usually this will be passively correctible and there will be no signs of Dupuytren's. Later, the fingers will stiffen because of volar plate contractures. The cause should be evident, however, because of the presence of other ulnar nerve signs and symptoms (see Chapter 6).

Tendon Problems

Extensor Pollicis Longus (EPL)

Patients with EPL ruptures present with problems using their thumb in day-to-day activities. They have difficulties in adducting and extending their thumb. When combined, this may be described as retropulsion or retroposition. This inability leads to functional problems, as this is a requirement prior to grasping and gripping.

Extensor pollicis longus ruptures occur suddenly but, in the absence of a clear tendon trauma, a history of an underlying causal pathology should be sought. The rupture almost always occurs in the third extensor compartment, probably due to an interruption of the already poor tendon blood supply (watershed zone) at this level. This could be an inflammatory arthropathy and tenosynovitis. Also seek signs of a distal radial fracture, a malunion or scars from surgical intervention. A dorsal approach to fixation may result in metalwork being placed directly under EPL. A volar approach does not exclude metalwork protruding and damaging EPL. Screws and pegs from the volar side may be too long and prominent.

Look

On examination, look for the attitude of the thumb; normally, the thumb is held slightly abducted. With an EPL rupture, it may lie in a slightly adducted position. The distal phalanx may lie in flexion (Figure 5.25), but this is not always the case. The extensor pollicis brevis (EPB) may work through the sagittal hood to maintain extension of the DIP joint.

Look for signs of an underlying cause of the EPL rupture such as other inflammatory signs, deformity from malunion or scars from surgical fracture fixation.

Feel

On palpation, metalwork may be prominent, palpable and tender. Synovitis along the course of the tendon may feel boggy and tender. You may be able to feel the tendon stumps.

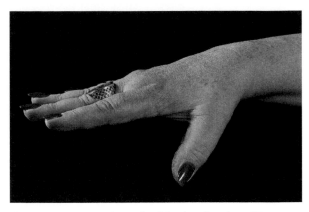

Figure 5.25 Abnormal attitude of the thumb with an EPL rupture.

Move

Ask the patient to perform a retropulsion movement and compare to the normal hand. An easy way to do this is to put the hand palm down on a table, and ask the patient to lift the thumb up off the table top. Retropulsion is elevation of the thumb in an extended position and isolates the action of EPL, excluding EPB's action. An EPL rupture makes it impossible to elevate the thumb in this way.

Special Tests

When a diagnosis has been made, it is then necessary to consider the management options. One of the options available is surgical reconstruction with EIP tendon transfer.[14] It is therefore necessary to determine whether this is present, as this is the tendon transfer of choice.

The technique for assessment of the presence of an EIP tendon is first to flex the MCP joints of all other fingers. This will defunction extensor digitorum communis (EDC). Then ask the patient to extend the index finger on its own (Figure 5.26). Any extension of the index finger MCP joint must therefore be the result of a present EIP. When palpating for EIP, it is found on the ulnar side of the EDC to index tendon.

Finger Extensor Tendon Problems

This is commonly an attritional rupture or direct tendon trauma (laceration). Effects will be loss of active extension of the affected digit. Remember that the index and little fingers have two extensor tendons each (EIP and EDM in addition to EDC).

81

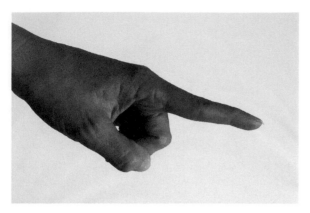

Figure 5.26 Testing for EIP. Ask the patient to point with the index finger. The effect of the EDC tendons is removed by asking the patient to flex the other fingers.

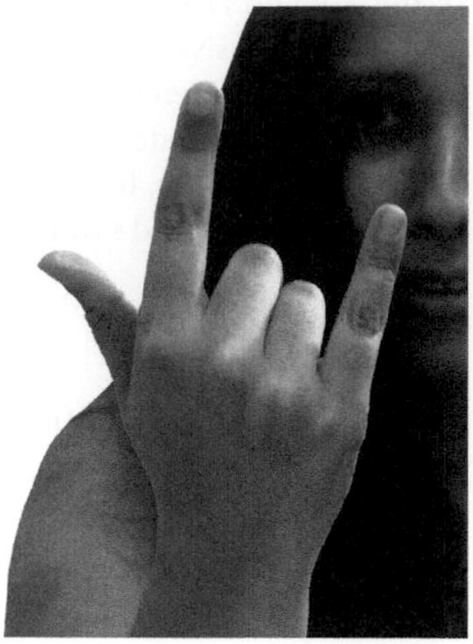

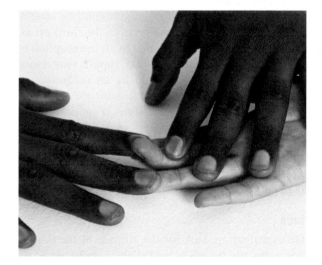

Figure 5.27 Testing EIP and EDM together. The 'rock-on' sign.

To simultaneously test the EDM with the EIP ask the patient to firstly flex all fingers then extend the little finger with the index – **'rock-on' sign** (Figure 5.27).

Flexor Digitorum Profundus (FDP) and Superficialis (FDS)

Loss of FDP or FDS function may occur from a direct injury or from tendon adhesions secondary to an injury, surgery, inflammatory synovitis or infection. With delayed presentation, patients may complain of loss of active movement or that the finger lies in an abnormal position.

Examination starts with inspection, which will provide clues to the underlying problem. Attention should be paid to the normal cascade of the fingers from both the dorsal and palmar aspect. If there is a break in the cascade, then this suggests the possibility of a tendon injury.

Look for any obvious signs as to the cause of the FDP or FDS injury. Scars along the finger, palm and forearm may suggest a laceration or an operation in the past. Swellings or a thickness along the course of the tendon may point towards the location of the terminal stump of the tendon. It may also be the location of scarring of the tendon to adjacent tissues such as the sheath.

On palpation, scarring may be felt as thickening along the flexor tendon sheath and in the palm. An ongoing inflammatory process may be tender.

Assessing movement is all about isolating the tendon to be tested and determining whether and to what extent it is working.

Figure 5.28 Testing FDP function.

To test FDP, isolate the DIP joint by holding the PIP joint in extension and asking the patient to flex at the DIP joint (Figure 5.28). Assess the strength with resistance against flexion. Compare to the other DIP joints.

To test FDS, FDP needs to be excluded; it traverses the PIP joint and may act upon and flex this joint. As the FDP tendons have a common belly, the FDP can be prevented from contracting by holding all the other fingers in extension (Figure 5.29). This prevents FDP flexing the finger being tested. The only movement that will occur will be flexion of the PIP

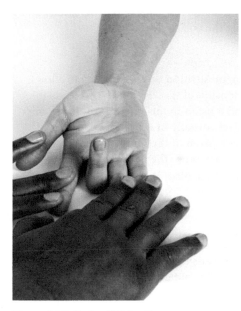

Figure 5.29 Testing FDS function.

joint if the FDS is intact. The distal phalanx will not move and, in fact, remains quite floppy. If the FDS is absent, then PIP joint flexion will not occur

Quadrigia Effect

When one FDP tendon is anchored down for any reason, e.g. adhesion, scarring, bony injury, it will impact on the ability of the other FDP tendons to contract because they all share a common muscle belly. This leads to loss of flexion of the remaining fingers.

Lumbrical Plus

The characteristic feature of this problem occurs when attempting active flexion of a finger. In the lumbrical plus finger, active flexion of the MCP joint results in paradoxical extension of the PIP joint. It occurs when the FDP tendon is damaged distal to the origin of the lumbrical muscle on the FDP. This may be because of a divided tendon or one that has been repaired with a graft that is too long. Division of the tendon may be the result of an amputation of the distal phalanx.

In these situations, the FDP tendon retracts proximally, taking with it the origin of the lumbrical muscle. This effectively tightens the lumbrical muscle. When flexing the fingers, active contraction of the FDP tightens the lumbrical further. The action of this tightened lumbrical through its insertion to the

radial side of the lateral band is then to extend the PIP joint when the patient is trying to flex the finger. Passive flexion of the MCP joint (as in Bunnell's test) will not give rise to the same problem.

Intrinsic Minus and Intrinsic Plus

Intrinsic minus position is similar to a claw hand and is therefore seen in ulnar/median nerve injuries or Volkmann's ischaemic contracture. This is characterised by MCP joint hyperextension and IP joint flexion as a result of an imbalance of forces across these joints.

The intrinsic plus hand is caused by intrinsic tightness (see section on intrinsic tightness above). The typical position of the hand is MCP joint flexion and IP joint extension.

Trigger Finger/Thumb

This is a constriction of the flexor tendon by narrowing of the flexor tendon sheath A1 pulley. Patients complain of a very characteristic symptom. The finger gets stuck with the PIP joint flexed (or the IP joint of the thumb). It may spontaneously reduce with voluntary extension with the sensation of a sharp movement and click. With more severe disease, the patient may need to reduce the finger with the other hand, forcing it into extension. The same sharp snapping sensation and click may be felt. This may also be painful. In the most severe cases, the finger may be locked in flexion and may be impossible to reduce without surgery. The previous history of intermittent locking would point towards this most severe form of triggering rather than a fixed flexion deformity secondary to other causes. With even the early stages, some, though not all, patients have significant levels of pain extending from the palm into the finger.

Observation may identify the snapping of the finger from the flexed position back into extension. If a finger is placed over the A1 pulley, a thickening or nodule may be palpated, which moves suddenly on reduction of the finger. This nodule may be tender, and the tenderness may extend along the flexor tendon sheath distally.

Multiple trigger fingers may occur (exclude diabetes in these situations) and all the fingers should be assessed during the consultation. Trigger thumb is a similar process to that which results from the FPL catching at the entrance of its flexor tendon sheath, resulting in clicking or locking of the IP joint of the thumb.

Other Pathologies

Flexor Tendon Sheath Infection

It is important that diagnosis of this condition is made correctly, as urgent treatment (often washout) is required to prevent long-term damage and adhesions to the flexor tendons within the sheath.

The main symptom is pain, with associated swelling and loss of movement in the affected finger. The classic history is of a small cut to the finger, often when gardening.

Kanavel's four cardinal signs[15] help to make the diagnosis:

- Fusiform 'sausage-like' swelling.
- Finger held in a semi-flexed position.
- Pain on passive extension.
- Percussion tenderness along the course of the flexor tendon.

Swan Neck Deformity

This is a characteristic deformity with hyperextension at the PIP joint and flexion at the DIP joint (Figure 5.30). There are five causes of swan necking, which can be divided up by the location of the primary pathology.

DIP Joint

- A mallet injury releases the distal attachment of the extensor mechanism. This allows retraction and excess tension in the central slip. This, over

time, can pull the PIP joint into hyperextension by stretching the volar plate.

PIP Joint

- Injury to, or attrition of, the volar plate allows hyperextension of the PIP joint. This leads to decreased tension in the extensor mechanism (particularly distally in the lateral bands) and increased tension in the FDP tendon, leading to secondary flexion of the DIP joint.
- A similar mechanism is responsible for swan necking after an FDS tendon rupture/avulsion.

MCP Joint

- Volar subluxation (e.g. in rheumatoid) of the MCP joint leads to excessive tension in the extensors, as the patient desperately tries to extend the finger. PIP joint hyperextension, and secondary DIP joint flexion ensue.
- Intrinsic tightness can cause swan necking, via the lumbricals' PIP joint extensor function.

Swan necking can be described according to severity:

- Actively reducible
- Passively reducible
- Locked

Gamekeeper's Thumb/Skier's Thumb

This is an ulnar collateral ligament (UCL) injury of the thumb MCP joint. Gamekeeper's thumb probably describes a more chronic attrition injury to the collateral ligament as a result of repetitive actions. Skier's thumb demonstrates clearly how an abduction injury to the thumb MCP joint can lead to an acute tear or avulsion of the UCL.

Palpation will often demonstrate tenderness at the origin, path and insertion of the UCL on the ulnar side of the joint. Examining range of movement may not demonstrate any problems with flexion or extension of the MCP joint.

To test the UCL, the MCP joint should be stressed radially, opening up the ulnar side. This is carried out with the joint slightly flexed (10°–15°). Even with a torn UCL, in full extension the tensioned volar plate and accessory collaterals will stabilise the joint. With radial deviation the MCP joint will open up. A comparison with the normal side will highlight this more clearly. A firm endpoint should be sought.

A longitudinal line may be drawn along the metacarpal, continuing along the proximal phalanx.

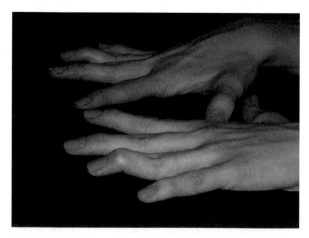

Figure 5.30 Swan neck deformity.

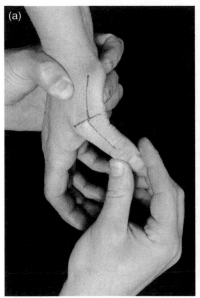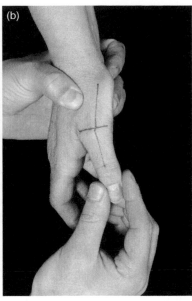

Figure 5.31a,b Stressing the MCP joint to reveal an UCL rupture.

A transverse line perpendicular to this on the dorsum of the MCP joint may also be drawn. On stressing the joint, these lines may make more obvious to the clinician how much angular deformation occurs (Figure 5.31a,b).

Swellings/Lumps

The diagnosis of a swelling in the hand depends to a large degree on its *location*. Assess any lump in the hand according to the same system as for a lump anywhere else.

Remember that ganglia (by far the most common non bony swelling) are synovial cysts arising from an underlying joint or tendon sheath pathology.

Volar

- Inclusion dermoid cysts.
- Ganglion of A1 pulley. Also called a pearl ganglion.
- Giant cell tumour of the flexor sheath. Usually located in relation to the proximal phalanx but can occur anywhere along the length of the sheath. Similar histologically to pigmented villonodular synovitis. This is the second most common benign soft tissue mass in the hand after ganglion.
- Volar wrist ganglion. These come from the STT joint. If considering surgery, remember to perform Allen's test (see below) to check for perfusion from the radial and ulnar arteries. A better strategy, however, is to address the underlying STT joint pathology.

Dorsal

- Radial-sided wrist ganglia often arise from scapholunate joint or radioscaphoid.
- Ulnar-sided wrist ganglia arise from DRUJ or TFCC commonly.
- Rheumatoid nodules on the extensor surface.
- Gouty tophi. Classically with chalky contents.
- Heberden's nodes. Osteophytes from the DIP joint.
- Bouchard's nodes. Osteophytes from the PIP joint.
- Garrod's pads. Over the PIP joints, in association with Dupuytren's disease.
- Carpometacarpal boss. A bony overgrowth of the dorsal aspect of the index and middle CMC joints, often presenting in the third and fourth decades. Sometimes occurs in repetitive sports, e.g. tennis or golf, although the exact cause is uncertain.

Nail Problems

- Subungual exostosis. An exostosis from the tip of the distal phalanx, causing nail deformity.
- Mucous cyst. Arising from the DIP joint, almost always with an underlying osteophyte. Sometimes causes deformation of the nail fold and subsequent nail ridges.
- Glomus tumour. A benign, but very painful, vascular tumour in the nail bed (although sometimes it can be at the fingertip). Often has a characteristic bluish tinge.

- ○ *Love test* – exquisite pain to pinhead pressure.
- ○ *Hildreth test* – pain and tenderness (including Love test) reduced by tourniquet inflation.
- ○ Both tests have high sensitivity and specificity.

- Melanoma. A common story is of a 'subungual haematoma' that doesn't resolve. Unfortunately, metastasises early.

Evaluation of Vascular Supply in the Hand

Vascular integrity of the hand can be assessed using Allen's test. This can be performed on the whole hand or on individual digits. An example of where it is important to test the whole hand is with excision of a volar ganglion or a surgical approach to the scaphoid tubercle where there is a chance of damaging the radial artery. In this case, the presence of a good ulnar artery supply to the hand should be established before embarking on surgery. In cases of revision surgery for Dupuytren's disease, a digital Allen's test should be performed.

Allen's test[16] is performed with the patient's elbow flexed and the forearm supinated (Figure 5.32a). Next, the ulnar and radial arteries are palpated with the fingers of the examiner's hands. Ask the patient to open and close the fists a few times before keeping them clenched. This action exsanguinates the blood from the hand. The radial and ulnar arteries are then simultaneously compressed by the examiner's fingers. The patient is then instructed to open the hand. It should appear blanched because the arterial supply is occluded. Next, release compression from one of the arteries and observe the colour to the hand. If the released artery is contributing significantly to perfusion, the normal colour should return to the palm and fingers within a few seconds. If it does not, then it is likely that perfusion via that artery is reduced. The test is repeated, this time releasing the other artery. In 75% of patients, the ulnar artery predominates over the radial artery. However, either artery should be able to perfuse the hand on its own in the majority of patients.

The **digital Allen's test** is performed in a similar manner.[17] The finger is flexed first to exsanguinate it. Then the digital arteries are occluded on either side of the finger being tested. Note the digital arteries are on the volar side of the finger. The finger is extended, and the pressure of the digital arteries is released in turn. (Figure 5.32b,c).

Advanced Corner

Palmaris Longus

The palmaris longus (PL) tendon has at least three main uses in orthopaedics:

1. As a surgical landmark to identify the median nerve
2. In interposition arthroplasty procedures, e.g. for Kienböck's disease
3. In tendon transfers

The PL is used in a variety of tendon transfers, e.g. in FPL ruptures, which are seen in rheumatoid patients and in patients following volar plating of the distal radius.

It can also be used as a graft for abductor pollicis brevis to augment elevation of the thumb in situations of low median nerve palsy.[18]

The PL is, however, not present in all individuals with an incidence of absence of 1.5% to 63% (average

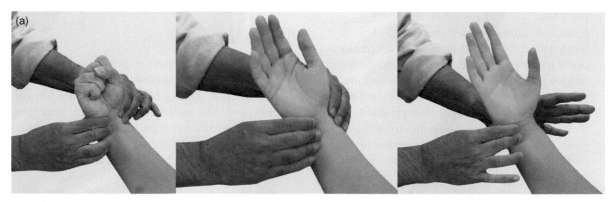

(a)

Figure 5.32a Allen's test. Testing the contribution of the radial and ulnar arteries to the hand.

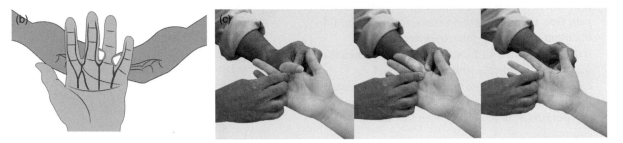

Figure 5.32b,c Digital Allen's test. Testing for the presence of the digital arteries to both the radial and ulnar side of the digit. Note that the vessels are occluded on the volar side of the digit.

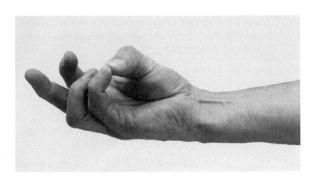

Fig 5.33 Schaeffer's test for palmaris longus. Oppose the thumb to the little finger and flex the wrist.

25%) in different populations.[19] It therefore needs to be tested for prior to surgery.

To Test for Palmaris Longus

Oppose the thumb to the little finger and flex the wrist. This is Schaeffer's test (Figure 5.33) and is the most commonly used test. In the Mishra test, passively hyperextend the MCP joints of the patient's fingers and then ask them to flex their wrist.

Assessment of Acute UCL Injury of Thumb MCP Joint

In an acute setting, the joint will be too painful to carry out the stress test described in this chapter. The options are then to let the injury and its discomfort settle down before reassessing or, if a definite injury is suspected and there is no fracture on X-ray, local anaesthetic may be used to numb the area before stressing the joint.

Beware that excessive testing runs the risk of converting a simple avulsion into a Stener lesion, where the UCL stump (or avulsed insertion) displaces proximal to the adductor pollicis aponeurosis. Adductor pollicis then becomes interposed between the stump and its intended insertion, preventing healing. For this reason, many surgeons prefer to confirm the diagnosis with imaging, usually magnetic resonance imaging (MRI).

The same process may be carried out to assess the potential for other ligamentous injuries affecting the joints of the hand, whether radial collateral or ulnar collateral injuries of MCP, PIP or DIP joints.

Base of Thumb Arthritis: Assessment of the Adjacent MCPJ

When assessing patients with basal thumb arthritis (CMC joint) it is also important to carefully examine the adjacent MCP joint. Hyperextension of the MCP joint is quite common and is an adaptation because of stiffness and loss of abduction at the CMC joint. Over time, there has been a gradual attenuation of the volar joint restraining structures. Typically, the patient also gradually loses some of the range of flexion.

The MCP joint may also be arthritic, which would be suggested by tenderness and swelling at this level and a reduced arc of movement. Radiographs would confirm the situation.

It is important, therefore, to assess the MCP in the following respects:

1. The presence and severity of joint hyperextension
2. The overall range of motion
3. The presence of joint swelling and or tenderness

Surgical Considerations

If surgery is planned for the basal thumb arthritis, then the assessment of the MCP joint influences preoperative and intraoperative decision making as follows:

87

- If the MCP joint is normal in range of motion and is pain free, then there are no concerns that it should maintain its function after trapeziectomy.
- If the MCP joint is stiff, swollen and painful, then this may indicate arthritis within the joint and consideration should be given to MCP arthrodesis at the time of trapeziectomy. If this is associated with a hyperextension deformity, then this will be corrected.
- If the MCP joint is essentially pain free, hyperextends but has a well-preserved arc of movement, then this hyperextension may slowly improve once the trapezium has been excised. In this scenario, most surgeons would treat the basal joint in isolation in the first instance.
- If the MCP joint is pain free but has developed a fixed hyperextension deformity with a very limited range of motion, then this is unlikely to improve after trapeziectomy and the patient should be made aware of this. The patient would often be offered an option to try to improve the MCP alignment at the time of trapeziectomy with, as examples, either a joint release and temporary (K-wire) stabilisation or MCP fusion.

References

1. Kapandji A. Clinical test of apposition and counter-apposition of the thumb. *Ann Chir Main* 1986;**5**(1):67–73.

2. Nalebuff EA, Millender LH. Surgical treatment of the Boutonniere deformity in rheumatoid arthritis. *Orthop Clin North Am* 1975 Jul;**6**(3):753–763.

3. Nalebuff EA, Millender LH. Surgical treatment of the swan neck deformity in rheumatoid arthritis. *Orthop Clin North Am* 1975 Jul;**6**(3):733–752.

4. Nalebuff EA. Diagnosis, classification and management of rheumatoid thumb deformities. *Bull Hosp Joint Dis* 1968;**29**:119–137.

5. Mannerfelt L, Norman O. Attrition ruptures of flexor tendons in rheumatoid arthritis caused by bony spurs in the carpal tunnel. A clinical and radiological study. *J Bone Joint Surg Br* 1969;**51**:270–277.

6. Vaughan-Jackson OJ. Rupture of extensor tendons by attrition at the inferior radio-ulnar joint. *J Bone Joint Surg Br* 1948;**30B**:528.

7. Alinaghi F, Calov M, Kristensen LE, et al. Prevalence of psoriatic arthritis in patients with psoriasis: A systematic review and meta-analysis of observational and clinical studies. *J Am Acad Dermatol* 2019 Jan;**80**(1):251–265.

8. Roberts ME, Wright V, Hill AG, Mehra AC. Psoriatic arthritis: follow-up study. *Ann Rheum Dis* 1976;**35**:206–212.

9. Hueston JT. The table top test. *Hand* 1982;**14**:100–103.

10. James JI. The assessment and management of the injured hand. *Hand*. 1970;**2**:97–105.

11. Elson RA. Rupture of the central slip of the extensor hood of the finger. A test for early diagnosis. *J Bone Joint Surg Br* 1986;**68B**:229–231.

12. Doyle JR. Extensor tendons – acute injuries. In Green DP, Hotchkiss RN, Pederson WC (eds), *Green Operative Hand Surgery*, 4th ed. Philadelphia: Churchill Livingstone, 1999; pp. 1962–1971.

13. Bunnell S. Ischaemic contracture, local, in the hand. *J Bone Joint Surg Am* 1953;**35A**:88–101.

14. Magnussen PA, Harvey FJ, Tonkin MA. Extensor indicis proprius transfer for rupture of the extensor pollicis longus tendon. *J Bone Joint Surg Br* 1990;**72B**:881–883.

15. Kanavel AB. *Infections of the Hand*, 7th ed. London: Baillière, Tindall & Cox, 1939.

16. Elson RA. Rupture of the central slip of the extensor hood of the finger. A test for early diagnosis. *J Bone Joint Surg* 1986;**68B**:229–231.

17. Ashbell TS, Kleinert HE, Putcha SM, Kutz JE. The digital Allen test. *Plast Reconstr Surg* 1967;**39**(3):311–312.

18. Berger P, Duerincx J. Flexor pollicis longus tendon rupture after volar wrist plating: reconstruction with palmaris longus interposition graft. *Acta Orthop Belg* 2017;**83**:467–472.

19. Ioannis D, Anastasios K, Konstantinos N, Lazaros K, Georgios N. Palmaris longus muscle prevalence in different nations and interesting anatomical variations: review of the literature. *J Clin Med Res* 2015;**7**(11):525–830.

Examination of the Peripheral Nerves in the Hand and Upper Limb

Kate Brown, L. Chris Bainbridge and John E. D. Wright

Assessment of the Peripheral Nerves in the Hand and Upper Limb

A. History

B. Clinical Examination

Step 1
Look

Step 2
Quick screen of nerves

Step 3
Feel

Step 4
Move

Step 5
(Provocation tests if necessary)

After inspection, a quick screen for assessing the peripheral nerves to the hand may be useful. This might be especially so in children. It can also provide a further clue as to which peripheral nerve it will be best to examine first.

Ask the patient to 'point your finger' (radial nerve), 'cross your fingers' (ulnar nerve), 'make an "O"' (median nerve).

On assessing each peripheral nerve, the examiner must have a system that allows them to determine whether the lesion is proximal (high) or distal (low). Clues are obtained from looking, feeling and moving. Therefore, the sites and sequence chosen to test sensation and muscles should allow the examiner to differentiate between the two. These are summarised in Tables 6.1, 6.2 and 6.3.

Median Nerve

Table 6.1 Median Nerve

Look	Scars, thenar wasting
Screen	OK sign – 'Make an O'

Table 6.1 (cont.)

Feel	Tip of index finger; base of thenar eminence
Move	FCR (flexor carpi radialis) FDS (flexor digitorum superficialis) to index APB (abductor pollicis brevis) OP (opponens pollicis) OK sign (AIN – anterior interosseous nerve)
Provocation	Ligament of Struthers / lacertus / PT (pronator teres) / FDS – pronator syndrome Tinel's / Phalen's carpal tunnel syndrome

Regarding sensory function, in the low lesion the thenar crease area will have preserved sensation as the palmar branch of the median nerve is superficial to the transverse ligament and is therefore not involved in carpal tunnel syndrome (low median nerve).

The motor sequence above allows differentiation between a high median nerve palsy and a low median nerve palsy. In a high median nerve lesion, both sensory and motor deficit will be present in all the groups. In low median nerve lesions, flexor digitorum superficialis (FDS) and flexor carpi radialis (FCR) will be preserved.

In anterior interosseous nerve (AIN) palsy, the patient will be unable to perform the OK sign as he or she will be unable to use flexor pollicis longus (FPL) and flexor digitorum profundus (FDP) to the index finger, both of which are supplied by the AIN.

Radial Nerve

Table 6.2 Radial Nerve

Look	Scars, wrist drop, splint
Screen	Extend index finger – 'point your finger'
Feel	Dorsum of first web space
Move	BR (brachioradialis) ECRL (extensor carpi radialis longus)

Table 6.2 (cont.)

	ECU (extensor carpi ulnaris)
	EIP (extensor indicis proprius) or EDC (extensor digitorum communis)
	EPL (extensor pollicis longus)
Provocation	Radial tunnel tenderness
	Resisted supination

Sensation is preserved in a PIN palsy but lost in the first web space in a high radial nerve palsy.

To differentiate high radial nerve palsy from a posterior interosseous nerve (PIN) palsy – in a high radial nerve injury the power in all these muscles groups will be affected, whereas in a PIN palsy the power in brachioradialis and extensor carpi radialis longus (ECRL) will be intact.

Ulnar Nerve

Table 6.3 Ulnar Nerve

Look	Scars. Wasting first dorsal interosseous. Guttering. Hypothenar wasting, claw deformity. Wartenberg's sign
Screen	Interossei muscles. 'cross your fingers'
Feel	Tip of little finger. Dorsum of fifth metacarpal
Move	FCU (flexor carpi ulnaris) FDP to little finger (flexor digitorum profundus) ADM (abductor digiti minimi) First dorsal interosseus Froment's sign
Provocation	Tinel's sign Elbow flexion test

Differentiation between high and low lesions can also be suspected on inspection. In lower lesions the clawing is much more pronounced than in high ulnar nerve lesions (due to the loss of the FDP to the little and ring fingers in the high lesion). This is called the ulnar paradox.

In high ulnar nerve palsy, such as injury around the medial epicondyle, sensation in both areas is affected, whereas in low ulnar nerve problems, such as compression in Guyon's canal, the dorsal branch is preserved, resulting in no loss of sensation in the region of the fifth metacarpal.

In a high ulnar nerve lesion the motor power in all muscle groups is affected and Froment's test is positive. In the lower lesion the power in FDP to the little finger and flexor carpi ulnaris (FCU) are both preserved.

Introduction

Productive examination of the peripheral nerves in the upper limb is based on a comprehensive knowledge of the anatomy of the brachial plexus and the course of the nerves as they pass distally. Examination of the terminal components of the nerves informs us of the proximal pathology. Knowledge of dermatomal and specific sensory nerve cutaneous supply is essential (Figure 6.1).

History

Examination is guided by a full history. The patient's age, hand dominance, main occupation, hobbies, past injuries and any neurological disorders should be documented. Age significantly affects both the quality and quantity of nerve recovery following injury. It is better in children and young adults; the rate of nerve regeneration in children is 2–3 mm per day, compared with 1–2 mm in adults.

The nature of the injury, e.g. sharp laceration or crush, should be clearly documented, as this will have a profound impact on the results of nerve surgery. In the elective situation, localisation of the site of injury along the course of the nerve may be comparatively difficult. However, enquiry should be made about previous injuries or operations in the upper limb. One should note whether there is any evidence for nerve recovery, especially if there has been a significant time lapse since the initial event. This will typically follow the proximal to distal innervation of the musculature from the nerve trunk: e.g. in a radial nerve injury distal to the spiral groove, the first muscle to be reinnervated is brachioradialis and the last is extensor indicis. This helps in counselling the patients if some recovery is already observed.

The timing of injury or the evolution and duration of a compressive neuropathy are important. For example, if the duration of carpal tunnel compression symptoms is less than 10 months, there is significant chance of recovery utilising conservative measures.[1] Enquire as to whether the symptoms are exacerbated by anything in particular such as driving (compression of the median nerve in the carpal tunnel) and holding a phone to the ear for prolonged periods of time (compression of the ulnar nerve in the cubital tunnel). Clearly document any treatments to date, and their success, such as steroid injections for the compressive

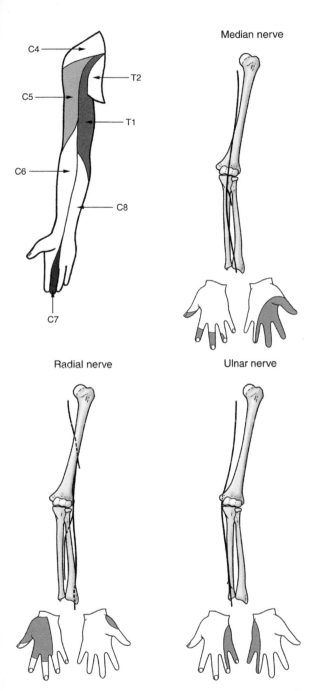

Figure 6.1 Dermatomes of the upper limb and the sensory supply of the median, radial and ulnar nerves. Note the general course of the nerve in the arm.

neuropathies or any formal surgical procedures. Patients who have responded well to steroid injections for carpal tunnel syndrome typically do well after a formal release.

A simple question to ask patients with possible cubital tunnel syndrome is whether they can read a magazine/broadsheet holding it up in the air or whether they need to put it on a table. For the millennial, enquire as to how long they can hold their phone in the air whilst looking at social media!

Co-morbidities (especially diabetes, thyroid disease and other endocrine disease) should be elicited, as compression syndromes (in particular, carpal tunnel syndrome) are commonly associated with systemic disease. Pregnancy is associated with carpal tunnel syndrome – it may or may not be obvious to the examiner! Smoking and alcohol intake may influence the outcome of surgery. The pattern and frequency of analgesic usage, including neuralgic medications, will forewarn the surgeon about the severity of the problem and provide information on diurnal variation in symptoms. Some hobbies are associated with the compression neuropathies such as cyclist palsy (compression of the ulnar nerve in Guyon's canal).

Some medications may cause peripheral neuropathy, examples including cisplatin (cancer medications), disulfiram (anti-alcohol) and dapsone (for dermatological disorders). A full drug history should be documented in order to ascertain whether there are any that need to be managed should an operative course be pursued (such as anticoagulant therapy). Folate and B12 deficiencies can be manifested as peripheral neuropathies.[2]

On the rare occasion, there may be a family history of polyneuropathy such as hereditary neuropathy with pressure palsies (HNPP). Enquiries should be made as to whether there are other members of the family with similar issues.

Specific Symptoms of Nerve Disease

Patients sometimes find it difficult to localise neurological symptoms specifically. Patients may describe pain along the course of a specific nerve, and the distribution of tingling, paraesthesia and numbness can be diagnostic, but there may be significant variation. Symptoms in the radial three digits are strongly suggestive of carpal tunnel compression, but symptoms may be just in the middle finger (these fibres are most superficial in the median nerve). It is also important to differentiate whether symptoms are in the distribution of a specific nerve or the radicular distribution of a cervical root.

Symptoms of nerve compression are often exacerbated at night and the temporal pattern of symptoms should be elicited. Night pain, unrelieved by analgesia, can be indicative of a sarcoma. Ongoing pain not relieved by adequate analgesia after an acute event (neurostenalgia), such as in the immediate post-operative period, should be addressed immediately. It may be secondary to compression of the nerve and increasing the time delay until the compression is relieved is deleterious to the nerve recovery.

Difficulty with fine tasks, like buttons or dropping objects, is often described: sensory loss and muscle weakness both contribute to a lack of dexterity. However, alternative pathologies, such as pain secondary to basal thumb arthritis, need to be excluded as the underlying cause of poor hand function.

Attention should be paid to exact nature of the patient's description of the pain. Different terms can be confusing but it is important to be precise. A brief synopsis is given here.[3]

- **Allodynia:** Perception of an ordinarily non-noxious stimulus as pain
- **Dysaesthesia:** Unpleasant or abnormal sensation with or without a stimulus
- **Hyperalgesia:** Increased response to noxious stimulation
- **Hyperpathia:** Presence of hyperalgesia and allodynia usually associated with over-reaction and persistence of the sensation after the stimulus
- **Neuralgia:** Pain in the distribution of a nerve or group of nerves
- **Neuropathic:** Persistent intractable pain disproportionate between the extent of the lesion and the severity of the pain
- **Neurostenalgia:** Neuropathic pain that results from continuing irritation of an anatomically intact nerve by a noxious agent

Examination of Specific Nerves

Compression neuropathy and traumatic injury are the two main causes of peripheral nerve symptoms in the upper limb. However, other causes such as iatrogenic or tumours should not be forgotten. Knowing a logical sequence of examination for each of the three main nerves and their branches will enable the examiner to identify the site of pathology in the course of the nerve. With knowledge from the elicited history, examination should follow the following pattern: inspection, sensory testing (including two-point discrimination), palpation, motor testing, presence or absence of sweating and provocation tests including a Tinel's test (see 'Advanced Corner').

There are common sites of compression for compressive neuropathies, and the syndromes for each nerve are described in Table 6.4. The aim of examination for traumatic injuries is to identify which parts of the nerve are injured, which are still functioning and, later on, assessment of recovery. Following on from a nerve injury, an early sign of muscle reinnervation is the **tender muscle sign** which manifests before motor recovery (see 'Advanced Corner').[4]

Median Nerve

The common syndromes associated with compression of the median nerve are pronator syndrome, AIN syndrome and carpal tunnel syndrome. It is important to know the common sites of pathology so that they can be examined specifically. Remember that the site of compression may be in the proximal forearm, but the diagnostic testing is in the function of the hand.

Table 6.4 Compression syndromes of peripheral nerves in the hand and upper limb

	Median nerve	Radial nerve	Ulnar nerve
Proximal – sensory	Pronator syndrome	Radial tunnel syndrome	Mild cubital tunnel syndrome
Proximal – motor	Anterior interosseous nerve syndrome	Posterior interosseous nerve syndrome	Severe cubital tunnel syndrome
Distal	Carpal tunnel syndrome	Wartenberg's syndrome*	Guyon's canal compression

*Wartenberg's syndrome is a compression of the superficial radial nerve branch rather than the radial nerve proper.

Potential Sites of Injury/Compression

Pronator Syndrome

Sites of proximal median nerve compression from proximal to distal are as follows:

- *Ligament of Struthers:* This is an aberrant ligament which, when present, lies between the medial epicondyle of the humerus and a bony spur located 5 cm proximally on the humeral shaft. The median nerve, along with the brachial artery and vein, runs between the ligament and the humerus where it is liable to compression (Figure 6.2a).
- *Lacertus fibrosus (bicipital aponeurosis):* Along its course from the elbow into the forearm, the median nerve runs beneath the thick lacertus fibrosus (extending from biceps tendon to the forearm fascia) (Figure 6.2b).
- *Pronator teres (PT):* Between the superficial and deep heads.
- *Fibrous arch of the FDS* muscle.
- Any one or combination of these are possible sources of compression.

Carpal Tunnel Syndrome

The site of compression of carpal tunnel syndrome is within the carpal tunnel beneath the transverse carpal ligament.

Anterior Interosseous Nerve Compression

The AIN can be compressed at similar sites to the median nerve or from additional sites as it branches off

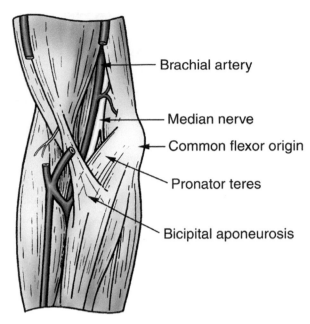

Figure 6.2b Bicipital aponeurosis (lacertus fibrosus) and its relationship to the median nerve.

the median nerve. Note that the AIN compression results in motor signs only as the AIN has no sensory component. If there are incomplete signs of an AIN palsy, suspect a Martin–Gruber anastomosis (see below).

Sites of AIN compression:

- Tendinous edge of the deep head of pronator teres – most common site
- Lacertus fibrosus edge
- Accessory muscles – the most common one being the Gantzer muscle

Gantzer muscles are variant muscles in the anterior forearm inserting most frequently into the FPL and sometimes into the FDP. It can compress the AIN (Kiloh–Nevin syndrome) or sometimes the median nerve.

An important point to note about AIN compression is that it is very uncommon. Most of the time, when a patient develops AIN symptoms and signs it is because of AIN neuritis rather than compression. This typically resolves in about 18 months.

Examination Routine for the Median Nerve

Inspection (Look)

Look for wasting of the thenar muscles, in particular abductor pollicis brevis (APB). This is best seen with

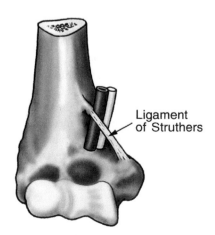

Figure 6.2a The ligament of Struthers and its relationship to the median nerve and the brachial artery.

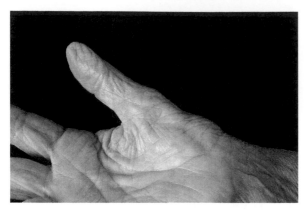

Figure 6.3 Gross wasting of the thenar muscles in a patient with median nerve palsy.

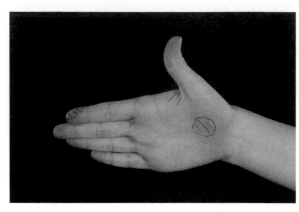

Figure 6.4 The two areas to test for median nerve sensation. In low lesions, the sensation in the base of the thenar eminence is preserved.

the hand in profile (Figure 6.3). The scar of a previous carpal tunnel decompression may not be obvious unless specifically sought.

Feel

Sensation: The median nerve terminal branch can be tested by sensation at the tip of the index finger. The presence or absence of sensation over the base of the thenar eminence will differentiate between proximal compression and compression within the carpal tunnel. The palmar cutaneous branch of the median nerve arises about 3–5 cm proximal to the wrist crease and runs superficial to the transverse carpal ligament. Consequently, in classical carpal tunnel syndrome, normal sensation is expected in the skin over the thenar eminence. Numbness at this site indicates a more proximal level of nerve compression (Figure 6.4). There are no cutaneous sensory fibres in the AIN.

Palpation: Tenderness over the median nerve in the proximal forearm can sometimes be elicited at one of the anatomical sites of compression described above.

Motor Testing (Move)

Table 6.5 presents median nerve motor testing. A logical sequence of testing is to examine the more proximally innervated muscles first and then test the muscles supplied by the AIN (Figure 6.5). The FCR and FDS are supplied by the median nerve in the forearm, proximal to the carpal tunnel. The APB and opponens pollicis (OP) are supplied by the median nerve distal to the carpal tunnel. Testing these four muscles in sequence will identify the level

of pathology. The classic test for the AIN is the **OK sign** or Kiloh–Nevin sign.[5] The patient is asked to make a circle with the thumb and index finger and pinch the tips together; if the AIN-innervated FPL and FDP are deficient, the patient extends at the interphalangeal (IP) joints and pinches with the thumb and finger pulps (Figure 6.6).

Provocation Tests

It is good practice to perform these at the end of the examination, as they can cause discomfort to the patient. The sites of specific compression syndromes and provocation tests for them are outlined below.

Pronator Syndrome

1. The patient's elbow is flexed and the forearm pronated. The patient is then instructed to supinate the forearm forcibly, against resistance. The biceps tendon and lacertus fibrosus become taut and may exacerbate the symptoms (Figure 6.7).
2. The patient's forearm is placed in full supination and the patient is instructed to pronate the arm forcibly against resistance. This will tighten PT and increase any median nerve entrapment.
3. Forceful flexion of the proximal interphalangeal (PIP) joint of the middle finger against resistance will similarly increase any compression of the median nerve by the arch of the FDS.

Carpal Tunnel Syndrome

1. *Phalen's test* – placing the patient's wrists in a maximally flexed position reproduces the patient's

Table 6.5 Median nerve

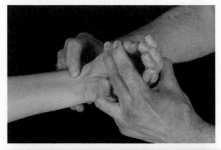

FCR – Ask patient to flex wrist against resistance, observe and palpate tension in the FCR tendon.

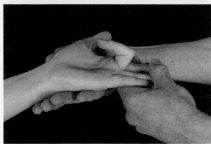

FDS – Place hand in palm or on table, hold fingers in extension except middle finger and ask the patient to bend the finger. Active flexion at PIPJ demonstrates FDS function.

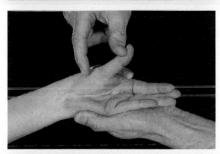

APB – Cradle the patient's hand in yours or place it on the table. Ask the patient to raise/abduct the thumb towards the ceiling and maintain it against resistance. Feel the APB, which is the most radial of the thenar muscles.

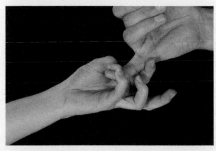

OP – Ask the patient to touch tip of thumb to little finger and ask them to resist you pulling fingers apart.

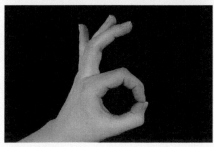

OK sign – Ask the patient to make a circle with the thumb and index finger and pinch the tips together; if the AIN innervated flexor pollicis longus and flexor digitorum profundus are deficient, the patient extends at the interphalangeal joints and pinches with the thumb and finger pulps.

FCR, flexor carpi radialis; FDS, flexor digitorum superficialis; APB, abductor pollicis brevis; OP, opponens pollicis

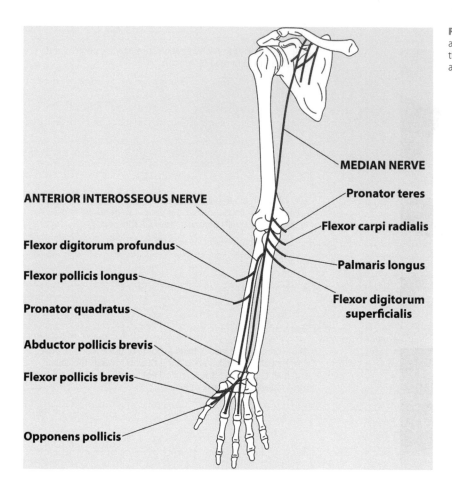

ANTERIOR INTEROSSEOUS NERVE

Flexor digitorum profundus

Flexor pollicis longus

Pronator quadratus

Abductor pollicis brevis

Flexor pollicis brevis

Opponens pollicis

MEDIAN NERVE

Pronator teres

Flexor carpi radialis

Palmaris longus

Flexor digitorum superficialis

Figure 6.5 Median nerve with its anterior interosseous branch showing the locations of their respective branches and the muscles they supply.

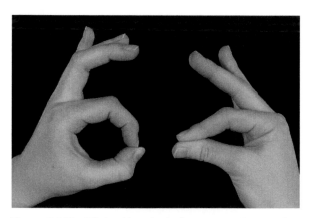

Figure 6.6 The OK sign. Note that in the presence of an anterior interosseous nerve palsy the FDP to the index finger and the FPL is affected, and therefore the patient is unable to make a complete 'O'.

symptoms. This is a time-dependent test, so the shorter the time it takes for the patient to notice symptoms the more sensitive the test (Figure 6.8a).

2. *Reverse Phalen's* – with the wrist maximally extended, the symptoms are reproduced (Figure 6.8b).

3. *Paley and McMurtry* – direct pressure applied over the median nerve at the level of the distal wrist crease reproduces the symptoms within 30 seconds to 2 minutes. There is no wrist movement involved in this test; therefore, it is a useful provocation test to employ among patients with painful wrist conditions or wrist stiffness.[6] Durkan described a modification of this, advising that pressure should be applied using both thumbs over the carpal tunnel itself (Carpal compression test, Figure 6.8d).[7]

4. Other less common tests include the *tourniquet test* and *straight arm raising* (SAR) test.[8] In these, the symptoms of nerve compression may be precipitated by increasing the nerve ischaemia by

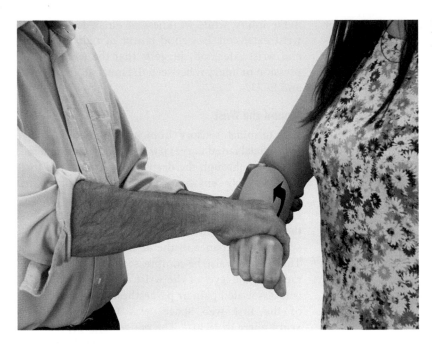

Figure 6.7 Test for pronator syndrome. The patient's elbow is flexed and forearm fully pronated. The patient is then asked to supinate against resistance. This results in pain if positive.

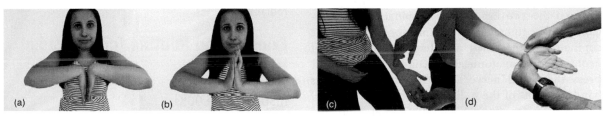

(a)   (b)   (c)   (d)

Figure 6.8a,b,c,d Testing for carpal tunnel syndrome. (a) Phalen's test for carpal tunnel syndrome. Wrists are in maximal palmarflexion. (b) Reverse Phalen's test for carpal tunnel syndrome. The wrists are placed in maximal extension (dorsiflexion). (c) Tinel's test. Light percussion over the site of compression stimulates 'pins and needles' in the cutaneous distribution. (d) Carpal compression test (Durkan) using both thumbs to compress the carpal tunnel.

either applying a tourniquet or simply elevating the arm above the head level with wrist in neutral position.

5. *Tinel's test* – percussion over the median nerve reproduces symptoms. The best place to percuss the nerve is just proximal to the wrist crease at the point at which the nerve enters the carpal tunnel (Figure 6.8c).

Radial Nerve

The radial nerve can be injured by trauma or compression. Classic sites of injury are either above the elbow (in the axilla or the spiral groove of the humerus), or below the elbow in the forearm. Trauma – blunt, penetrating

or iatrogenic – can injure the radial nerve as it passes around the humerus. The common compression syndromes are posterior interosseous nerve (PIN) syndrome, radial tunnel syndrome and Wartenberg's syndrome (compression of the superficial radial nerve).[9] Following the examination sequence of inspection, sensory testing, palpation, motor testing and provocation tests, the examiner should be able to identify the level of radial nerve pathology.

Potential Sites of Injury/Compression

Above the Elbow

Common causes of radial nerve injury are a spiral fracture of the distal humerus (Holstein–Lewis

97

injury), iatrogenic injury at the time of surgery for stabilisation of a humeral fracture and external pressure (including tourniquet injury). The examiner should be alerted to possible radial nerve pathology by scars in the upper arm, either from trauma or surgery. A high injury of the radial nerve before it divides will affect the brachioradialis and the ECRL as well as the superficial sensory branch and the PIN innervated musculature.

Around the Elbow

The two classic radial nerve compression syndromes described are **radial tunnel syndrome** and **PIN syndrome**. These are sometimes difficult syndromes to diagnose, and their exact aetiology and management are unclear. The major difference between the syndromes is the presence of pain and motor weakness in the PIN-innervated muscles with PIN syndrome, and the presence of pain but without weakness in radial tunnel syndrome.

The motor branch of the radial nerve divides above the supinator muscle and the PIN passes through the two heads of the supinator in the so-called radial tunnel. The proximal boundary of the supinator is thickened and termed the arcade of Frohse. Other anatomical structures that can compress the radial nerve are believed to be fibrous bands in front of the radiocapitellar joint, a leash of vessels from the anterior recurrent radial artery and the fibrous proximal edge of extensor carpi radialis brevis (ECRB).

The main differential diagnosis for these syndromes is lateral epicondylitis. In both diagnoses, the patient may report pain in the lateral aspect of the elbow, radiating to the forearm. Classically, the point tenderness for lateral epicondylitis (the insertion of ECRB just anterior to the lateral epicondyle) is more proximal and posterior than the tenderness of palpating the radial tunnel. It is possible for the two pathologies to co-exist and can make differentiation difficult. This is where targeted steroid injections may be helpful in the diagnostic workup.

It is important when examining for compression or injury to the PIN to assess for radial deviation on extension of the wrist. The reason for this is that the ECRL is supplied by the radial nerve and ECRB by the PIN, before it enters the radial tunnel. However, extensor carpi ulnaris (ECU) is supplied by the PIN after entry to the radial tunnel. Therefore, complete weakness of wrist extension suggests a very high radial nerve injury, while weakness of ulnar deviation and wrist extension, but good power of radial deviation and wrist extension, suggests that the level of compression or injury is between the innervation of ECRL and ECU.

Around the Wrist

The terminal sensory branch of the radial nerve (superficial radial nerve) passes under brachioradialis to emerge through the deep fascia in the distal forearm to supply sensation over the dorsum of the first web space. The nerve is vulnerable when an anterior Henry approach is used to plate a radial fracture, and the scar for this should alert the examiner to possible sensory disturbance in the distribution of the nerve. The nerve can also be compressed as it passes over the radius at the level of the wrist. Trauma at this level, with associated pain or paraesthesia over the dorsum of the first web space, was first described by Wartenberg in 1930.[10] The patient may report a history of wearing a new watch or having been handcuffed, as both can cause irritation of the superficial radial nerve.

Examination Routine for the Radial Nerve

Inspection (Look)

Observe the posture of the wrist and identify any potentially relevant scars. Inspection may reveal a 'dropped wrist' posture and possibly the use of a wrist extension splint.

Feel

Sensation: Testing for sensation in the first web space in the dorsum of the hand will identify whether there is pathology either in the main radial nerve trunk or in the superficial sensory branch (Figure 6.9). There are no cutaneous sensory fibres in the PIN, so, if there is weakness of PIN-innervated muscles but normal sensation in the superficial sensory branch distribution, the pathology is distal to the bifurcation of the radial nerve.

Palpation: If lateral epicondylitis or compression in the radial tunnel is suspected, then palpation for tenderness on the lateral side of the elbow will be helpful in differentiating between them. Distally, examination may reveal tenderness along the course of the superficial sensory nerve with a positive Tinel's

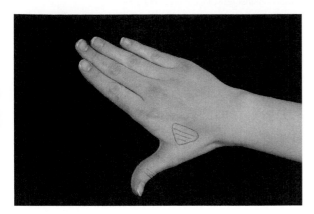

Figure 6.9 Area to test for radial nerve sensation.

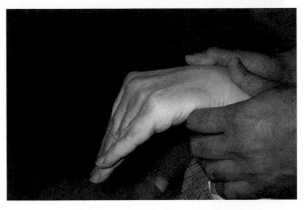

Figure 6.10 Inability to extend the fingers at the MCP joints in a patient with radial nerve palsy.

test. This must be differentiated from the tenderness of De Quervain's disease, which is slightly more distal.

Motor Testing (Move)

Table 6.6 presents radial nerve motor testing. The radial nerve supplies the wrist extensors and extensors of the metacarpophalangeal (MCP) joints of the fingers (Figure 6.10). It is logical to examine the muscles in the order in which they are innervated (Figure 6.11). The most proximal muscle to be tested is brachioradialis, which is visualised and palpated by asking the patient to flex the elbow against resistance when held at 90°. Then the muscles ECRL and ECU are tested as described above to identify whether the pathology is above or below the bifurcation of the radial nerve. The more distally innervated muscles of the PIN are the extensor pollicis longus (EPL) and extensor indicis (EI), which can be tested by demonstrating retropulsion of the thumb or index finger pointing.

A common error is to believe incorrectly that the patient can fully extend their fingers, when the extension is only at the IP joints, but not the MCP joints. Therefore, care should be taken to observe that the extension of the index finger (extensor indicis proprius, EIP) or the other fingers (extensor digitorum communis, EDC) is actually coming from the MCP joint. Interphalangeal joint extension is a function of the median and ulnar nerves through the intrinsic muscles.

Provocation Tests

If compression within the radial tunnel is considered, provocation is performed. Resisted active supination with the elbow in extension will increase the pressure beneath the arcade of Frohse. This will increase the pain if the PIN is already being compressed. A positive test is indicated by reproduction of pain in the proximal forearm.

Ulnar Nerve

The ulnar nerve may be injured by trauma or primary neurological disease, but the most common cause for dysfunction is compression either in the cubital tunnel behind the medial epicondyle (cubital tunnel syndrome) or compression in Guyon's canal at the wrist.

Detailed knowledge of the anatomy and a structured examination can identify the level of pathology along the course of the nerve (Figure 6.12).

Classically, examination is aiming to identify whether there is a 'high' or 'low' lesion of the ulnar nerve. In a high, or proximal, lesion, the extrinsic and intrinsic muscles are affected. In a low, or distal, lesion, only the intrinsic muscles are involved.

The last muscles to be innervated by the ulnar nerve via its deep branch are the first dorsal interosseus and the adductor pollicis muscles. Hence these are the last muscles to recover following an ulnar nerve lesion.

Potential Sites of Injury/Compression

Around the Elbow

Compression around the elbow can be caused by the following structures:

- *The arcade of Struthers:* a fascial band extending from the medial intermuscular septum to the medial head of triceps

Table 6.6 Radial nerve

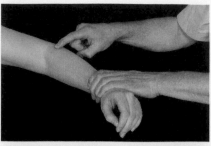

BR –Visualised and palpated by asking the patient to flex the elbow against resistance when held at 90°.

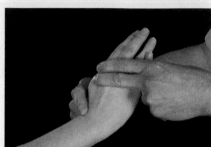

ECRL – The patient is asked to extend and radially deviate their wrist against resistance.

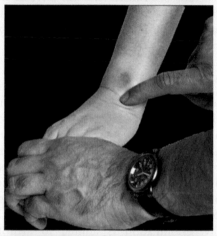

ECU – The patient is asked to extend and ulnar deviate the wrist against resistance.

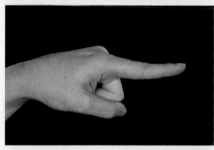

EIP – The patient is asked to flex the ulnar three fingers and point with the index finger.

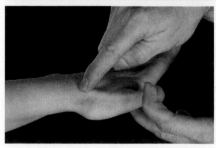

EPL – The patient is asked to place the hand palm down on the table and then lift the thumb, called retropulsion of the thumb. Palpate the EPL.

BR, brachioradialis; ECRL, extensor carpi radialis longus, ECU, extensor carpi ulnaris; EIP, extensor indicis proprius; EPL, extensor pollicis longus

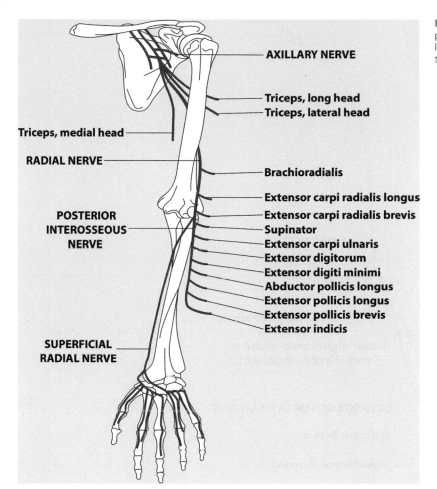

AXILLARY NERVE

Triceps, long head
Triceps, lateral head

Triceps, medial head

RADIAL NERVE

POSTERIOR INTEROSSEOUS NERVE

Brachioradialis

Extensor carpi radialis longus
Extensor carpi radialis brevis
Supinator
Extensor carpi ulnaris
Extensor digitorum
Extensor digiti minimi
Abductor pollicis longus
Extensor pollicis longus
Extensor pollicis brevis
Extensor indicis

SUPERFICIAL RADIAL NERVE

Figure 6.11 Radial nerve with its posterior interosseous branch showing the locations of their respective branches and the muscles they supply.

- The medial intermuscular septum itself
- Exostoses or osteophytes of the medial epicondyle
- The cubital tunnel and Osborne's ligament: a fascial band bridging the two heads of FCU muscle
- Anconeus epitrochlearis: an accessory muscle

At the Wrist

Compression at the wrist is in Guyon's canal. Here the ulnar nerve passes between the transverse carpal ligament and the volar carpal ligament before passing around the hook of hamate.

Examination Routine for the Ulnar Nerve

Inspection (Look)

The appearance of a hand with severe ulnar nerve pathology is usually easy to identify from the combination of muscle wasting and finger posture. The **rectangle palm sign** has been described, showing that the normal square palm shape becomes rectangular with severe wasting of the hypothenar eminence and first dorsal interosseous muscle.[11] Proximal dysfunction can cause wasting of the volar ulnar side of the forearm – FCU and FDP. Sometimes the wasting of the interossei (guttering), the hypothenar eminence and the first dorsal interosseous can be subtle (Figure 6.13). Screening with the shoulders and elbows flexed 90° may reveal the wasting of the hypothenar eminence. However, further inspection with elevation of the elbows is required to fully inspect the posterior aspect of the elbow for the scars of cubital tunnel decompression (Figure 6.14).

Wartenberg's sign (1930), or 'little finger escape sign', is considered one of the earliest signs. In this the little finger adopts an abducted posture – due to weakness of the third palmar interosseous muscle, and its

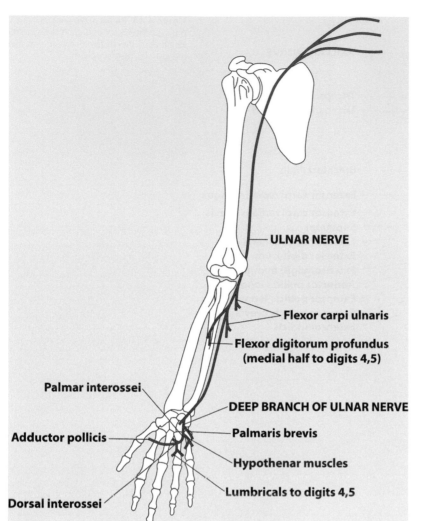

Figure 6.12 Ulnar nerve anatomy showing the location of the branches and the muscles they supply.

ULNAR NERVE

Flexor carpi ulnaris

Flexor digitorum profundus (medial half to digits 4,5)

Palmar interossei

DEEP BRANCH OF ULNAR NERVE

Adductor pollicis

Palmaris brevis

Hypothenar muscles

Lumbricals to digits 4,5

Dorsal interossei

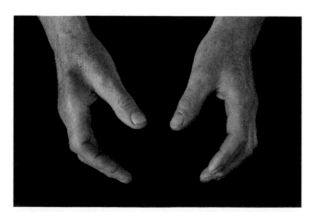

Figure 6.13 Ulnar nerve palsy resulting in gross wasting of the first dorsal interosseous muscle of this patient's right hand.

function being overpowered by the extensor digiti minimi (EDM), which is PIN-innervated (Figure 6.15).

'Clawing' of the fingers or 'benediction hand' (Duchenne's sign, which was first described in 1867) is a classic feature of ulnar nerve dysfunction. It is important to identify hyperextension at the MCP joint in association with flexion at the PIP joint – the opposite of lumbrical function. The index and middle fingers are less affected, as the median nerve innervates the first two lumbricals.

Unlike any other peripheral nerve lesions, the claw deformity is exaggerated with more distal ulnar nerve lesions, as FDP to the little and ring fingers (which are partly responsible for the clawing) are innervated in the proximal forearm. This is called the 'ulnar

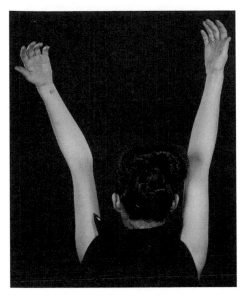

Figure 6.14 When inspecting it is useful to ask the patient to lift the arms so that the elbows can be inspected for scars. In this case, there is suggestion of a significant cubitus valgus.

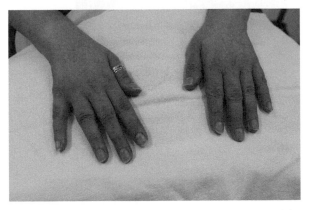

Figure 6.15 Wartenberg's sign. Note the abducted position of the little finger due to weakness of the third palmar interosseous muscle. The extensor digiti minimi (EDM) pulls the finger into an extended position.

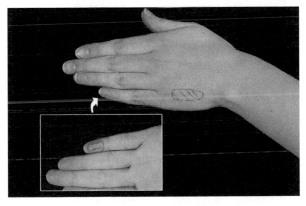

Figure 6.16 Areas to test for ulnar nerve sensation. In low lesions, the sensation on the dorsal surface of the fifth metacarpal is preserved.

paradox'. The paradox also manifests after a high ulnar nerve injury. In this instance, the claw deformity initially worsens as the nerve recovers and starts to reinnervate the FDP.

Feel

Sensation: Sensory testing can differentiate between a 'high' and a 'low' ulnar nerve lesion. The ulnar nerve gives off a sensory branch 5 cm proximal to the wrist, whose cutaneous territory is over the dorsum of the fifth metacarpal (Figure 6.16). If sensation is altered here, it suggests that the pathology is more proximal, usually at the cubital tunnel. In this case, sensation at the tip of the little finger is also altered. If sensation is intact over the dorsum of the fifth metacarpal, but altered in the tip of the little finger, the pathology is most likely to be in Guyon's canal (a low lesion).

Palpation: Tenderness may be elicited over either the cubital tunnel or Guyon's canal. The former should be differentiated from medial epicondylitis, which can coexist.

Motor Testing (Move)

Table 6.7 presents ulnar nerve motor testing. The only muscles supplied by the ulnar nerve in the forearm are FCU and FDP to the little and ring fingers. These will be intact with a low lesion and can be tested by resisted wrist flexion, palpating the tendon of FCU, followed by resisted flexion of the distal interphalangeal (DIP) joint of the little finger. Inability to flex the DIP joint of the little and ring finger was described by Pollock in 1919. The same information can be gained by asking a patient to make a fist and observe whether they are able to tuck the little finger into the palm.

There are numerous ways of testing the intrinsic muscles of the hand innervated by the ulnar nerve. Simply crossing the fingers (middle over index) is an easy test and very useful in children. Alternatively, asking the patient to press their abducted little fingers together can easily demonstrate unilateral weakness of the hypothenar eminence. Rarely, only the deep

103

Table 6.7 Ulnar nerve

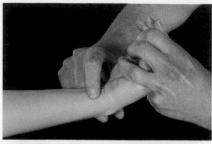

FCU – The patient is asked to flex the wrist against resistance; the tension in the tendon of FCU can be seen and palpated.

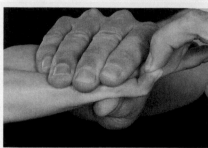

FDP (little finger) – Stabilise the patient's little finger PIPJ in extension and feel for active flexion of the DIPJ against resistance.

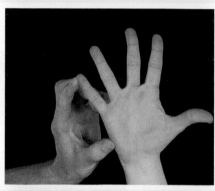

ADM – Ask the patient to hold their hands with palms facing their face and spread open their fingers. Push the little finger towards the ring finger. Weakness results in the inability of the little finger to maintain its position.

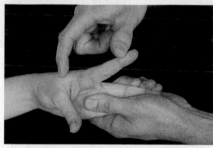

First dorsal interosseous – Hold the patient's hand with the index finger uppermost. Ask them to lift the finger (abduct), then resist your pressure as you span the finger with your other hand as you palpate the muscle belly.

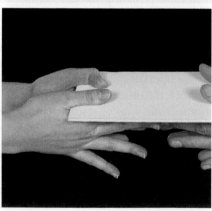

Froment's test – The patient is asked to grasp a piece of paper in the first web space, between their extended thumb and extended fingers. Normally, the first dorsal interosseous and adductor pollicis would be able to resist the examiner pulling the paper out and the thumb would remain extended. However, if the ulna nerve is deficient, the patient will recruit the AIN innervated FPL to grasp the paper and the thumb IP joint will flex.

FCU, flexor carpi ulnaris; FDP, flexor digitorum profundus; ADM, abductor digiti minimi branch of the ulnar nerve is compromised, and in this situation the hypothenar muscles are spared but the rest of the intrinsic muscles are affected. The first dorsal interosseous can be tested for power and the muscle belly palpated by holding the patient's hand, asking them to abduct their index finger; resist the movement with your middle finger and palpate the muscle with your thumb.

Provocation Tests

Forced flexion of the elbow can increase pressure in the cubital tunnel and cause sensory disturbance in the ulnar nerve distribution. Tinel's test with percussion of the ulnar nerve over the cubital tunnel and over Guyon's canal can be helpful; however, in many 'normal' subjects, percussion over the ulnar nerve at the elbow can cause sensory disturbance into the little and ring fingers – the 'funny bone'!

The classical test for the ulnar nerve was described by **Froment** (1915). The patient is asked to grasp a piece of paper in the first web space, between their extended thumb and extended fingers. Normally, the first dorsal interosseous and adductor pollicis would be able to resist the examiner pulling the paper out and the thumb would remain extended. However, if the ulnar nerve is deficient, the patient will recruit the AIN innervated FPL to grasp the paper and the thumb IP joint will flex (Figure 6.17).

Martin–Gruber Anastomosis

Contrary to popular teaching, the innervation pattern in the hand and forearm is not sacrosanct. Crossover of nerve fibres between the three major nerves in the upper limb is possible. The most common exchange of fibres is between the median and ulnar nerves in the forearm. This is called the Martin–Gruber anastomosis.[12] It is believed to be present in 15–20% of individuals. In this, motor fibres from the median nerve cross over to the ulnar nerve in the proximal forearm. Clinically, this becomes significant, as normal intrinsic muscle function may exist in spite of the ulnar nerve being injured above the level of the anastomosis.

A similar sharing of sensory fibres in the hand can exist between these two nerves. This is due to the *Riche–Cannieu anastomosis*.

Other Peripheral Nerves

The other terminal nerves of the brachial plexus that supply the upper limb are the axillary nerve and the musculocutaneous nerve.

Axillary Nerve

This nerve supplies the deltoid muscle as well as teres minor. It is vulnerable following anterior dislocation of the shoulder (although one should not miss a more widespread infraclavicular plexopathy, although it is

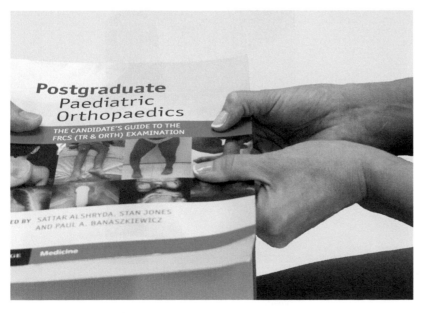

Figure 6.17 Froment's test. The patient is asked to grasp a piece of paper or thin book between extended finger and thumb. Because adductor pollicis (ulnar nerve) is not working, FPL is recruited to perform the task.

often missed in the acute stage). Rarely, compression of the axillary nerve (with its accompanying posterior circumflex humeral artery) can occur in the quadrangular space usually secondary to trauma but occasionally due to a space-occupying lesion or fibrous bands.[13,14]

To assess this nerve, sensation is tested in the region of the deltoid insertion, the 'regimental badge' area. Motor function is mainly by testing the deltoid muscle. Passively abduct the shoulder to 90° and then extend it. Ask the patient to resist as you push downward on the arm. Feel the muscle. This tests the posterior deltoid. The central and anterior fibres of the deltoid can be tested by placing the abducted arm in neutral and flexed positions, respectively (Figure 6.18).

The direction of travel for the nerve is from posterior, as it exits out of the quadrangular space, to anterior. Therefore, in the setting of a neurapraxia of the nerve, one expects the posterior fibres of deltoid to

recover before the anterior and it is useful to follow this during recovery.

Musculocutaneous Nerve

This nerve supplies the biceps brachii, coracobrachialis and the brachialis muscles. It enters the biceps 5–8 cm distal to the coracoid process. It is the most lateral branch of the plexus and runs perilously close to the conjoint tendon and therefore is vulnerable during any operation using the standard deltopectoral approach to the shoulder. Like the axillary nerve, it can be involved in an infraclavicular plexopathy following anterior dislocation of the shoulder.

Testing the biceps is sufficient to assess the motor function of this nerve. The supinated forearm is placed in 90° of elbow flexion. Further active flexion is resisted by the examiner and the strength of the biceps assessed. To test supination, the forearm is

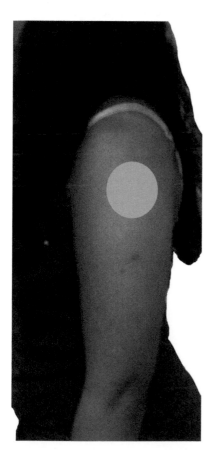

Figure 6.18 Test deltoid for the axillary nerve. The 'regimental badge' area is marked out.

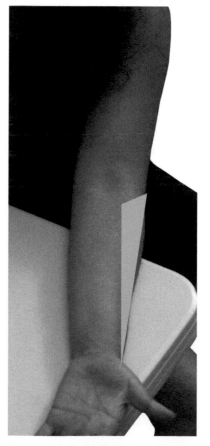

Figure 6.19 Testing the musculocutaneous nerve. Test biceps flexion and supination strength as well as sensation of the lateral forearm

pronated with the elbows flexed to 90° and held firmly at the sides. Active supination is then resisted by the examiner. The musculocutaneous nerve continues as the lateral cutaneous nerve of the forearm. Therefore, sensation can be tested along the lateral aspect of the forearm (Figure 6.19).

Thoracic Outlet Syndrome

Neurogenic thoracic outlet syndrome (nTOS) is by far the most common of the thoracic outlet syndromes (95% of cases). Five per cent are vascular, with venous compression being more common than arterial. Symptoms are elicited due to compression of the brachial plexus as it passes through the posterior triangle of the neck and the subcoracoid space (Figure 6.20).[15]

Causes can be secondary to trauma, anatomy or functional overuse. With regard to anatomy, there are bony or soft tissue structures that can cause compression. This is most commonly in conjunction with repetitive overuse. Bony structures include: a cervical rib (from C7 vertebra), large transverse process of C7, first rib, corocoid process and clavicle. Soft tissue structures include: scalenus anterior and medius, pectoralis minor or aberrant scalene musculature or connective tissue.

Symptoms are typically reproducible, most notably when performing overhead activities. The most common compression is of the lower plexus (C8, T1) and patients present with paraesthesia along the inner aspect of the arm and into the little and ring fingers.[15]

Potential Sites of Compression

- Within the 'interscalene triangle' bordered by the scalenus anterior, the scalenus medius and the first rib inferiorly.
- In the 'costoclavicular space' bordered by the subclavius muscle anteriorly, the first rib and scalenus anterior muscle inferoposteriorly and the clavicle superiorly.
- In the 'subcoracoid space' bordered by the pectoralis minor anteriorly, ribs two–four posteriorly and the coracoid superiorly.

Examination

A thorough examination of C5–T1 is required.

Inspection: Look for any gross muscle wasting as well as more subtle signs of differences in colour compared to the contralateral arm. There may be a fullness in the supraclavicular fossa and look for the

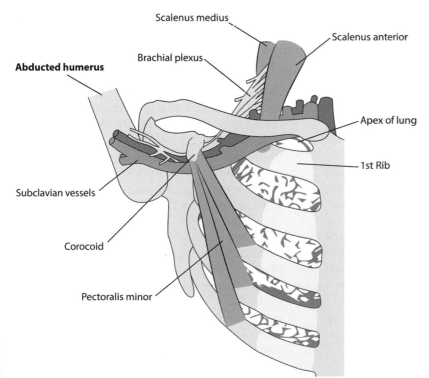

Figure 6.20 Anatomy of the thoracic outlet. Note the scalene muscles, clavicle, first rib, corocoid, pectoralis minor and the position of the arm as potential sources of symptoms in thoracic outlet syndrome. Wright's hyperabduction test is demonstrated by the position of the arm.

Scalenus medius

Scalenus anterior

Brachial plexus

Abducted humerus

Apex of lung

1st Rib

Subclavian vessels

Corocoid

Pectoralis minor

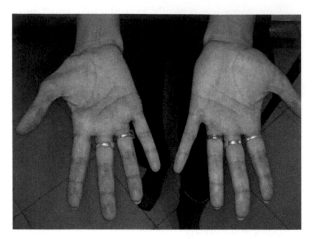

Figure 6.21 Gilliatt–Sumner hand (patient's right hand). Note the wasting of the intrinsic muscles but especially abductor pollicis brevis.

Gilliatt–Sumner hand (wasting of all of the intrinsic musculature of the hand, but particularly marked for APB) (Figure 6.21).

Sensation: Sensation is tested in a dermatomal distribution (Figure 6.1). Typically, there is an alteration in sensation in the C8/T1 distribution (note this differs from the high ulnar nerve lesion in that it also includes the medial forearm). Make a note of any differences in temperature between the two arms.

Palpation: Palpate for a cervical rib in the supraclavicular fossa and for alteration in the strength of the radial pulse both in the normal and elevated position of the arm.

Motor: Test for motor power looking for weakness in a cervical root distribution (see Chapter 7, Figure 7.11) Weakness tends to be confined to the T1 distribution with weakness of *all* the intrinsic musculature of the hand (this differentiates from either a median or an ulnar neuropathy).

Provocation tests: A number of tests have been described. They are all based on impingement of the nerves and/or vessels as they pass through the thoracic outlet. The following describe the most commonly used. Broadly speaking, Adson's manoeuvre assesses the vascular component of a thoracic outlet syndrome and Roos test assesses the neurological component:[16]

1. **Adson's test**. Evaluates the 'interscalene space' as described above. The affected arm is abducted to 20° at the shoulder while maximally extended. While extending the neck and turning head towards ipsilateral shoulder, the patient inhales

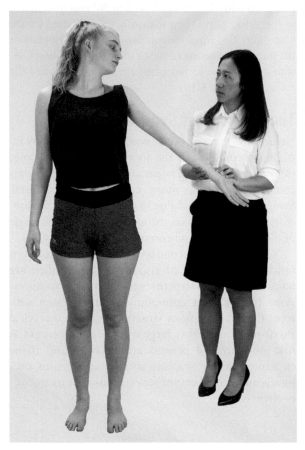

Figure 6.22 Adson's test. The radial pulse reduces with deep inspiration.

deeply (and therefore inflates the lungs), causing a reduction or elimination of the ipsilateral radial pulse (Figure 6.22).[17]

2. **Roos test** (elevated arm stress test). Evaluates the entire thoracic outlet. In this test the arms are placed in the surrender position with shoulders abducted to 90° and in external rotation, with elbows flexed to 90°. The patient slowly opens and closes hand for 3 minutes precipitating pain, paraesthesia and heaviness in ipsilateral arm (Figure 6.23).[18]

3. **Elevated arm pulse oximetry test.** This is similar to the Roos test except that the patient wears a pulse oximeter on the thumb of the affected limb. The patient is asked to repeatedly open and close their hand for 3 minutes or until the discomfort becomes too severe to carry on. A positive test occurs when oxygen saturation

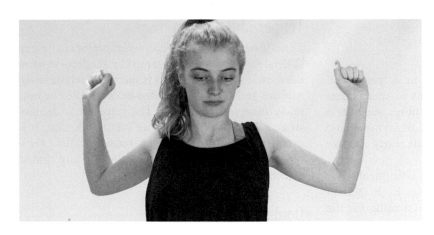

Figure 6.23. Roos test. Tingling in the fingers on opening and closing the fist suggests the diagnosis.

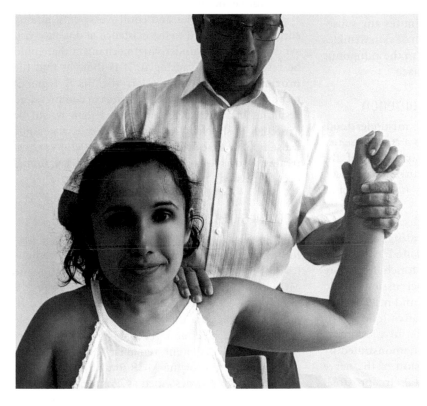

Figure 6.24 Wright's test. The shoulder is externally rotated and hyperabducted. In a positive test, there is a reduction of the pulse.

drops below 87% for a sustained period of time.[19]

4. A combination of the Adson's and the Roos test increases the specificity to 82% when both are positive.[20]

5. **Wright's test** (hyperabduction test). Evaluates the 'subcoracoid space' as described above, as the pectoralis minor contracts and reduces the space. In this test, the examiner externally rotates the shoulder and maximally abducts it whilst palpating the radial pulse. A reduction in the pulse will indicate a positive result (Figures 6.24 and 6.20). Note up to 7% of a normal population will have a positive result.

Advanced Corner

Autonomic Nerves

Sympathetic unmyelinated fibres in a peripheral nerve are among the most resistant to mechanical trauma. As such, damage to these fibres suggests a more severe injury. Disturbance of sympathetic function is therefore an important early feature of nerve damage.

Testing autonomic function can be difficult, and several methods are in common use. Each method relies on either directly or indirectly testing for the presence of sweat.[21]

Ballpoint test: This relies on the loss of tactile adherence in an anhydrotic area when a ballpoint pen is lightly drawn across the skin.

Skin wrinkle test: By wrapping the traumatised digit in a wet swab, within a few minutes any subsequent examination of the distribution of skin wrinkles will show whether any serious injury to the autonomic (and hence other) fibres has taken place.

Tinel's Sign and Valleix Phenomenon

The Tinel's sign is commonly misunderstood. Described by Jules Tinel (1915), it is a *tingling sensation* referred to the *cutaneous* distribution of the nerve, similar to that of an electric current, produced by slight percussion of a nerve trunk. It should not be painful.

It is thought to be a result of the decrease in action potential threshold of the regenerating nerve and therefore of good prognosis. It is elicited by stimulation of nerve branches in which touch fibres are regenerating. The intensity of the percussion should be just enough to generate the 'pins and needles'.

It is pathognomic of a degenerative lesion. It is useful not only in identifying a degenerative lesion but also to follow any regeneration, as demonstrated by the **advancing Tinel's sign**. Percussion of the nerve trunk should move from a distal to proximal direction.[22]

On light percussion, *retrograde radiation of pain* from a distal nerve compression neuropathy is called the **Valleix phenomenon**. This should not be confused with the Tinel's sign. A *Valliex point* is any tender area along the course of the nerve that is mainly seen at the points where the nerve emerges from a bony canal or pierces a muscle or aponeurosis.

Tender Muscle Sign

The reinnervation of nociceptive receptors in human skeletal muscle results in cramp-like tenderness when the muscle is squeezed. This is specific to reinnervated muscles and cannot be elicited in denervated or normally innervated muscles. The response is demonstrated before any recovery of motor function. It is useful in monitoring motor recovery after nerve regeneration, as it can be present before any clinical evidence of motor recovery.[4]

Double Crush

Symptoms resulting from two or more sites of compression along a peripheral nerve is called a 'double crush' syndrome, e.g. a cervical radiculopathy and a carpal tunnel or cubital compression.

Numerous theories and controversy exist among surgeons with regard to the existence of double crush syndrome and the underlying mechanism that could be responsible for causing it. It is thought that the proximal compression renders the distal segment more prone to injury by a second area of compression, resulting in more severe symptoms than would be expected. It should also be recognised as a possible cause for failure of relief of symptoms after surgical treatment of one area (e.g. failure of carpal tunnel decompression).[23]

Bouvier's Test

With an ulnar claw hand, Bouvier's test can be performed. It tests the integrity of the extensor mechanics over the digits. It involves passively correcting the MCP joint hyperextension. If the patient's flexed PIP joint posture improves and there is improved PIP joint extension then the clawing is defined as simple (PIP joint capsule and mechanism working normally). If the PIP joint remains flexed even after passive correction of the MCP joint hyperextension then the clawing is described as complex (with attrition of central slip, adherent central slip at the PIP joint or volar subluxation of the lateral bands).[24]

This test helps in the decision-making for surgery for claw correction. It guides whether a procedure to prevent hyperextension at the MCP joint would be sufficient or more extensive procedures such as augmentation of the extensor apparatus or joint contracture surgery is needed.

References

1. Kaplan SJ, Glickel SZ, Eaton RG. Predictive factors in the non-surgical treatment of carpal tunnel syndrome. *J Hand Surg Br* 1990;**15**:106–108.

2. Reynolds EH. The neurology of folic acid deficiency. *Handb Clin Neurol* 2014;**120**:927–943.

3. Birch R, Bonney G, Wynn-Parry CB (eds). *Surgical Disorders of the Peripheral Nerves.* Edinburgh: Churchill Livingstone, 1998.

4. Lee EY, Karjalainen TV, Sebastin SJ, Lim AYT. The value of the tender muscle sign in detecting motor recovery after peripheral nerve reconstruction. *J Hand Surg Am* 2015;**40**(3):433e437.

5. Kiloh LG, Nevin S. Isolated neuritis of the anterior interosseous nerve. *Br Med J* 1952;**1**(4763):850–851.

6. Paley D, McMurtry RY. Median nerve compression test in carpal tunnel syndrome diagnosis reproduces signs and symptoms in affected wrist. *Orthop Rev* 1985;**14**:411.

7. Durkan JA. A new diagnostic test for carpal tunnel syndrome. *J Bone Joint Surg Am* 1991;**73**:535–538.

8. Gilliat RW, Wilson TG. A pneumatic-tourniquet test in the carpal-tunnel syndrome. *Lancet* 1953;**265** (6786):595–597.

9. Sarhadi NS, Korday SN, Bainbridge LC. Radial tunnel syndrome: diagnosis and management. *J Hand Surg Br* 1998;**23**:617–619.

10. Dellon AL, Mackinnon SE. Radial sensory nerve entrapment in the forearm. *J Hand Surg Am* 1986;**11**:199–205.

11. Lloyd N, Sammut D. The rectangular palm sign in ulnar nerve paralysis. *Eur J Plastic Surg* 2012;**35** (7):569–570.

12. Leibovic SJ, Hastings H. Martin–Gruber revisited. *J Hand Surg Am* 1992;**17**:47–53.

13. Cahill BR, Palmer RE. Quadrilateral space syndrome. *J Hand Surg Am* 1983;**8**, 65–69.

14. Hangge PT, Breen I, Albadawi H, et al. Quadrilateral space syndrome: diagnosis and clinical management. *J Clin Med* 2018 Apr 21;7(4):pii:E86.

15. Jones MR, Prabhakar A, Viswanath O, et al. Thoracic outlet syndrome: a comprehensive review of pathophysiology, diagnosis, and treatment. *Pain Ther* 2019;**8**:5–18.

16. Povlsen S, Povlsen B. Diagnosing thoracic outlet syndrome: current approaches and future directions. *Diagnostics (Basel)* 2018 Mar 20;**8**(1):21.

17. Adson AW, Coffey JR. Cervical rib: a method of anterior approach for relief of symptoms by division of the scalenus anticus. *Ann Surg* 1927;**85**:839–857.

18. Roos DB. Transaxillary approach for first rib resection to relieve thoracic outlet syndrome. *Ann Surg* 1966;**163**:354–358.

19. Braun RM, Rechnic M, Shah KN. Pulse oximetry measurements in the evaluation of patients with possible thoracic outlet syndrome. *J Hand Surg Am* 2012 Dec;**37**(12):2564–2569.

20. Gillard J, Pe´rez-Cousin M, Hachulla E, et al. Diagnosing thoracic outlet syndrome: contribution of provocative tests, ultrasonography, electrophysiology, and helical computed tomography in 48 patients. *Joint Bone Spine* 2001;**68**(5):416–424.

21. Phelps PE, Walker E. Comparison of the finger wrinkling test results to established sensory tests in peripheral nerve injury. *Am J Occup Ther* 1977 Oct;**31** (9):565–572.

22. Moldaver J. Tinel's sign. Its characteristics and significance. *J Bone Joint Surg Am* 1978;**60**(3):412–414.

23. Kane PM, Daniels AH, Akelman E. Double crush syndrome. *J Am Acad Orthop Surg* 2015 Sep;**23** (9):558–562.

24. Bouvier Note sur une paralysie partielle des muscles de la main. Bull Acad Nat Med (Paris) 1851;18:125.

Examination of the Adult Spine

Chapter

7

Antonia Isaacson, James Tomlinson and Neil Chiverton

Assessment of the Lumbar Spine

A. History

B. Clinical Examination

Step1

Stand the patient and look

Step 2

Feel

Step 3

Move

Step 4

Screen tests – squat and then get up (L3), stand on heel(L4), tiptoe (S1), one leg (L5)

Step 5

Walk

Step 6

Lie patient down and complete neurological examination

Tone, sensation, power, reflexes

- Provocation tests – straight leg raise (SLR), cross sciatic stretch, bowstring, Lasègue's, femoral stretch
- Perianal sensation and rectal examination (PR) (if indicated)

Stand and Look

Clinical examination of the lumbar spine starts with standing the patient and looking from the back, assessing any curves, scars and any other stigmata of spinal disease such as café-au-lait spots or spinal dysraphism. Look from the side for lumbar lordosis, thoracic kyphosis and cervical lordosis. Then look from the front.

Feel

Palpate down the bony prominences and paraspinal area of the spinal column.

Move

Movements are forward flexion (assessed qualitatively by fingers to knees, ankles, etc., or quantitatively by Schober's test), lateral flexion, extension and rotation. Forward flexion is probably the most useful clinically, with lateral flexion and rotation rarely adding much information. Rotation is performed by fixing the pelvis (by holding it securely) or by asking the patient to sit and rotate.

Screen Tests

Before walking the patient, perform a quick screen for the lower lumbar nerve roots by asking the patient to squat and get up (L3), to walk on heels (L4), to stand on one leg (Trendelenburg test (L5)) and to walk on tiptoes (S1).

Walk

Ask the patient to walk, assessing the gait and looking for any neurological pattern of gait.

Lie Patient Down: Neurological Examination

A complete neurological examination is performed, including sensation, tone, power and reflexes.

- Tone – Passively roll the hips into internal and external rotation.
- Sensation – Remember that sensation around the kn*ee* is L3 (thr*ee*)
- With regard to the myotomes (American Spinal Injury Association (ASIA) system), an easy way to remember the nerve root level for the movements is that all the movements on the anterior aspect of the lower limb are in sequence – hip flexion L2, knee extension L3, ankle dorsiflexion L4, big toe extension L5.
- In addition, all the movements on the posterior aspect of the lower limb are essentially S1, i.e. hip extension, knee flexion, ankle plantar flexion and big toe flexion.
- Lower limb reflexes – knee jerk L3/4 (hamstring jerk L5), ankle jerk S1.

Provocation Tests

For the lumbar spine: sciatic stretch test, Lasègue's test, bowstring test, cross sciatic stretch test, femoral stretch test.

Assessment of the Cervical Spine

The process is similar to a lumbar spine examination.

A. History
B. Clinical Examination

Step1

Sit/Stand the patient and look

Step 2

Feel

Step 3

Move

Step 4

Screen tests – Romberg's test

Step 5

Walk

Step 6

Lie patient down and complete neurological examination. **Upper and Lower limb**

Tone, sensation, power, reflexes

• Tests for cervical myelopathy – Hoffman's test, inverted radial reflex
• Provocation tests – Spurling's, L'hermitte's
• Perianal sensation and PR (as indicated)

Stand and Look

Clinical examination of the cervical spine starts with sitting the patient and looking from the back, assessing for scars and any other stigmata of spinal disease such as café-au-lait spots or low hairline. Look from the side at the cervical lordosis, thoracic kyphosis and lumbar spine lordosis. Look from the front.

Feel

Palpate down the bony prominences and paraspinal area of the spinal column.

Move

Movements are forward flexion, lateral flexion, extension and rotation.

Screen Tests

Before walking the patient, do a screen by performing Romberg's test.

Walk

Then ask the patient to walk, assessing the gait and looking for any neurological pattern of gait, e.g. seen with cervical myelopathy.

Neurological Examination

Neurological examination should include both the upper and lower limbs (for cervical myelopathy).

• Tone, sensation, power, reflexes
• Sensation – Remember middle finger is C7 and work around that
• Myotomes (ASIA system): Elbow flexion C5; elbow extension C7; wrist extension C6; finger flexion C8; finger abduction, especially little (spread the fingers) T1
• Reflexes: Biceps jerk (C5), brachioradialis reflex (C6), triceps jerk (C7)
• For upper motor neuron lesions, e.g. cervical myelopathy, include Hoffman's test, inverted radial reflex

Provocation Tests

Provocation tests include Spurling's test for radicular pain and L'hermitte's manoeuvre for cervical myelopathy.

History

General

Most adult patients with problems of a spinal origin present with complaints of pain in the back and/or limbs. Commonly, lower back pain is associated with leg pain and neck pain is associated with arm pain. Both can be associated with a resultant loss of function.

It is therefore as important to understand and record the impact of the perceived pain on the patient's daily work, activities of daily living and recreational activities as it is to enquire about the nature of the pain itself.

One should begin with the patient's occupation, social circumstances and sporting activities. Then enquire about the limitations on all these aspects of daily living with particular reference to days taken off work, periods of relative immobility and problems coping with household duties. Specific disability scoring systems[1,2,3] can be used if wished. The patient's age should always be used to help steer thoughts towards a likely diagnosis. Be careful not to reach a diagnosis of new onset mechanical back pain in patients outside the age range of 20–55 years without appropriate investigation, particularly in the presence of non-mechanical or other atypical symptoms.

With regard to **pain**, its site, radiation, any precipitating or relieving factors (e.g. posture, cough/sneeze, physical activity), causation, duration and any pain-free intervals should be documented. It is essential to distinguish between back pain and leg pain. Grade these on a scale of 0–10 and determine which troubles the patient more.

It is essential to enquire directly about **bowel or bladder dysfunction**. A useful catch-all question is to ask whether the patient has experienced any recent change in bladder or bowel function, and then ask more detailed questions if indicated. More detailed questions should include whether the patient has the urge to urinate, if they can feel urine passing, if they are aware when they have finished urinating and if it feels numb when wiping. It is also important to ask about episodes of incontinence and sexual dysfunction.

Additionally, it is important to take note of whether the patient considers their back problem to be work related and whether any legal proceedings are pending, as this has been shown to have a negative impact on recovery.[4,5,6]

The requirements for analgesics and their effectiveness are a useful guide for the clinician as to the degree of pain perceived by the patient. Also ask about any previous episodes of back pain and treatments received such as physiotherapy or chiropractic therapy, and what treatment they have offered.

Specific Pathologies and Their Related Symptoms

Degenerative Disease of the Cervical Spine

Pain in the neck may be a symptom of cervical spondylosis. Other causes of referred pain to the neck such as shoulder girdle pathology and cervical soft tissue tumours should be considered. Neck stiffness is often reported. Patients may also present with dual pathology (i.e. shoulder and cervical spine pathology).

In advanced cases of spondylosis, patients can present with symptoms of compressive cervical myelopathy, cervical radiculopathy or a mixture of both.

Myelopathy usually presents with the initial loss of fine hand function that may be reported as clumsiness,

e.g. dropping a mug, difficulty picking up change, doing up buttons and a change in handwriting, combined with some unsteadiness of gait. They may report tripping yet being unable to explain why. This is often more noticeable in poor lighting, e.g. when going to the bathroom at night. A patient may also describe furniture surfing; walking around their home holding on to furniture for balance. Patients will commonly report an episodic rather than a gradual deterioration.

A thorough history will be required if metabolic, rheumatological and primary neurological disorders are not to be overlooked as potential causes of these symptoms.

Acute cervical disc protrusion may cause myelopathic symptoms, but more typically will present with neck and arm pain (brachialgia), the latter resulting from cervical nerve root compression that is the most troublesome to the patient. It is usually described as a burning/toothache type pain. Sensory disturbance is frequently associated. The site of the upper limb pain varies according to the disc level involved. The most common are the C5/6 and C6/7 disc levels affecting the C6 and C7 nerve roots, respectively. Root compression from C6 gives rise to pain and paraesthesiae along the radial aspect of the forearm and into the radial two digits. The pain from C7 root compression gives rise to pain which is typically described as being deep within the forearm and sensory disturbance affecting the middle finger. differential diagnosis based on these symptoms will include peripheral nerve entrapment syndromes, thoracic outlet syndrome, tumours abutting the brachial plexus, idiopathic brachial neuritis and spinal tumours.

A painless but progressive flexion deformity (loss of lordosis) of the cervical spine progressing from a limitation of the forward field of view to difficulty with jaw opening characterises the cervical spinal manifestations of ankylosing spondylitis.

Degenerative Disease of the Lumbar Spine

A history of low back pain proportional to activity level with periods of exacerbation lasting 2–6 weeks and with radiation into the gluteal and thigh regions only is indicative of referred pain from degenerative lower lumbar motion segments. Any associated pain or sensory disturbance in the lower leg or foot suggests the coexistence of a compressive radiculopathy. If the cause of this is an acute intervertebral disc protrusion, the leg pain tends to be severe, unilateral and exacerbated by posture.

Any reported perianal or genital sensory disturbance or bowel or bladder disturbance necessitates urgent further investigation, with a definitive diagnosis only being possible with magnetic resonance imaging (MRI) scanning (or computed tomography (CT) +/− myelography if MRI scanning is contraindicated).

Neurogenic bladder dysfunction culminates in painless overflow incontinence.[7] Symptoms of prostatic hypertrophy in men and stress or urge incontinence in women are not consistent with a cauda equina syndrome, and careful differentiation is essential before urgent investigations are requested unnecessarily.

Back pain with leg pain after a certain length of time, walking or standing is suggestive of **spinal claudication**. Leg symptoms are commonly bilateral (but not a red flag symptom in this scenario), and the reported distribution is less specific than isolated nerve root compression.

Patients with spinal claudication will frequently report improvement in symptoms when sitting and leaning on a walking stick or shopping trolley or when walking uphill as these flexed postures increase spinal canal diameter. Complete relief is achieved by sitting for several minutes. In the more severe cases rest and night symptoms are present and neurogenic bladder dysfunction can occur.

The differential diagnosis of vascular claudication can be difficult to exclude on history alone, but this condition is usually relieved by stopping walking without sitting, and symptoms resolve more rapidly. The walking distance required to induce symptoms is said to be more consistent and symptoms are often described as starting distally before becoming more proximal.

Other differential diagnoses include diabetic or alcoholic peripheral neuropathy and spinal tumours. A combination of radicular and stenotic symptoms as outlined above should raise the possibility of degenerative lumbar spondylolisthesis in which both spinal canal compromise and nerve root entrapment result from the forward slip of one complete vertebra on another.

Degenerative Disease of the Thoracic Spine

Pathology involving the thoracic spine is rare, with only 0.5% of all disc protrusions occurring in this region. However, they should be considered in anyone complaining of interscapular back pain. The pain has the same nature and precipitating factors as are found in equivalent conditions of the lumbar spine. Radicular symptoms are felt around the chest wall in the distribution of the corresponding intercostal nerve. Patients may develop lower limb myelopathic symptoms and report an unsteady gait. In late stages bladder and bowel function may also be affected.

Differential diagnoses include herpes zoster, mediastinal or abdominal pathology and, as always, spinal tumours.

Examination

Inspection (Look)

Examination of any localised spinal disorder requires inspection of the entire spine. All patients must undress to their underwear for this to be possible (Figure 7.1a). The patient should be offered a gown and a chaperone.

The usual format for inspection should be followed, first noting any obvious swellings or surgical scars. The erect spinal profile must be assessed for any deformity in the coronal and sagittal planes. Scoliosis will be the result of either a previous congenital or developmental deformity, or degenerative disease of later onset, or both (Figure 7.1b).

An **'Adams forward bend test'** may reveal the presence of a rib prominence (never use the term 'hump') due to spine rotation, and thus a structural curve.[8] Kyphosis in the region of the cervicothoracic junction is typically seen with ankylosing spondylitis, whereas in the thoracic region it is more likely to represent either previous Scheuermann's disease or multiple osteoporotic wedge fractures.

Loss of lordosis in the lumbar spine is commonly seen in association with either long-standing degenerative structural changes or acute paravertebral muscle spasm secondary to acute regional pain. Hyperlordosis should raise the suspicion of a high-grade spondylolisthesis, or may be compensatory for a fixed flexion deformity in the hip. A compensatory lumbar hyperlordosis may also be found below a primary thoracic kyphotic deformity. Prominent buttocks, shortened trunk and flexed hips and knees may be seen with severe slips.

One should follow this assessment with a check for leg length, pelvic tilt and shoulder and waist asymmetry. A plumb line can be placed on the C7 spinous process to quantify any coronal imbalance.

Palpation (Feel)

Palpation along the line of the spine over the paravertebral muscles on both sides is very non-specific

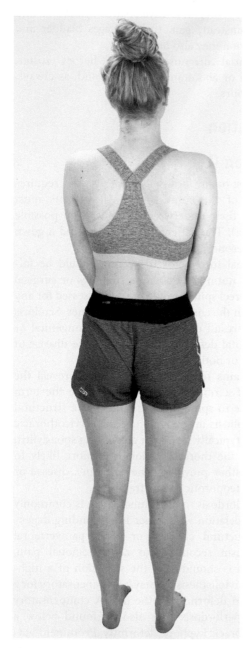

Figure 7.1a Stand patient and inspect the entire spine from the back, sides and front. Look for other stigmata associated with spinal disease.

but helps to localise the level of the spine involved (Figure 7.2). Often a region of tenderness on deep palpation is found. Very localised points of tenderness on deep muscle palpation are suggestive of fibromyalgia.

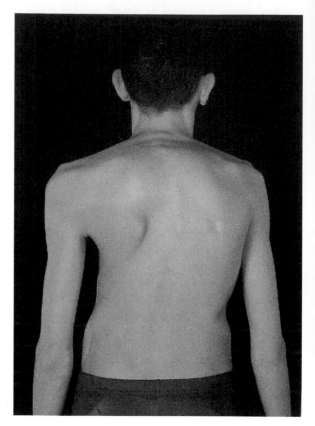

Figure 7.1b Lateral curvature of the spine or scoliosis.

Occasionally one may encounter marked superficial tenderness, or a non-anatomic distribution of tenderness that may be non-organic in nature.[9,10] This is further discussed in the 'Advanced Corner' of this chapter.

Palpation should be completed with an abdominal examination to identify any masses, especially a distended neurogenic bladder and the obligatory PR examination of sensation, anal tone and prostate.

Movement (Move)

All spinal movements are best assessed actively by instructing the patient on the movements required, but some passive movements are useful.

For the cervical spine, movements of flexion, extension, rotation and lateral flexion should be assessed (Figure 7.3). Flexion and extension are mostly affected by spondylosis. A tendency to hold the head to one side with radicular arm pain when the neck is gently passively laterally flexed to the other side suggests a cervical disc prolapse (on the contralateral side to the active lateral flexion).

Normally, only 40% of rotational movement occurs in the subaxial spine so this movement is well preserved in most degenerative disorders. Movement

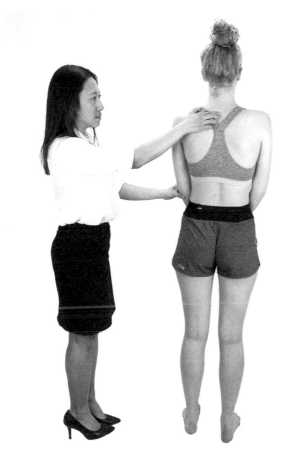

Figure 7.2 Palpate the central bony prominences and the paraspinal areas.

is difficult to quantify numerically, and descriptors are more useful, e.g. flexion chin to chest and look up towards the ceiling.

Facet joint orientation and the splinting effect of the thoracic cage allow for essentially only rotational movement in the thoracic spine. Assessment of this movement is, however, of little diagnostic significance. Conversely, because of the orientation of the facet joints in the lumbar spine, little rotation is possible and flexion/extension movements are examined.

Asking the patient to try and touch their toes allows measurement of forward bending. Record the amount of flexion achieved using anatomical landmarks (e.g. fingers to thigh, knees, midshin, toes). One should ensure by inspection that the movement is achieved by flexion of the lumbar spine and not the hips only.

Schober's test[11,12,13] can be used to provide a more quantitative evaluation of lumbar spine flexion. Mark a horizontal line at the level of the posterior superior iliac spines (PSISs) and a second at a distance of 10 cm above this. On forward flexion this distance should increase by at least 5 cm (Figures 7.4a and 7.4b).

A modification of this test uses a distal fixed point 5 cm below the PSIS line and the same point 10 cm above.[14] The increase using the modified test should be 6–7 cm.

Limitation of flexion is caused by pain protection or ankylosing spondylitis. The test may also be positive in elderly patients in the absence of pathology.

When testing extension, stand behind the patient while supporting and reassuring them. The limitation here can be more marked than the limitation of flexion in degenerative disease and is said to indicate facet joint arthrosis.

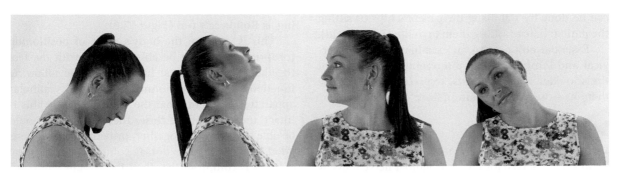

Figure 7.3 Movements of the cervical spine include flexion, extension, rotation and lateral flexion as shown here.

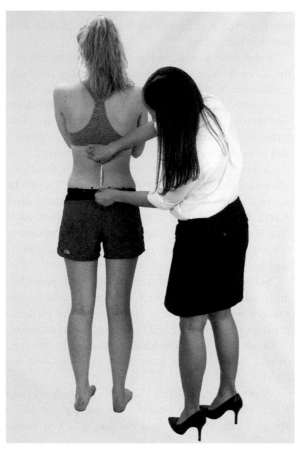

Figure 7.4a Forward flexion of the lumbar spine can be quantified by Schober's test. A 10 cm line is drawn from a point midway between the posterior superior iliac spines.

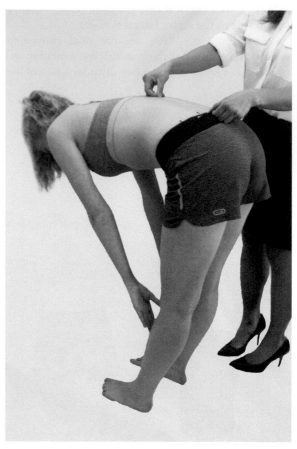

Figure 7.4b With flexion, in a normal spine, the length of this line should increase by at least 5 cm.

Lateral flexion can be quantified by recording how far down the legs the tips of the fingers can reach (e.g. to the knee or upper leg) (Figure 7.4c). Alternatively, the distance from the tip of the fingers to the ground can be measured.

Rotation is performed by fixing the pelvis. This can be done by stabilisng the patient's hips or sitting the patient before asking them to rotate (Figure 7.4d).

Essential adjuncts to an examination of the cervical and lumbar spine are screening movements of the shoulder and hip joints, respectively, to exclude them as a cause of the pain in these regions.

Screen

Before walking the patient, it may sometimes be helpful to do a quick screen for the lower lumbar nerve roots by asking the patient to squat and get up (assessing quadriceps function, L3), to stand on heels (dorsiflexion of ankles, assessing L4), to stand on one leg (and perform Trendelenburg test, assessing the hip abductors, L5) and finally asking them to stand on tiptoes (assessing plantar flexion of ankle, S1) (Figure 7.5).

The screen test for the cervical spine, before walking, is **Romberg's test** (Figure 7.6).

This is a test of the body's sense of positioning (proprioception). To be able to stand with the feet together, a patient must have two of the following functioning: dorsal column, eyesight and vestibular apparatus. Assuming that the vestibular apparatus is intact, then if a patient closes their eyes, they should be able to stand, feet together, providing that there is good function of the dorsal column. If the dorsal column is compromised, then the patient will overbalance. This is a 'static Romberg's test'.

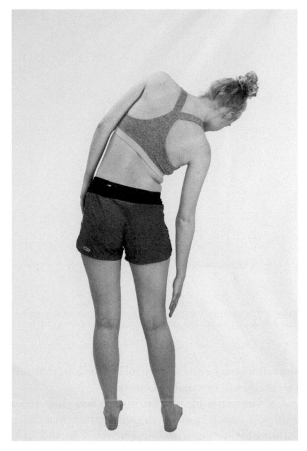

Figure 7.4c Lateral flexion.

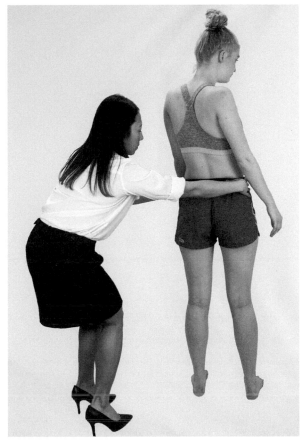

Figure 7.4d Rotation is performed with the pelvis fixed.

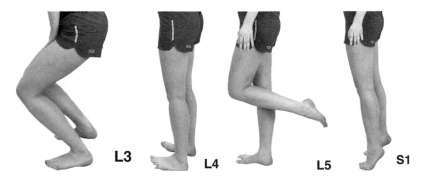

Figure 7.5 Screening tests for the lower lumbar nerve roots (**L3**), (**L4**/5), (**L5**), (**S1**).

Should the patient be able to perform this test ('Romberg's negative'), they can be further tested by being asked to walk with closed eyes to see whether they overbalance ('dynamic Romberg's test'). This needs to be done with caution as there is the risk of the patient falling if the test is strongly positive.

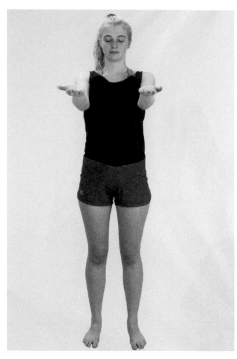

Figure 7.6 Romberg's test. Ask the patient to close their eyes with their feet together. If the dorsal column is compromised, the patient will overbalance.

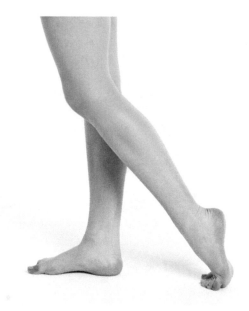

Figure 7.7 Walking is an essential part of the examination of the cervical, thoracic and lumbar spines.

Walk

Following the screen test, the patient must be observed walking; any neurological gait should be sought (Figure 7.7). An antalgic gait is often noted in the presence of lumbar radiculopathy secondary to disc prolapse. A high stepping gait may indicate a foot drop. A broad-based unsteady gait can be seen in advanced cervical myelopathy. Sometimes a compensatory scoliosis may be the result of a leg length discrepancy, and this may manifest in a short leg gait.

Neurological Examination

A thorough, orderly examination of tone, sensation, power and reflexes must be performed to all four limbs for problems with the cervical spine and on the lower limbs for thoracolumbar disease. This is most conveniently done with the patient sitting for the cervical spine or lying down for the lumbar spine.

Muscle tone can best be assessed by feeling the muscle's resistance to passive stretch. In the upper limb, to do this, support the elbow with one hand and with the other flex and extend the fingers, wrist and elbow in one smooth movement. In the lower limb, tone can be assessed by rolling the hip (passively internally and externally rotating it).

A summary of muscle innervation and reflex values (Tables 7.1a and 7.1b) and dermatomal distributions for testing sensation (Figures 7.8a and 7.8b) are given.

The American Spinal Injury Association have developed the **ASIA chart** and scoring system.[15] It provides guidance and is a very useful adjunct, allowing quick, clear documentation. (Figure 7.9) shows the ASIA worksheet. Further information about the worksheet and scoring system is available on the ASIA website.

The Muscle Research Council (MRC) booklet on neurological testing[16] or Chapter 1 will give a more detailed description of assessing muscle power. There is a logical sequence to assessing the myotomes of the lower limb (Figures 7.10 and 7.10a) and upper limb (Figure 7.11).

When testing reflexes (Figures 7.12a and 7.12b) it is important to remember to examine the abdominal reflexes (Figure 7.13), especially for thoracic spine pathology.

This **abdominal reflex test** is performed by stroking the abdomen radially out from the umbilicus in four directions (e.g. 2, 4, 8 and 10 o'clock positions). Normally, the underlying muscles will contract involuntarily, resulting in the umbilicus moving in the direction of the quadrant being stroked. Absence of

Table 7.1a The muscle innervation and reflex values of the upper limb muscles

Action	Principle muscles	Major root values
Shoulder abduction	Supraspinatus / deltoid	C5
Elbow flexion	Brachialis / biceps brachii	**C5**, C6
Wrist extension	Extensor carpi radialis / ulnaris	**C6**, C7
Elbow extension	Triceps	C6, **C7**, C8
Finger extension	Extensor digitorum / pollicis / indicis	C7, C8
Finger flexion	Flexor pollicis / digitorum communis	**C8**
Finger abduction	Dorsal interossei	C8, **T1**
Finger adduction	Palmar interossei	C8, T1

Table 7.1b The muscle innervation and reflex values of the lower limb muscles

Action	Principle muscles	Major root values
Hip flexion	Iliopsoas	L1, **L2**
Hip adduction	Adductor longus / magnus	L2, L3
Knee extension	Quadriceps femoris	**L3**, L4
Ankle dorsiflexion	Tibialis anterior	**L4**, L5
Toe extension	Extensor digitorum / hallucis	**L5**
Hip abduction	Gluteus medius / minimus	L4, **L5**
Hip extension	Gluteus maximus	L5, **S1**
Knee flexion	Hamstrings	**S1**
Foot plantar flexion	Gastrocnemius and soleus	**S1**, S2
Toe flexion	Flexor digitorum / hallucis longus	**S1**, S2

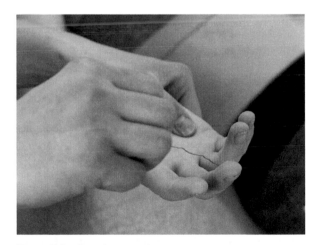

Figure 7.8a Assessing sensation.

the normal response indicates possible spinal cord pathology on the side of the diminished reflex (note: this may be physiological). Remember that the level of the umbilicus is supplied by T10.

All peripheral pulses need to be checked, as vascular claudication in the upper or lower limbs can mimic symptoms of radiculopathy or canal stenosis.

Lumbar Disc Protrusion

This is a common presentation to the orthopaedic surgeon. Interpreting the findings on neurological examination will give an idea of the location of the disc protrusion (Figures 7.14a and 7.14b).

If the protrusion is between the pedicle and the centre of the spinal canal (most common location), it is referred to as a *posterolateral disc protrusion*, and will impinge on the traversing nerve root (e.g. at the L4/5 disc, this will be the L5 nerve root).

If the prolapse is lateral to the foramen it is termed a *far lateral prolapse*. The disc will impinge on the exiting nerve root (e.g. at the L4/5 disc, this will be the L4 nerve root).

The spinal cord ends at approximately L1. Below that is the cauda equina. A large central disc protrusion in the lower lumbar region will therefore compress the cauda equina and may result in a compressive *cauda equina syndrome*. This condition is characterised by:

- Motor and sensory deficit at and below the level of the disc protrusion*
- Neuropathic leg pain (often severe)*
- Perianal or genital sensory disturbance (S2–S5)*, 'saddle anaesthesia' (Figure 7.15)

121

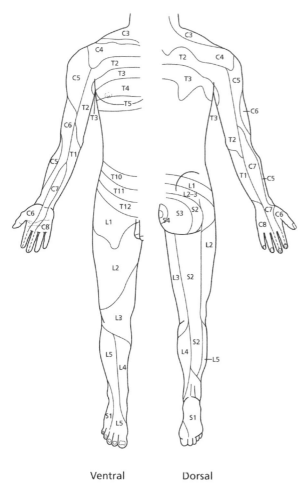

Ventral   Dorsal

Figure 7.8b Dermatomal distributions.

- Bowel and bladder dysfunction
  *(these features may be unilateral or bilateral)

Special Tests/Provocation Tests

Cervical Spine

Cervical Radiculopathy

Symptoms of cervical radiculopathy can be exacerbated by **Spurling's manoeuvre/test**.[17] The neck is loaded by axial pressure and then gently hyperextended. It is then laterally flexed and rotated to the side of the suspected lesion (Figure 7.16), thereby narrowing the involved neuroforamen. In a positive Spurling's sign, the pain arising in the neck radiates to the corresponding ipsilateral dermatome. The

sensitivity of Spurling's test is variable. However, its specificity is reported to be approximately 94%.[18,19] This test should never be performed if spinal instability is suspected.

Significant relief of symptoms with subsequent abduction of the ipsilateral shoulder (**shoulder abduction relief test**[20]) lends further support to the diagnosis of intervertebral disc herniation and is thought to result from a reduction in tension on the nerve root.

A positive **Tinel's sign** can sometimes be elicited over the exiting nerve root. This is where percussion of the affected nerve causes corresponding numbness, paresthesia and/or pain.

Cervical Myelopathy

Flexion of the neck that precipitates lightning pains or paraesthesia radiating down the back into the lower limbs represents **L'hermitte's sign**.[21] Although rarely elicited, it is characteristic of cervical spinal myelopathy (Figure 7.17).

Other important long tract signs in the assessment of cervical myelopathy are the following (Figure 7.18a,b,c):

The **plantar responses (Babinski sign)**: When performing this test, use a gentle stroke with your thumbnail or tendon hammer. A normal response is a downward contraction of the toes. An abnormal response is an upward contraction, especially of the great toe.

Clonus at the ankle or knee: More than three beats is an abnormal finding.

Hoffman's sign: Flick the distal interphalangeal joint of the index or middle finger into flexion and observe the thumb interphalangeal joint. In a positive test, this joint will flex. A positive test indicates an upper motor neuron lesion (test may be false positive in up to 25% of patients). This interphalangeal joint flexion of the thumb can be made more pronounced by asking the patient to flex and extend their neck at the same time ('dynamic Hoffman's').[22]

Inverted radial reflex: Finger flexion seen with the brachioradialis tendon reflex.

Finger escape sign: Ask the patient to hold fingers extended and adducted. The little finger spontaneously abducts due to weakness of the intrinsic muscles.

Grip and release test: Ask the patient to make a fist and release as quickly as they can. In cervical

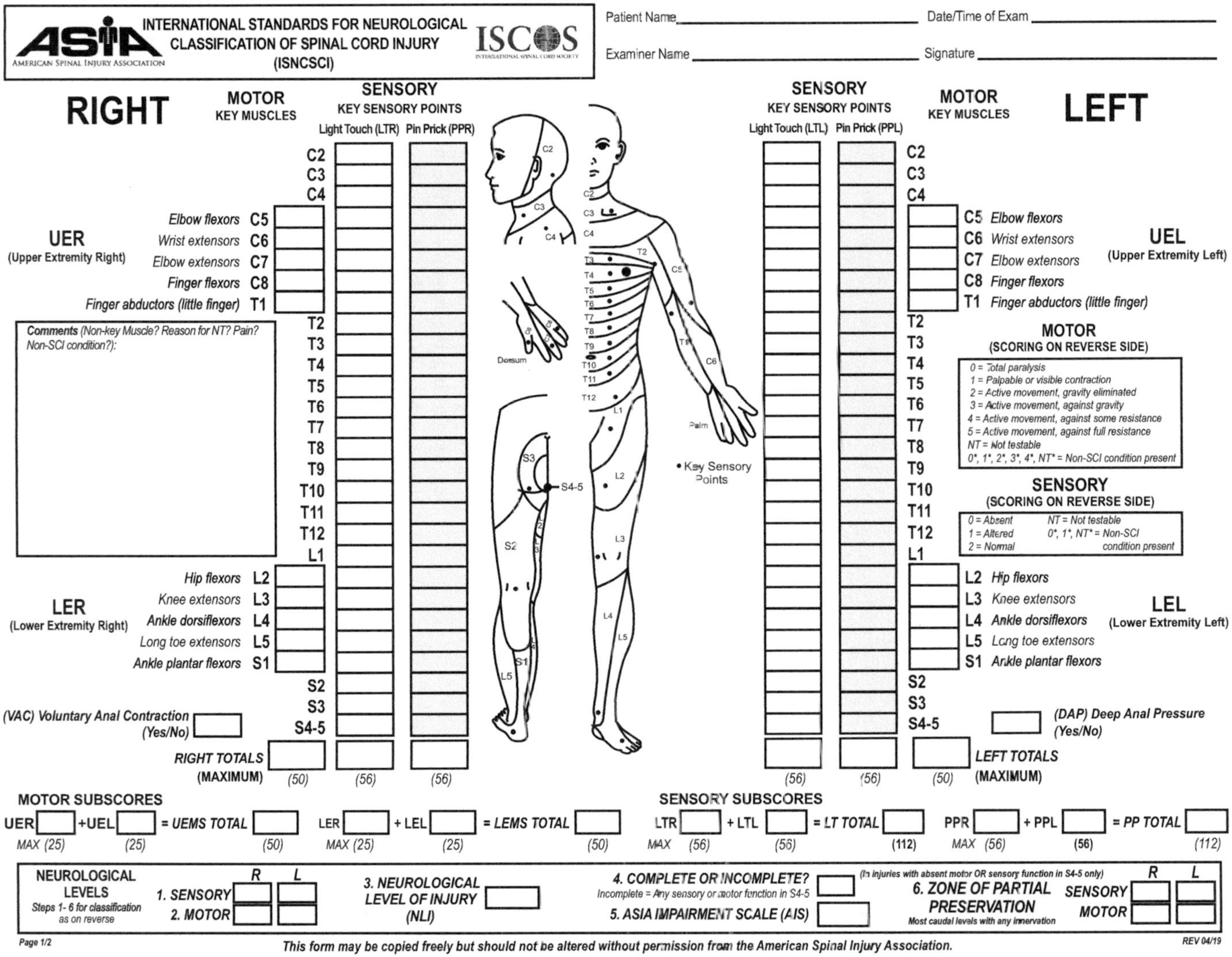

Figure 7.9 ASIA chart for documentation of neurology.

© 2020 American Spinal Injury Association. Reprinted with permission.

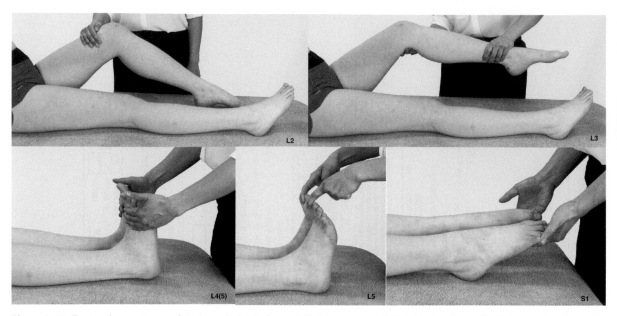

Figure 7.10 Testing the myotomes of the lower limb. Hip flexors (L2). Knee extensors (L3). Ankle dorsiflexors (L**4**/5). Big toe dorsiflexors (L5). Ankle plantarflexors (S1).

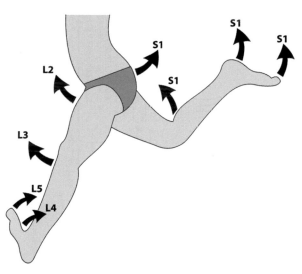

Figure 7.10a Illustration showing the myotomes of the lower limb.

myelopathy, the patient will be unable to do this 20 times in 10 seconds.

A positive test, together with the finger escape sign, is referred to as the '**Myelopathy hand**'.

Scapulohumeral reflex: Tap on scapula spine; scapula elevates or humerus abducts.

Heel-to-toe walk: Patient will be unable to do this in cervical myelopathy.

Note, as described before, the patient may also present with a positive Romberg's test, unsteady gait, clumsiness and loss of dexterity.

Lumbar Spine

Lumbar Radiculopathy

Signs of lumbar nerve root irritation, most commonly because of an intervertebral disc protrusion, may be observed when performing a series of tests. These tests rely on reproducing/exacerbating pain in the affected leg by altering the tension of the nerve and should therefore be performed at the conclusion of the examination and in the order described.

With the patient lying supine, slowly raise the affected leg; support it with the palm of the hand under the heel rather than grasping the ankle. Ensure there is no knee flexion. When the patient complains of pain (usually between 30°–60° of elevation), stop and ask whether the pain is being experienced in the back or down the leg (Figure 7.19a). This is the straight leg raise test (**sciatic stretch test**).

If the leg is then lowered a little to relieve the discomfort and the foot passively dorsiflexed, the pain may be reproduced again (Figure 7.19b). This is **Lasègue's sign.**[23]

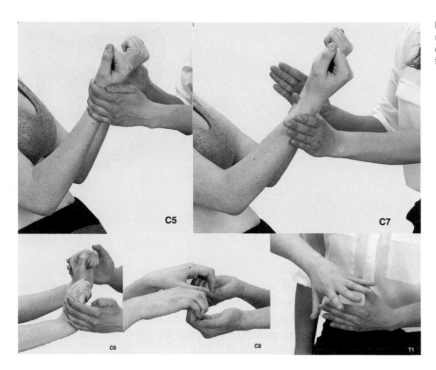

Figure 7.11 Testing the myotomes of the upper limb. Elbow flexors (C5). Elbow extensors (C7). Wrist extensors (C6). Finger flexors (C8). Intrinsics of the hand (T1).

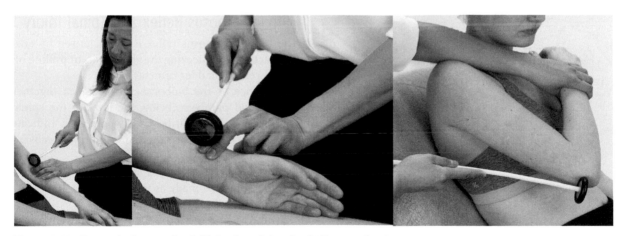

Figure 7.12a Testing the biceps reflex **C5**(6). Brachioradialis reflex C6. Triceps reflex C7.

Next, at the point where the sciatic stretch test is positive, flex the knee to 45°. This relieves the pain. The 'bowstring test' can be carried out by pressing behind the knee over the popliteal nerve with one's thumb. If leg pain is reproduced, this indicates sciatic nerve tension (Figure 7.19c). With true sciatic irritation, pressure over the medial or lateral hamstring tendons should not give a positive result.

Finally, with both legs again now flat on the couch and one hand placed gently on the knees to keep them in extension, the patient is asked to sit forwards. In the presence of nerve root tension, the patient will not be able to sit upright with the knees fully extended.

The 'flip test' is a variation of the last manoeuvre. Sit the patient upright with the knees flexed over the edge of the couch and actively extend the knees in turn (Figure 7.19d). This should produce the same response as the straight leg raise test in the genuine patient.

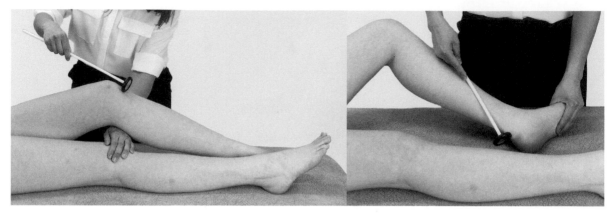

Figure 7.12b Testing the knee jerk reflex L3/4. Ankle jerk reflex S1.

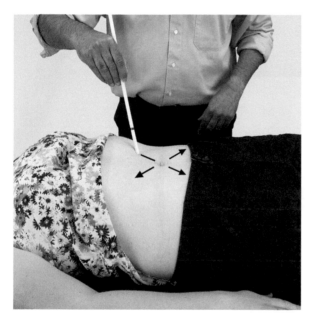

Figure 7.13 Testing of the abdominal reflexes should not be forgotten, especially when examining the thoracic spine.

A straight leg raise test performed on the unaffected leg may give rise to pain in the affected leg – the '**crossover sign**'. This has a high specificity in diagnosing a prolapsed disc. It has been reported that the disc protrusion lies in the axilla of the nerve root rather than in the more common lateral position; however, this correlation is not reliable.

Finally, with the patient now lying in the prone position, the **femoral stretch test** can be performed (Figure 7.19e). With the knee passively flexed to 90°

and a hand gently keeping the pelvis against the couch, lift the foot upwards and note the distribution of any pain provoked by this manoeuvre. A positive test usually represents an upper lumbar nerve root dysfunction (L2,3,4).

Advanced Corner

Bulbocavernosus Reflex and Spinal Injury

The bulbocavernosus reflex is characterised by anal contraction on squeezing the glans penis or pulling on an indwelling bladder catheter.

Absence of the bulbocavernosus reflex together with flaccid paralysis (below the level of the spinal cord injury), bradycardia and hypotension indicate **spinal shock**. Its return therefore indicates recovery from spinal shock.[24]

With the recovery from spinal shock, an assessment can then be made as to whether the injury was 'Complete' or 'Incomplete' (ASIA).[15]

Complete

- No voluntary anal contraction
- And, no perianal sensation
- And, Grade 0/5 power distally
- And, bulbocavernosus reflex present (patient not in spinal shock)

Incomplete

- Voluntary anal contraction (sacral sparing)
- Or, palpable or visible muscle contraction below the spinal level
- Or, perianal sensation present

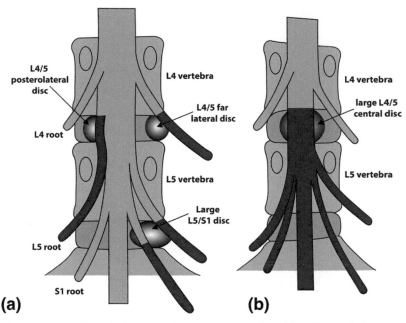

(a)   **(b)**

Figures 7.14a and 7.14b Illustration showing L4/5 posterolateral disc affecting the L5 nerve root. L4/5 far lateral disc affecting the L4 nerve root. A large L5/S1 disc affecting both the L5 and S1 roots. (b) Illustration showing L4/5 large central disc pressing on the nerve roots of the cauda equina bilaterally.

Tandem Spinal Stenosis (TSS)

- Concurrent cervical and lumbar stenosis.[25]
- Incidence averages 20% (0.12–28%)[26]
- A complex clinical picture (combined upper motor neuron and lower motor neuron signs).
- Cervical stenosis causes upper limb myelopathy and/or radiculopathy.
- Lumbar stenosis causes neurogenic claudication in the lower limbs.
- The dilemma is both in making the diagnosis and in the subsequent treatment. There is a high index of suspicion especially if the patient presents with mixed signs.
- Treatment is usually staged surgery, although single stage decompression is possible.

Waddell's Non-organic Signs

Waddell described a group of physical signs that indicated a non-organic or psychological component to lower back pain. Five categories of signs were described:[9]

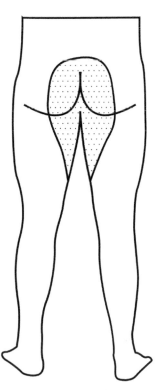

Figure 7.15 The site of 'saddle anaesthesia'.

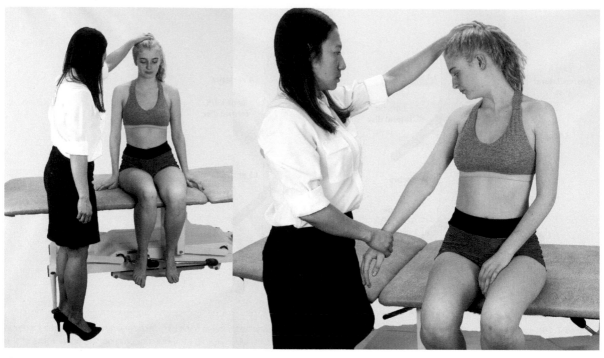

Figure 7.16 Spurling's test. A provocation test for cervical radiculopathy. This is performed with axial compression and neck extension. This is then combined with rotation and lateral flexion to the side of the symptoms. Relief of symptoms occurs with abduction of the ipsilateral shoulder (shoulder abduction relief test).

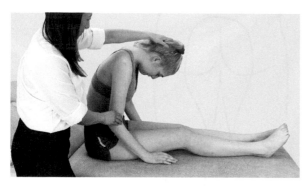

Figure 7.17 L'hermitte's sign. A provocation test for cervical myelopathy. Flexion of spine results in lightning pains down the legs.

1. **Overreaction:** This may take the form of a disproportional verbalisation, facial expression, muscle tension and tremor, collapse or sweating.
2. **Non-anatomical distribution** of signs and symptoms.
3. Regional disturbance: **'Glove and stocking'** weakness or sensory disturbance in a region of the body which deviates from accepted neuroanatomy, e.g. an entire leg.
4. **Simulation tests:** Simulation of a movement that would produce pain without actually causing the movement, e.g. axial loading of the spine and pain on passive rotation of the shoulders and pelvis.
5. **Distraction tests:** A positive physical finding is demonstrated in the normal way and then the finding is rechecked with the patient distracted. For example, a positive finding would be pain on straight leg raise whilst lying down; this can be rechecked by bringing the leg out straight whilst the patient is sitting and the plantar reflex is being performed.

Three or more signs were felt to be a positive finding. However, several studies have cast doubt as to the validity of these signs; as such, the test has limited use in current practice but is used in medico-legal situations and asked in examinations.[27,28]

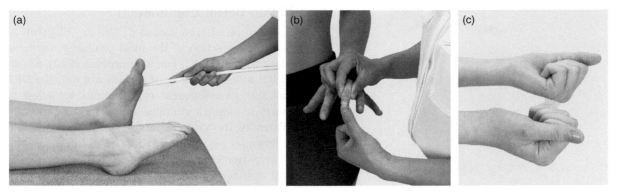

Figures 7.18a,b,c Some tests for cervical myelopathy: (a) Upgoing plantar response (positive Babinski sign) where the great toe extends on stroking the plantar aspect of the foot. (b) Hoffman's sign. Note that if the middle finger distal interphalangeal joint (DIPJ) is 'flicked', then the DIPJ of the index finger and the interphalangeal joint (IPJ) of the thumb will flex. (c) Grip and release test. An abnormal response is the inability to open and close the fist 20 times in 10 seconds.

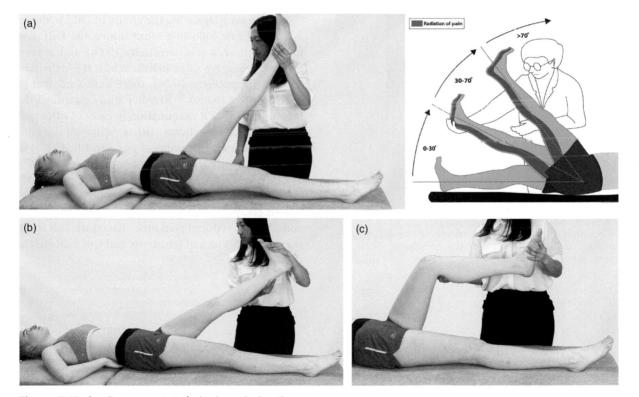

Figures 7.19a,b,c Provocation tests for lumbar radiculopathy.
(a) The straight leg raise test (sciatic stretch). The palm is placed under the heel with the leg extended. Only a reproduction of pain down the leg with elevation is regarded as positive and not an exacerbation of back pain. The main pain is felt in an arc between 30° and 70° because the sciatic nerve is under the most tension between these points.
(b) Lasègue's sign. After lowering the leg, passive dorsiflexion of the foot increases root tension and reinforces a positive straight leg raise.
(c) Bowstring test. The hip and knee are flexed 45° with pressure in the popliteal fossa on the nerve. This increases root tension and results in pain.

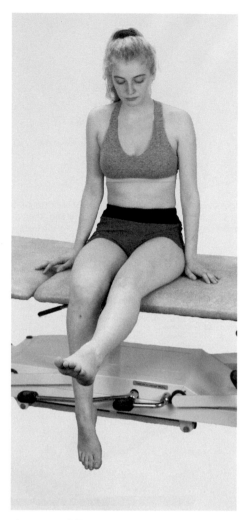

Figure 7.19d The Hip test. The patient sits upright on the examination couch with the knees flexed over the side. Active extension of the knee resulting in pain down the leg is a positive result, as this is equivalent to a straight leg raise test.

Digital Rectal Examination

A digital rectal examination ('DRE' or 'PR') aims to assess the function of the most caudal spinal nerve roots: S3, S4 and S5. For the purposes of any neurological assessment, it must include not only the DRE but also an assessment of cutaneous sensation to sharp or pinprick stimulus which must be assessed bilaterally, the S3 dermatomes being over the ischial tuberosities (or so-called saddle area) and the S4 and S5 dermatomes localised in target fashion around the anal sphincter. When performed, the DRE itself should assess both the resting and active motor function of the external anal sphincter and anal sensation.[29]

Although a DRE/PR examination has always been a necessary part of a complete spinal examination in suspected cauda equina syndrome (CES) and spinal cord injury (SCI), several studies have highlighted limitations with this examination.

In one study assessing the ability of DRE to detect SCI in patients following blunt injury, the DRE was found to have a low sensitivity (50%) and a poor positive predictive value (93%). Whilst it did demonstrate high specificity (97%), there were a number of false positives (6.8%).[30] Another study examined the role of the DRE/PR examination in cases of suspected cauda equina. In patients with a radiologically confirmed CES, saddle numbness was identified in 64%, whereas reduced anal tone was present in only 18% and 22% had a normal examination. Compared with these figures, in patients without radiologically confirmed compressive CES, 54% had saddle numbness and 21% had reduced anal tone. Therefore, this study suggests both a lack of sensitivity and specificity of the

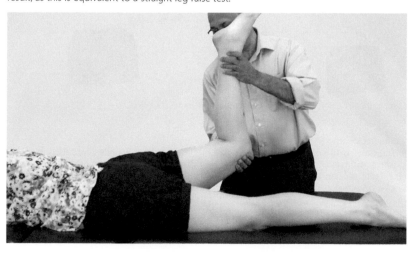

Figure 7.19e Femoral stretch test. The hip is extended with the knee extended or preferably flexed. Pain shoots down the front of the thigh in a positive test.

DRE/PR examination and its necessity in the assessment of a suspected CES prior to imaging is now increasingly being called into question.[31]

Rectal examination remains a critical part of spine examinations where there is a suspicion of sacral nerve root dysfunction, despite the shortcomings highlighted above. This must be carefully documented in the clinical notes.

Nerve Root Value Discrepancy (Ankle Dorsiflexion and Elbow Flexion)

In recent times, there has been some debate in the literature and amongst spinal surgeons on the true nerve root supply for ankle dorsiflexion and elbow flexion. A summary is presented here.

The nerve root value attributed to ankle dorsiflexion when performing a neurological examination is L4. However, foot drop is commonly attributed to an L5 radiculopathy.[32] In a recent study,[33] 59.6% of patients experiencing foot drop were caused by L5 radiculopathy, 38.5 % by an S1 radiculopathy and only 1.9 % by an L4 radiculopathy. In the first instance, this may seem contradictory, but in reality, dorsiflexion of the foot is caused by three muscles, tibialis anterior (**L4**, L5), extension hallucis longus (**L5**, S1) and extensor digitorum longus (**L5**, S1), and as a result the dominant contribution to dorsiflexion of the foot is L5. This emphasises the need to palpate the belly of the muscle being assessed to confirm findings. It should also be noted there is variation from person to person in the dominant nerve root contribution to the peripheral nerves.

Elbow flexion is another area of discrepancy where C5 or C6 may be considered the dominant nerve root. Elbow flexion is caused by three muscles, biceps, brachialis and brachioradialis. Both biceps and brachialis are supplied by the musculocutaneous nerve (C5, C6) and brachioradialis is supplied by the radial nerve (C5, **C6**). The discrepancy may result from individual variations in the dominant nerve root supplying the respective muscles. The position of the forearm will also alter the contribution of each of the three muscles to elbow flexion and will need to be controlled.

References

1. Fairbank JCT, Pynsent PB. The Oswestry Disability Index. *Spine (Phila Pa 1976)* 2000;**25**(22):940–953.
2. Childs JD, Piva SR, Fritz JM. Responsiveness of the numeric pain rating scale in patients with low back pain. *Spine (Phila Pa 1976)* 2005;**30**(11):1331–1334.
3. Hashizume H, Konno SI, Takeshita K, et al. Japanese Orthopaedic Association Back Pain Evaluation Questionnaire (JOABPEQ) as an outcome measure for patients with low back pain: reference values in healthy volunteers. *J Orthop Sci* 2015;**20**(2):264–280.
4. Gluck J V, Oleinick A. Claim rates of compensable back injuries by age, gender, occupation, and industry. Do they relate to return-to-work experience? *Spine (Phila Pa 1976)* 1998;**23**(14):1572–1587.
5. Murgatroyd DF, Harris IA, Tran Y, Cameron ID. The association between seeking financial compensation and injury recovery following motor vehicle related orthopaedic trauma. *BMC Musculoskelet Disord* 2016;**17**:282.
6. Sanderson PL, Todd BD, Holt GR, Getty CJM. Compensation, work status, and disability in low back pain patients. *Spine (Phila Pa 1976)* 1995;**20**(5):554–556.
7. Venkatesan M, Nasto L, Tsegaye M, Grevitt M. Bladder scans and post-void residual volume measurement improve diagnostic accuracy of cauda equina syndrome. *Spine (Phila Pa 1976)* 2019;**44**(18):13013–1308.
8. Adams W. Lectures on the pathology and treatment of lateral and other forms of curvature of the spine. *Br Med J* 1865;**1**:484–486.
9. Waddell G, McCulloch JA, Kummel E, Venner RM. Nonorganic physical signs in low-back pain. *Spine (Phila Pa 1976)* 1980;**5**(2):117–125.
10. Fairbank J. Historical perspective: William Adams, the forward bending test, and the spine of Gideon Algernon Mantell. *Spine (Phila Pa 1976)* 2004;**29**(17):1953–1955.
11. Schober P. Lendenwirbelsäule und Kreuzschmerzen. *Münch Med Wsclir* 1937;**84**:336–338.
12. Castro MP, Stebbings SM, Milosavljevic S, Bussey MD. Construct validity of clinical spinal mobility tests in ankylosing spondylitis: a systematic review and meta-analysis. *Clin Rheumatol* 2016;**35**(7):1777–1787.
13. Stolwijk C, Ramiro S, Vosse D, et al. Comparison of tests for lumbar flexion and hip function in patients with and without axial spondyloarthritis. *Arthritis Care Res* 2015;**67**(4):538–545.
14. Macrae IF, Wright V. Measurement of back movement. *Ann Rheum Dis* 1969;**28**(6):584–589.
15. American Spinal Injury Association. International Standards for Neurological Classification of SCI (ISNCSCI) worksheet, n.d. https://asia-spinalinjury.org/international-standards-neurological-classification-sci-isncsci-worksheet/ (accessed 26 March 2020)

16. *Aids to the Examination of the Peripheral Nervous System*. London: Her Majesty's Stationery Office, 1976.

17. Jones SJ, Miller J-M M. *Spurling Test*. StatPearls Publisher, 2019.

18. Tong HC, Haig AJ, Yamakawa K. The Spurling test and cervical radiculopathy. *Spine (Phila Pa 1976)* 2002;**27**(2):156–159.

19. Shabat S, Leitner Y, David R, Folman Y. The correlation between Spurling test and imaging studies in detecting cervical radiculopathy. *J Neuroimaging* 2012;**22**(4):375–378.

20. Davidson RI, Dunn EJ, Metzmaker JN. The shoulder abduction test in the diagnosis of radicular pain in cervical extradural compressive monoradiculopathies. *Spine (Phila Pa 1976)* 1981;**6**(5):441–446.

21. Marie P, Chatelin C. Sur certains symptômes vraisemblablement d'origine radiculaire chez les blessés du crâne. *Rev Neurol* 1917;**31**:336.

22. McRae R. (ed). *Clinical Orthopaedic Examination*, 6th ed. London: Churchill Livingstone, 2010; p. 41.

23. Lasegue C. Considerations sur la sciatique. *Arch Gen Med* 1864;**2**:558.

24. McLain RF, Dudeney S. Clinical history and physical examination. In Fardon DF, Garfin SR (eds), *Orthopaedic Knowledge Update: Spine 2*. Rosemont, IL: American Academy of Orthopaedic Surgeons, 2002; pp. 39–51.

25. Dagi TF, Tarkington MA, Leech JJ. Tandem lumbar and cervical spinal stenosis: natural history, prognostic indices, and results after surgical decompression. *J Neurosurg* 1987;**66**(6):842–849.

26. Krishnan A, Dave BR, Kumar Kambar A, Ram H. Coexisting lumbar and cervical stenosis (tandem spinal stenosis): an infrequent presentation. Retrospective analysis of single-stage surgery (53 cases). *Eur Spine J* 2014;**23**(1):64–73.

27. Fishbain DA, Cutler RB, Rosomoff HL, Rosomoff RS. Is there a relationship between nonorganic physical findings (Waddell signs) and secondary gain/malingering? *Clin J Pain* 2004;**20**(6):399–408.

28. Fishbain DA, Cole B, Cutler RB, et al. A structured evidence-based review on the meaning of nonorganic physical signs: Waddell signs. *Pain Med* 2003;**4**(2):141–181.

29. Çelik EC. Updates in ASIA examination: anorectal examination. *Turk J Phys Med Rehab* 2015;**61**(1):10–11. doi: 1 0.5152/tftrd.2015.00087.

30. Guldner GT, Brzenski AB. The sensitivity and specificity of the digital rectal examination for detecting spinal cord injury in adult patients with blunt trauma. *Am J Emerg Med*. 2006;**24**(1):113–117. doi: 10.1016/j.ajem.2005.05.012.

31. Hoeritzauer I, Pronin S, Carson A, et al. The clinical features and outcome of scan-negative and scan-positive cases in suspected cauda equina syndrome: a retrospective study of 276 patients. *J Neurol* 2018;**265**(12):2916–2926. doi: 10.1007/s00415-018-9078-2.

32 Carolus AE, Becker M, Cuny J, et al. The interdisciplinary management of foot drop. *Dtsch Arztebl Int* 2019;**116**(20):347–354.

33 Ma J, He Y, Wang A, et al. Risk factors analysis for foot drop associated with lumbar disc herniation: an analysis of 236 patients. *World Neurosurg* 2018;**110**:e1017–e1024.

Examination of the Hip

Paul Banaszkiewicz and Ian Stockley

Assessment of the Hip

A. History

B. Clinical Examination

Step 1

Stand the patient and look

Step 2

Walk the patient

Step 3

Trendelenburg test

Step 4

Lie the patient down and square the pelvis

Step 5

Thomas test and range of movement of hip

Step 6

Leg length measurement

Step 7

Special tests

Impingement: Anterior impingement test, Posterior impingement test and FABER test.

Contractures: Ely's test, Ober's test, Phelps' test.

Stand and Look

Expose the patient adequately, remembering to lift the underwear and look closely for any scars. Look at the general attitude of the lower limb. Look from the front, side, both laterally and medially, and behind. In particular, when looking from the side assess the degree of lumbar lordosis, and when looking from behind look for any associated scoliosis. An increased lumbar lordosis may indicate a fixed flexion deformity of the hip and a scoliosis may help to indicate a leg length discrepancy.

Walk

Whilst the patient is walking, it is important to comment on the gait. Knowledge of the stages of the gait cycle will help in this. Remember to look for walking aids.

Trendelenburg Test

In performing the Trendelenburg test, flexion should occur only at the knee. Demonstrate this to the patient. It is reassuring to hold on to the patient's waist and ask them to hold on to your shoulder or forearm, as many older patients may have difficulty balancing on one leg.

Lie Patient Down

Make sure the couch is flat and square the pelvis. Squaring the pelvis is very important as all assessments of deformity and leg length should be based on a squared pelvis. By squaring the pelvis, we mean that both anterior superior iliac spines are perpendicular to the side of the examination couch.

Thomas Test

Thomas test is performed to assess fixed flexion deformity of the hip. What it is actually achieving is obliterating the lumbar spine compensation that takes place when a patient has a fixed flexion deformity of the hip. As such, it gives the true measurement of the fixed flexion deformity.

Movements

First, ask the patient to actively flex the affected hip as far as it will go, and then passively take it beyond that point to see the full degree of flexion of the hip. Then perform other movements passively: abduction, adduction, internal rotation and external rotation.

Leg Length Measurements

Note that it is important to assess the contralateral hip movements prior to proceeding with leg length measurements, as both limbs need to be placed in exactly the same degree of deformity for the measurements to be accurate.

Real and apparent (not necessary to perform if the pelvis is squared) lengths are measured and these can be fine-tuned by doing Galeazzi's test to assess whether shortening is above or below the knee. Bryant's triangle or Nelaton's line will make clear whether the femoral shortening is above or below the trochanter.

Then, if necessary, stand the patient and perform the block test.

Special Tests

These are mainly for soft tissue pathology. There are many described, but the important ones are indicated in the 'Summary' box above.

History

Presenting complaints in hip pathology may include pain, limp and stiffness. Patients may not complain of stiffness per se but of the disability produced by it (e.g. the inability to put shoes and/or socks on). In trying to evaluate a patient's symptomatology, it is important to know what effect, if any, the symptoms have on the patient's ability to undertake activities of everyday living. Mechanical symptoms such as locking, clicking, catching or popping can also be presenting symptoms in their own right.

It is important to ask patients whether they have had any previous problems with their hips. Childhood conditions affecting the hip may cause symptoms in early adult life because of the development of secondary degenerative changes. In addition, a history of previous surgery is very important when contemplating further surgical procedures, as consideration needs to be given to previous scars and the surgical approach. These may cause an increased risk of complications such as infection, dislocation and sciatic nerve injury with arthroplasty surgery.

Several validated hip assessment scores are now available, and these allow for a more objective assessment of hip function. The Harris Hip Score is scored by the examiner and emphasises range of motion, pain and function. The Oxford Hip Score and the WOMAC Osteoarthritis Index are scored by the patient and so remove any potential clinician bias. These scores, if re-administered after treatment, are useful in objectively quantifying both how patients perceive the results of that treatment modality and whether it led to improved wellbeing and functional ability.

Patient Reported Outcome Measures (PROMs) are now widely used for hip arthroplasty surgery. PROMs assess the quality of care delivered to patients from the patient's perspective. They calculate the health gains after surgery using pre- and post-operative scoring systems.

Soft tissue hip pathology can be associated with specific sports, so it is important to determine the type, intensity and frequency of any sporting activity performed both currently and in the past. Ask about

locking, snapping or other mechanical symptoms that are common complaints associated with soft tissue hip pain. Ask about the inciting movements/activities that can provide clues to a possible diagnosis. With femoroacetabular impingement (FAI), patients may complain of anterior groin pain that is worse on hip flexion or groin pain on prolonged sitting. Other important factors to elicit include exact location of pain and any associated paraesthesia or neurological deficit.

Pain

Pain is the most important symptom. Pain felt in the groin or thigh region will most likely be from hip disease and is thought to arise from the joint capsule, synovial lining and labrum. Radiation to the anterior, medial or lateral thigh is common, as is pain referred to the knee. Obviously, patients may have symptoms related to the knees as a direct consequence of knee pathology, but referred pain from above always needs to be considered. A common symptom of intra-articular soft tissue pathology is the so-called C sign, where the patient demonstrates the location of their pain by cupping the lateral aspect of the hip in their hand, fingers anteriorly and thumb posteriorly.[1]

Hip pain localised to the gluteal region is often referred pain from lumbosacral pathology and there may be associated radicular symptoms and signs. Pain felt below the knee is suspicious for spinal pathology. Differentiation between hip and back pain can usually be made on the basis of history, clinical examination and X-rays, but, if in doubt, an injection of local anaesthetic into the hip joint can be very useful. The presence of inguinal herniae, or the so-called sportsman's groin, produces groin symptoms that may be increased by coughing, sneezing and the Valsalva manoeuvre.

Pain as a consequence of arthritis is usually exacerbated by exercise and relieved by rest. However, as the pathology progresses, pain at rest becomes a feature.

The differential diagnosis of a patient presenting with hip pain should always include infection. Pyogenic infection of the hip presents as pain localised to the groin or inner thigh. Pain secondary to infection is constant and unrelenting in character. The patient will experience pain with weightbearing but will also have pain at rest. When pain is caused by haematogenous spread, the onset is often acute and caused by distension of the joint capsule and secondary muscle spasm. A more insidious onset is the norm when the infection is by direct extension, as there is no dramatic increase in intra-articular pressure.

Claudication-like pain may also be present in degenerative hip pathology, and a differential diagnosis should consider neurogenic (presence of stenosis of the spinal canal) or vascular (presence of peripheral vascular disease) causes. With neurogenic causes, when the patient bends forwards, the pain decreases. Meanwhile, with a vascular cause, the patient reports distal rather than proximal pain and needs to sit for a while.

Stiffness and Limp

Patients do not often complain of stiffness but complain of the difficulties they have undertaking activities of everyday living as a consequence of the stiffness, i.e. going up stairs, cutting toe nails and putting on socks. The term *stiffness* usually includes some loss of range of motion; it is a feeling experienced by the patient.

Limping can result from a variety of reasons, including pain, limb length inequality, muscle weakness and bone and joint deformity. If the hip is very stiff, then patients often complain of a limp and not necessarily pain.

Snapping and Clicking Hips

Snapping and clicking hips tend to occur in adolescents and young adults.[2] Patients often reproduce the symptoms and demonstrate the physical signs on demand, and so these tend to become habitual in nature. Intra-articular and extra-articular pathologies have been described, although often there is no obvious abnormality detected either clinically or by investigation. Pain can be associated with the mechanical symptoms and radiates to the groin or laterally towards the greater trochanter area.

Examination

Examination starts as soon as the patient walks into the room. Are any special shoes, use of a walking frame or orthosis noted? Is a cane or crutches needed? Is there a limp? Are they in pain? Often, there are many clues that can be explored later during the formal examination.

Inspection (Look)

With the patient adequately exposed, muscle wasting and scars can be seen and posture is noted for the presence of contractures, spinal deformity and the ability to stand with feet flat on the ground (Figure 8.1).

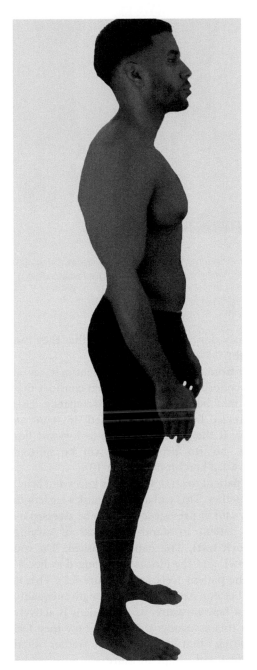

Figure 8.1 Stand the patient and look from the front, side and back. Observe the spine and knees to see if they may be compensating for hip pathology.

When looking from the side, look for an increased lumbar lordosis. This can signify a fixed flexion deformity of the hip, as up to 30° of fixed flexion deformity of the hip can be compensated for by increasing the lumbar lordosis. This is

135

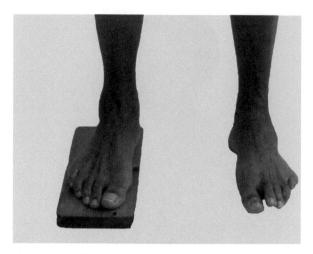

Figure 8.2 Block test. This is a useful test for leg length discrepancy that can be done whilst the patient is standing. It involves placing blocks of different thicknesses under the foot of the patient's affected leg and then asking them if they feel balanced.

spontaneously done by the patient so that they can stand upright.

Looking from the back of the patient may reveal a postural scoliosis. If this is seen, then consider that the patient may have a leg length discrepancy. This can be corrected by asking the patient to stand on blocks. Also, if the patient is asked to forward flex their spine, no rib prominence will be noticed (Adam's forward bend test, Chapter 13).

Ask the patient to straighten their knees and bring both feet together. This will again unmask a leg length discrepancy and, if present, could also be assessed by asking the patient to stand on blocks of varying heights (**block test**). The patient is asked, 'Do you feel level now?' and the blocks are changed as necessary until the patient feels level (Figure 8.2). This is probably a better assessment of leg length inequality than using a tape measure, as the patient is actively involved in this assessment, and it is how they feel when standing that is important rather than a measurement with a tape measure.

Looking at and palpating the iliac crests gives an assessment of pelvic obliquity, which will be corrected if the obliquity is caused by leg length inequality. However, fixed obliquity resulting from lumbosacral disease cannot be compensated for in this manner.

Gait (Walk)

Abnormal pathology in the lower limb is often demonstrated by changes in the gait pattern, whether it is

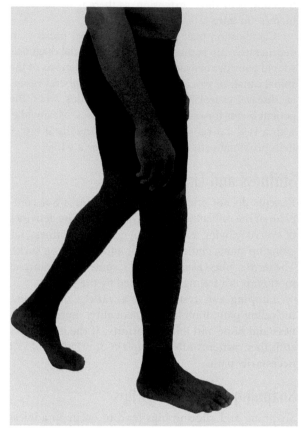

Figure 8.3 Walk the patient and observe the gait.

a compensatory adaptation to pain, loss of motion or weakness (Figure 8.3). Common gait patterns include:

- **Antalgic gait:** Pain in the hip on weightbearing can be diminished by reducing the time spent on the affected leg (stance phase) and by leaning the trunk over to the symptomatic side when in stance phase. It also involves an excessive drop in the centre of gravity as a means of reducing peak loading on weightbearing. This produces an uneven stance period, which is the characteristic feature of an antalgic gait.
- **Short-leg gait:** This involves excessive shift of the centre of gravity towards the short side, with a drop of the centre of gravity. It differs from the antalgic gait in that the stance period is equal.
- **Trendelenburg gait:** This is indicated by a drop of the pelvis on the opposite side to the stance limb. However, to maintain centre of gravity above the stance limb, it is not unusual for the trunk to lurch towards the ipsilateral stance limb.

- **Gluteus maximus gait:** Hip extensor weakness (gluteus maximus) necessitates a forward thrust of the pelvis and backward thrust of the trunk. This position places the centre of gravity posterior to the hip, tenses the iliofemoral ligament and stabilises the situation.

Trendelenburg Test

Hip abductor function can be assessed by the Trendelenburg test. In 1895 Trendelenburg recorded observations describing the gait of patients with congenitally dislocated hips (CDH). He described how the upper body swings to the side of weightbearing in a child with CDH. Later he went on to describe the pelvic inclination on single leg weightbearing, which became known as the Trendelenburg sign. This was originally described with the examiner standing behind the patient so that the dimples overlying the posterior superior iliac spines could be seen to move up and down when the test was being performed.

The Trendelenburg test can be performed either with the examiner in front or behind the patient. It is our experience, however, that unless the examiner is actually facing the patient, they are reluctant to stand on one leg, particularly if the hip is painful. In addition, it is easier to give verbal instructions to the patient and be able to anticipate any loss of balance.

When assessing the patient, ask them to face the examiner and then ask them to place their forearms on the examiner's, thereby giving support and, hopefully, a feeling of confidence. The patient is then asked to stand on one leg and bend the opposite knee to 90° without flexing the hip. This action eliminates the role of hip flexors as they play a role in pelvic stability and may affect the Trendelenburg sign (Figure 8.4). The test is then repeated by standing on the other leg. The sign is deemed negative, i.e. the abductor mechanism is normal, when the pelvis remains level. A positive result indicates abductor mechanism dysfunction and the pelvis on the unsupported side will descend. A patient standing on his right leg would be Trendelenburg-positive for the right if the left side dipped.

A Trendelenburg test can be positive for three main reasons: (1) power failure, (2) lever arm failure and (3) fulcrum (pivot) failure.

A power failure can be secondary to generalised muscular or neurological weakness or paralysis or abductor dysfunction. A lever arm failure occurs with a fractured neck of femur or short neck in coxa

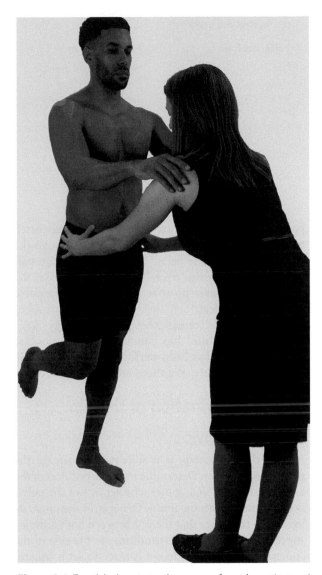

Figure 8.4 Trendelenburg test – the surgeon faces the patient and asks them to stand on one leg. The opposite knee is flexed behind to 90°. The pelvis should remain level or rise. In a positive result, the pelvis dips on the unsupported side.

vara. A fulcrum failure occurs when there is absence of a stable fulcrum. This typically occurs with destruction of the femoral head secondary to infection, tuberculosis and developmental dysplasia of the hip.

It is important to be aware that patients who have a weakened abductor mechanism may not descend on one side when assessing for the Trendelenburg sign, as they can compensate by leaning over the affected hip to shift the body's centre of gravity in that direction. This is called a *Trendelenburg lurch*. However,

137

Table 8.1 Causes of false positive and false negative results for the Trendelenburg test[3]

False positive	False negative
Pain	Leaning beyond the hip on the standing side
Lack of cooperation from patient	Use of muscles above and below the pelvis
Impingement between rib cage and iliac crest	Adduction deformity of the hip
Abduction deformity of hip	
Severe genu varum	

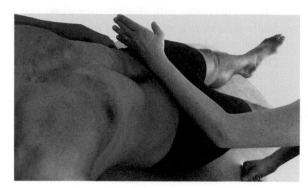

Figure 8.5a Lie the patient on the couch and square the pelvis. The examiner's arm, which is placed over both anterior superior iliac spines, should be perpendicular to the side of the couch.

patients with advanced arthritis of the hip may lurch towards the ipsilateral stance limb simply because the arthritis prevents the pelvic tilt and, to maintain balance, the patient leans over. Table 8.1 summarises the causes of a false positive and a false negative Trendelenburg test.[3]

The *delayed Trendelenburg sign* is really non-specific. Any painful hip condition will be positive after the patient has been performing the test for 30 seconds to a minute. We therefore question its value.

Supine Examination of the Hip

Square the Pelvis

As a preliminary step, it is important to square the pelvis (Figure 8.5a). Determine from the position of the anterior superior iliac spines whether or not the pelvis is lying square with the limbs. One way of demonstrating this is to ensure that the line between both anterior superior iliac spines is perpendicular to the side of the couch. If it is not, an attempt is made to set it square.

If the pelvis cannot be squared up, then there is a fixed adduction or abduction deformity of one or both hips. Fixed adduction will cause an apparent shortening (10°, causing 2.5 cm apparent shortening) and the opposite is true for a fixed abduction (Figure 8.5b).

Palpation

The hip joint is too deep to assess for the presence of an effusion or synovial thickening. Bony landmarks can be palpated and include the anterior superior iliac spine, the ischial tuberosity and the greater trochanter.

Thomas Test

Contracture of the joint capsule will cause deformity. Fixed flexion, fixed adduction and external rotation

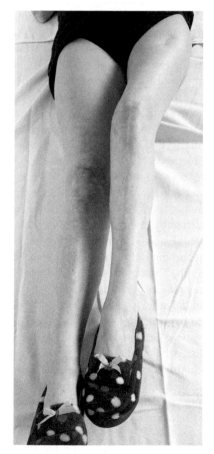

Figure 8.5b This patient has a fixed adduction deformity of the left leg, resulting in pelvic obliquity and apparent leg length discrepancy.

are the common deformities.[4] A fixed flexion deformity is best determined by performing the Thomas test.

Hugh Owen Thomas described this test in 1876. A positive Thomas test probably had more relevance in the 1920s when a fixed flexion contraction of the hip was a common occurrence secondary to tuberculosis.

A patient with a fixed flexion deformity at the hip will compensate, when lying on their back, by arching the spine and pelvis into an exaggerated lordosis. This is because the patient would want to lie flat on the couch. If they had a fixed flexion deformity of the hip, then the only way they could accomplish this would be to arch their back and increase their lumbar lordosis. Up to 30° of fixed flexion deformity can be compensated for by increasing the lumbar lordosis.

Technique

A hand placed under the back will assess the lumbar lordosis. If the hip not being measured is flexed to its limit, the pelvis rotates and the lordosis is eliminated. During this manoeuvre, the other hip, if in fixed flexion, is passively lifted from the couch. The angle through which it is raised is the fixed flexion deformity (Figure 8.6a,b).

An alternative way of assessing fixed flexion deformity is to start with both hips in the knee–chest position. Each hip can be extended separately, and the angle from the horizontal to the thigh is the flexion deformity. This alternative method is most suited for a younger, active patient and best avoided in an elderly patient with significant bilateral hip disease.

It is also important to ensure that there is no fixed flexion deformity of the knee before doing a Thomas test, as this will give a false positive result (Figure 8.6c). In this situation, it would be necessary to hang the lower leg off the side of the couch (with the knee on the edge), so that the thigh is flat on the couch, before performing the Thomas test.

The Thomas test is either omitted or done with extreme care ('patient controlled') if the patient has a total hip arthroplasty on the opposite side for fear of causing a dislocation. Also, be careful when flexing up the opposite hip if there is significant arthritis present (on that side) for fear of hurting the patient.

See Chapter 1, 'Advanced Corner' for more examples.

Movements

Hip movements are probably the most important clinical sign and the key to the diagnosis of hip disease. For ease of examination purposes, hip movements are best

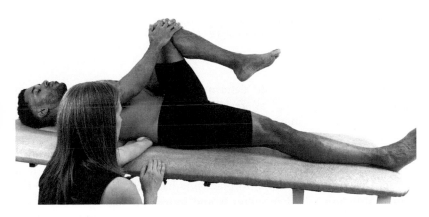

Figure 8.6a Thomas test for a flexion deformity of the hip. The hand placed under the lumbar spine confirms the lumbar lordosis has been eliminated. Any persistent elevation or flexion of the thigh relative to the examination couch represents the flexion deformity.

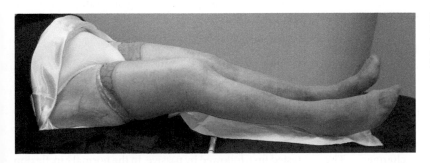

Figure 8.6b This patient with a fixed flexion deformity of her right hip is unable to place her leg flat on the bed unless she compensates by increasing her lumbar lordosis.

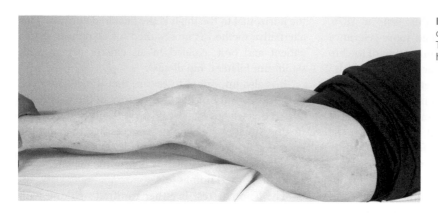

Figure 8.6c Patient with a fixed flexion deformity of the knee. To perform the Thomas test, the leg would have to be hanging over the side of the couch.

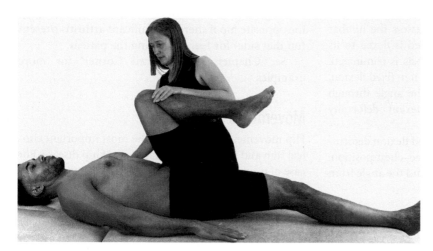

Figure 8.7 Hip flexion is best assessed with the ipsilateral knee flexed to relax the hamstrings.

demonstrated by testing active movements first and then following on with passive movements (rather than an artificial separation of active and passive movements).

If movements are severely restricted in all directions, think of rheumatoid arthritis, tuberculosis, septic arthritis. If hip movements are reasonably well preserved but there is pain and terminal limitation of movement, think of osteoarthritis. One or more movements may be more limited than others if the head is deformed in such cases as Perthes disease or avascular necrosis.

Measurements should include flexion and extension, abduction and adduction, internal and external rotation both in flexion and extension. There is considerable variation in the 'normal' range of motion among individuals. The patient with hip pathology may well have significant reduction in movement secondary to pain, bony abnormalities and degenerative changes. The accurate determination of hip movements needs care, as restriction of hip movement is easily masked by movement of the pelvis. This is particularly important with adduction and abduction as the pelvis easily moves and you can significantly overestimate degrees of movement. As such, it is essential to place one hand on the pelvis while the other supports and moves the leg.

Hip extension is important for various athletic activities such as sprint running and jumping. A lack of hip extension may lead to an over-striding gait and increased impact forces during running.

Flexion

The examination process flows best if hip flexion is tested immediately after a Thomas test.

Hip flexion is normally tested in the supine position with the knee flexed to prevent hamstring tightness restricting movement (Figure 8.7). Active flexion is tested first, followed by passive. In the normal hip, flexion

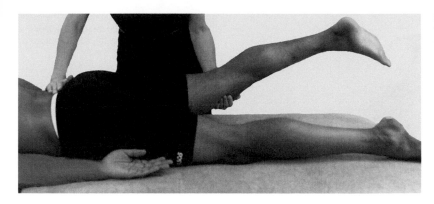

Figure 8.8 Hip extension. Performed in the prone position. It is best to have the knee flexed when performing this manoeuvre.

is limited by the soft tissues of the thigh and abdomen. Tilt of the pelvis increasing the range of flexion is best detected by grasping the crest of the ilium. Normal flexion is recorded from 0° to between 100° and 135°.

The primary flexor of the hip is the iliopsoas muscle. Iliopsoas power is assessed by having the patient sit on the edge of the examination couch with the legs dangling down. The patient is then asked to raise the thigh from the table. The examiner places their hands on the distal thigh and assesses muscle power.

Extension

Extension is not commonly tested except in the more athletic patient. However, when tested it is best measured in the prone position with the knee either flexed or straight (Figure 8.8). The natural tendency is for the patient to augment hip extension by hyperextending their spine. Therefore, maximum extension is assessed when the pelvis begins to rotate. The normal range is reported to be from 0° to between 15° and 30°. Extension, especially in the older arthritic patient, is painful and does not need to be tested.

The main hip extensor muscle is gluteus maximus, with contributions from the hamstrings. Power of gluteus maximus is best assessed by asking the prone patient to lift the leg off the couch with the knee flexed. This minimises the effect of the hamstring muscles.

Abduction

Hip abduction is measured with the patient lying supine and the pelvis stabilised with the examiner's hand on the opposite anterior superior iliac spine (ASIS) (Figure 8.9a,b). There are other ways described for fixing the pelvis:

1. Examiner's hand can be on the ipsilateral ASIS – especially useful in a large patient.

2. The contralateral leg can be placed to hang over the other side of the couch to fix the pelvis – difficult if that hip is also arthritic.

Normal ranges are from 0° to between 40° and 45°. False abduction is detected when the contralateral ASIS moves.

Abductor strength is assessed by one hand stabilising the pelvis while the other applies resistance to the lateral thigh as the patient abducts. Alternatively, with the patient lying on the side, they can be asked to abduct against resistance. Flexing the knee relaxes the iliotibial band and isolates the abductors.

An abduction deformity is present when the angle between the transverse axis of the pelvis and the limb is greater than 90°. Abduction in flexion is often the first movement to be restricted in osteoarthritis of the hip. The patient flexes their hips and knees by drawing the heels towards the buttocks. The knees are then allowed to fall away towards the couch. The normal range is approximately 70°.

Adduction

True adduction can only be measured if the contralateral leg is in a position of abduction (Figure 8.10). If it is in a neutral position, then a degree of pelvic tilt comes into play as the examined leg crosses over the contralateral static leg. Hip adduction is measured with the patient lying supine and, as with abduction, the pelvis needs to be stabilised when measuring the range of movement. Normal ranges are from 0° to between 20° and 30°.

Adductor strength is measured by resisting adduction of the abducted leg in the supine position. The examining hand is placed on the medial side of the knee. Alternatively, in the lateral position the patient can be asked to adduct against resistance.

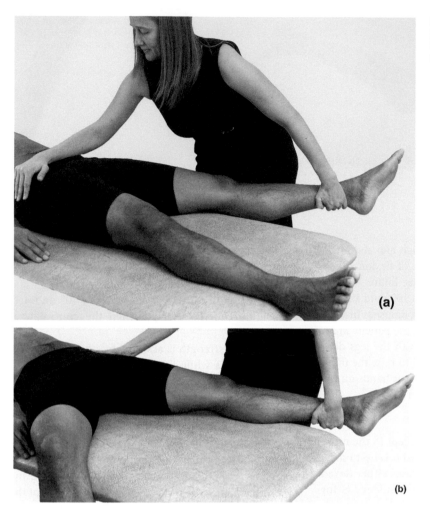

Figure 8.9a,b Hip abduction. The pelvis is stabilised either by (a) the examiner's hand or (b) hanging the contralateral leg over the side of the couch.

(a)

(b)

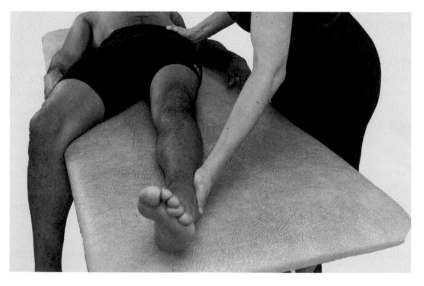

Figure 8.10 Hip adduction. This is best performed if the contralateral leg is first abducted out of the way.

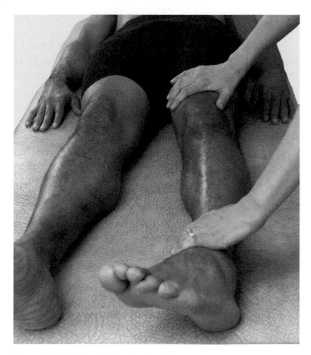

Figure 8.11 Hip rotation in extension.

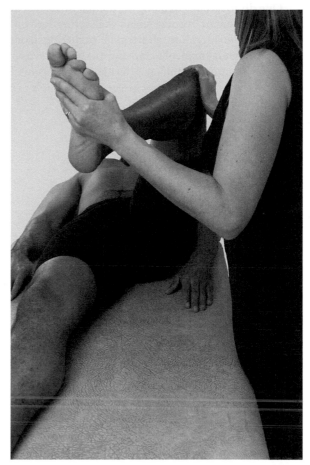

Figure 8.12 Hip external rotation in flexion.

Rotation in Extension

Internal rotation is considered normal if the hip rotates from 0° to between 30° and 40°. External rotation is slightly greater and is recorded from 0° to between 40° and 60° (Figure 8.11). It is preferable to use an imaginary line from the patella, as opposed to the foot, to act as a pointer for measurement. Alternatively, rotational movements can be measured with the patient lying prone with the hip extended and the knee flexed at 90°. This method would be less suitable for the older or more obese patient.

Rotation in Flexion

Early signs of hip pathology (e.g. an irritable hip) can be picked up by evaluating rotation in flexion. External rotation is usually greater except in cases of excessive femoral neck anteversion. The range for internal rotation is from 0° to between 30° and 40°, with external rotation from 0° to between 40° and 50° (Figure 8.12).

Historically, one of the reasons why rotation is performed both in flexion and extension is that (especially in the young patient) a significant difference in movement between the two may give an indication of an abnormally shaped femoral head.

Measurements of Leg Length

It is important to know whether any leg length inequality present is 'real' or 'apparent' (Figure 8.13). Although it is usually necessary to measure for real discrepancy, it is not so for apparent inequality, unless there is fixed pelvic obliquity. However, *if the pelvis is squared, it then takes out of the equation an abduction or adduction deformity (apparent discrepancy), and therefore any leg length discrepancy now seen is 'real' or 'true'.*

Ideally, for **true leg length** it would be best to measure from the centre of the femoral head, the normal axis of hip movement. However, as there is no surface landmark, then the nearest fixed point, the ASIS, is chosen. Distally, real leg length measurements are taken to the medial malleolus (Figure 8.14a).

143

One disadvantage of using the medial malleolus as the distal extent of 'true leg length' is that this does not take into consideration shortening occurring from below the medial malleolus for example with previous calcaneal fractures, subtalar arthritis and congenital

talipes equinovarus (CTEV). In these cases, it would be more accurate to use the block test.

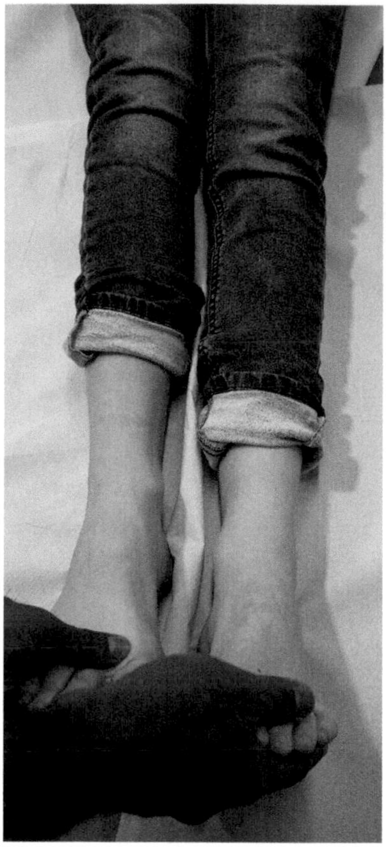

If there is a fixed deformity, the good leg must be placed in a comparably deformed position relative to the pelvis before measurements are taken. If this is not done, measurements will be inaccurate, as the angle between the leg and pelvis will be different on the two sides. *For this reason, it is better to assess leg length measurements after hip movements and any fixed deformities are noted.*

In some other fixed deformities such as a varus or valgus knee, true leg length has to be assessed in segments, as the degree of deformity is unlikely to be the same on both sides. In addition, the examiner will not be able to recreate the deformity on the contralateral side. In such a case, prominent bony landmarks should be used to assess leg length in segments (Figure 8.14b). These landmarks are usually the ASIS, the medial condyle and the medial malleolus.

Apparent shortening is measured from a fixed midline point in the body, usually the bony xiphisternum (Figure 8.14c). The umbilicus may not be central or may be diseased so is probably best avoided. Remember, adduction makes the limb appear shorter – each 10° of fixed adduction adds a further 2.5 cm of apparent shortening to any real shortening that the disorder may have caused.

If there is shortening of the limb, decide if the shortening is above or below the knee. If both knees

Figure 8.13 Patient with an obvious leg length discrepancy. The next step will be to square the pelvis and quantify with a tape measure.

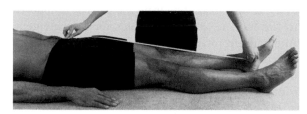

Figure 8.14a Real leg length measurements. The unaffected side is placed in the same position as the affected in order to compare.

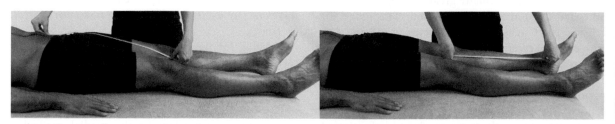

Figure 8.14b Measuring leg length in segments using ASIS, medial condyle and medial malleolus as the bony landmarks. Useful for measuring leg length if there is significant knee varus or valgus.

are flexed while the heels remain together on the couch, it can be seen whether shortening is in the femur or tibia (Figure 8.15). This is called the **Galeazzi's test**. It is best to assess for femoral shortening by looking from the side and to assess for tibial shortening from looking from the foot of the bed.

Having determined that the limb length inequality is in the femur, then decide if the shortening is coming from above the trochanter (suggesting a problem in or near the hip joint) or below the trochanter.

X-rays would obviously tell the answer, but there are clinical measurements that can be taken. However, in everyday clinical practice they are not often used. The tests described for shortening above the greater trochanter include Bryant's triangle, Nelaton's line and Schoemaker's line.

Bryant's Triangle

With the patient lying supine, a perpendicular line is dropped from the anterior superior spine of the ilium; this meets a second line projected upwards from the tip of the greater trochanter. The length of this second line is compared between the two sides (Figure 8.16). Relative shortening on one side indicates that the femur is displaced upwards as a consequence of a problem in or near the hip joint. If the pathology is bilateral, Bryant's triangle is not helpful.

Nelaton's Line

The patient lies with the affected side uppermost. A tape measure or string is stretched from the ischial

tuberosity to the anterior iliac spine. Normally, the greater trochanter lies on or below the line; if the trochanter lies above the line, the femur has been displaced proximally.

Schoemaker's Line

A line is projected on each side of the body from the greater trochanter through and beyond the anterior superior iliac spine. Normally, the two lines meet in the midline above the umbilicus. If there is a proximal femoral problem, the lines will meet away from the midline on the opposite side. If the problem is bilateral,

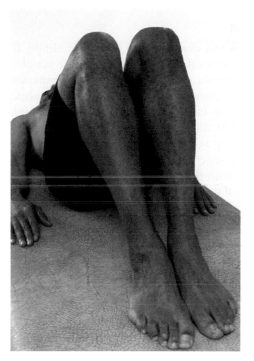

Figure 8.15 Galeazzi's test. Placing both heels together on the examination couch allows the examiner to determine whether a leg length discrepancy is above or below the knee. Tibial shortening causes the affected knee to lie lower than the unaffected side. Femoral shortening causes the knee to adopt a more proximal position.

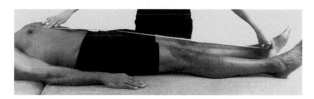

Figure 8.14c Apparent leg length measurements are taken from the medial malleolus to a midline structure such as the umbilicus or xiphisternum.

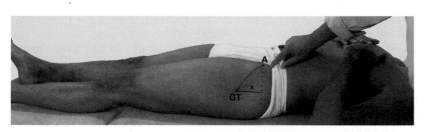

Figure 8.16 Bryant's triangle. A perpendicular line is drawn downwards from the ASIS. A second line is drawn proximally from the tip of the greater trochanter. The length of this second line is compared to the contralateral side.

A, anterior superior iliac spine; GT, greater trochanter; x, distance to be compared to contralateral side the lines will meet at or near the midline but below the umbilicus.

Special Tests

Soft Tissue Evaluation of the Hip

General

Joint hypermobility should be assessed with the Beighton score. The performance of a single leg squat, which activates gluteal musculature, can be used to assess subtle abductor weakness or irritation associated with (FAI or intra-articular pathology.

Log-Roll Test

The log-roll test evaluates hip joint pain simply by moving the femoral head in relation to the acetabulum and the joint capsule. The patient lies supine, and the examiner places their hands on the limb, gently rolling the hip into internal and external rotation. A positive test elicits pain, but its absence does not exclude the hip as a source of symptoms.

Capsular laxity and instability of the hip can also be assessed with this test. The examiner rolls the leg from internal to external rotation and then lets the leg rest in whatever position it naturally adopts. The test is positive when there is no obvious endpoint and the affected limb lies in more external rotation than the unaffected side. This indicates possible laxity of the iliofemoral ligament.

Impingement Tests

These are especially important to perform in the younger and more athletic patient that presents with hip or groin pain. **Femoroacetabular impingement (FAI)** is the encompassing diagnosis.[5] *It is important to understand what happens in FAI in order to perform the impingement tests.*

Femoroacetabular impingement is a movement-related problem of the hip involving premature contact between the acetabulum and the proximal femur which can result in pain.[6,7] FAI syndrome is associated with certain varieties of morphology of the hip joint (Figure 8.17a,b). Note that 30% of the population have either a cam or pincer morphology and are asymptomatic:

1. Cam morphology – a flattening or convexity of the femoral head–neck junction, e.g. aspherical femoral head, decreased head-to-neck ratio and

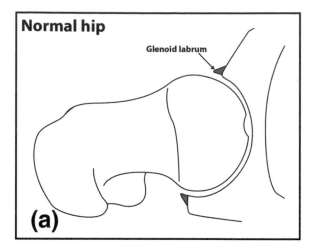

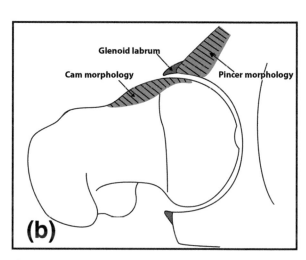

Figure 8.17 (a) Normal hip. (b) Hip with cam and pincer morphology.

femoral neck retroversion. This is more common in young males.

2. Pincer morphology – 'over-coverage' of the head by the acetabulum, e.g. acetabular protrusio, acetabular retroversion and coxa profunda. This is more common in middle-aged females.

3. Mixed cam and pincer – 80–85% of patients have a mixed morphology.

Both types of morphology can lead to damage of the articular cartilage and acetabular labrum due to impingement. This can eventually lead to osteoarthritis. This damage due to impingement can occur circumferentially but especially anteriorly and posteriorly.

The **anterior impingement test,** also known as the flexion, adduction and internal rotation (**FADIR**) test, is a moderately sensitive and specific test to reveal any intra-articular hip pathology, in particular a torn acetabular labrum or anterior rim FAI.[8] With the patient supine, the hip is flexed to 90°, then adducted and internally rotated (Figure 8.18). A positive test reproduces the patient's pain in the groin. A positive test may sometimes be accompanied by a clicking or popping feeling.

A posterior impingement test is useful to identify any conflict between the posterior acetabular wall and the femoral neck. For this test, the patient lies supine at the edge of the examination couch with the affected leg dangling. The contralateral leg is held in either extension or preferably in flexion while the examiner fully extends the affected hip while abducting and externally rotating the leg (Figure 8.19). Note this manoeuvre is the *opposite* to FADIR.

The Patrick or **FABER** (flexion, abduction, external rotation) test may be used to differentiate pathology within the sacroiliac joint from pain arising from the posterior aspect of the hip.[9] It is also a valuable test for posterior impingement. The patient lies supine, placing their ipsilateral foot on the contralateral knee. This is the so-called Figure-4 position. The ipsilateral leg is then allowed to relax, and the leg will be seen to drop outwards to a variable degree. When the endpoint of this manoeuvre has been reached, the examiner places one hand on the flexed knee and the other on the ASIS of the contralateral side and presses gently downwards on the flexed knee (Figure 8.20). Increased pain can be elicited but with different localisation of symptoms for the sacroiliac joint and posterior hip. The test is performed bilaterally.

The **FABER distance** is measured for both legs as the vertical distance between the knee and the examination table. It will be reduced in the presence of

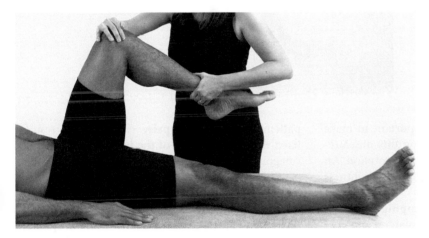

Figure 8.18 Anterior impingement test. Passive flexion of the hip to 90° with adduction and internal rotation.

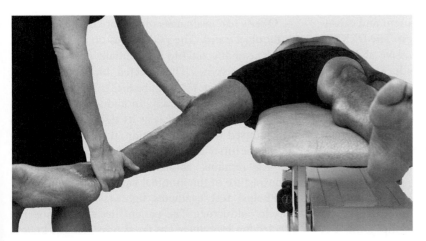

Figure 8.19 Posterior impingement test. The patient is positioned at the edge of the examination table and passive extension, abduction and external rotation of the hip are performed.

147

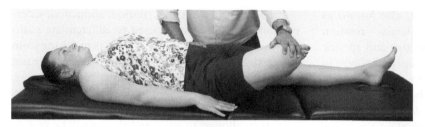

Figure 8.20 The Patrick (FABER) test. The patient lies supine while placing the ipsilateral foot on the contralateral knee, the Figure-4 position. The examiner places one hand on the flexed knee and the other on the ASIS of the contralateral side and presses gently downwards on the flexed knee.

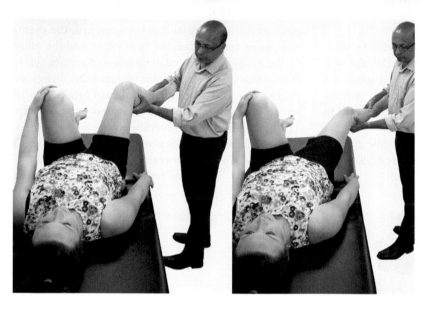

Figure 8.21 DEXRIT test. The hip is taken from 90° flexion or beyond and dynamically taken through a wide arc of abduction and external rotation to extension. The contralateral hip is fully flexed at the same time.

posterior hip impingement. It is important to make sure the pelvis does not rotate during this measurement to avoid overestimation of external rotation. An increased FABER distance suggests capsular tightness and irritation or psoas irritation

The dynamic external rotation impingement test (DEXRIT) is an assessment of superolateral and posterior femoroacetabular impingement. Patients with antero-inferior hip instability, antero-inferior acetabular hypoplasia, torn teres ligament and capsular laxity may also exhibit a positive test. The DEXRIT includes a wide-arc movement of passive abduction and external rotation that may reproduce a patient's pain. The patient lies supine and holds the contralateral leg in flexion to establish the zero set point of the pelvis. The examined hip is dynamically taken from 90° flexion or beyond through an arc of abduction and external rotation to extension (Figure 8.21).

Tests of Hip Contractures

These are useful tests to perform on patients who present with tightness around their hip joint, e.g.

patients with cerebral palsy. The Thomas test for fixed flexion deformity of the hip also falls into this category.

Ely's test is used to evaluate a tight rectus femoris. The patient lies prone, and the knee is passively flexed. If the rectus femoris is contracted, then the patient's hip, on the same side as the flexed knee, will spontaneously rise. Normally, the hip will remain flat against the examination couch (Figure 8.22).

Ober's test evaluates contracture of the fascia lata or iliotibial band. The patient lies on the unaffected side. The unaffected hip is maximally flexed to flatten the lumbar spine. The affected hip is flexed and abducted at least 45° (Figure 8.23). This hip is then slowly extended. Normally, in abduction and extension the ilio-tibial band is at its tightest. If the leg is now released from this position, it will be possible to adduct the hip to the midline. If this proves difficult or the leg remains abducted, this is indicative of a contracture of the iliotibial band.

Phelps' test evaluates tightness in the gracilis muscle (adductor). The patient lies supine, and the affected hip is abducted as far as possible. The knee is

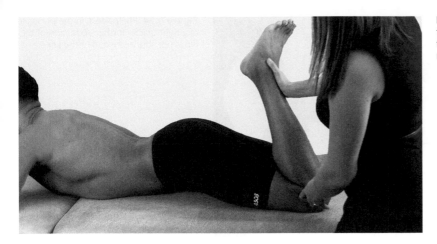

Figure 8.22 Ely's test. Passive flexion of the knee in the presence of a tight rectus femoris leads to the ipsilateral buttock rising.

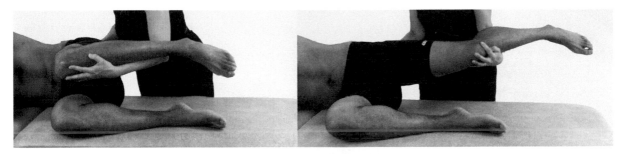

Figure 8.23 Ober's test. The patient lies on the unaffected side. The affected hip is flexed and abducted 45⁰. This hip is then slowly extended. Normally in bringing the hip into extension, it will be possible to adduct the hip to the midline. In the presence of a tight iliotibial band, the leg remains abducted.

then flexed over the side of the couch (Figure 8.24). If more abduction is possible by flexing the knee (and relaxing the gracilis), then this signifies that the gracilis is tight.

Neurovascular Examination

Finally, having examined the hip, it is important to carry out a vascular and neurological examination of the whole limb. This is especially important if any surgical procedure is to be performed on this limb.

Advanced Corner

Iliopsoas Test

Straight leg raise against resistance is also known as the **Stinchfield test**. It is an assessment of iliopsoas strength and also a sign of intra-articular pathology as the iliopsoas presses against the acetabular labrum during active resistance. The patient performs an active straight leg raise to 45° and is asked to resist as the examiner pushes downwards on the affected leg. A positive test is noted when pain is elicited or weakness of iliopsoas identified (Figure 8.25).

Hip Examination and Some Arthroplasty Considerations

- Patients with a loose hip arthroplasty often complain of 'start-up pain'. This is pain felt in the anterior thigh or knee at the beginning of ambulation. This pain often subsides after 5–10 minutes, only to recur later, resulting in the patient having to stop and rest. Patients with a loose femoral component often experience thigh pain when asked to perform an active straight leg raise in the supine position.
- When there is a reduced range of motion, hip arthroplasty surgery involves the release of

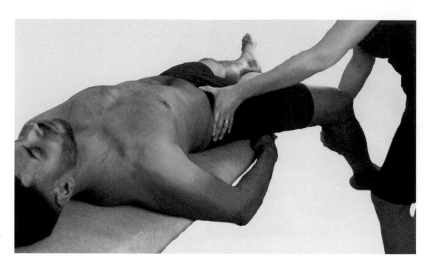

Figure 8.24 Phelps' test. In the presence of a tight gracilis further abduction of the hip is possible on flexion of the knee.

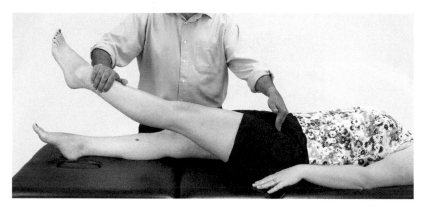

Figure 8.25 Stinchfield test to test for iliopsoas. The patient actively flexes to 45°, then resists a downward pressure by the examiner.

contracted soft tissue (periarticular adhesions) and muscle around the hip joint, excision of a thickened joint capsule and removal of any osteophytes. This improves range of movement, reduces apparent leg length discrepancy and leads to an improved functional outcome.

- When the Thomas test reveals a significant fixed flexion deformity of the hip, arthroplasty surgery is likely to be technically more difficult with more bleeding, difficulties with hip exposure, increased risk of dislocation and leg length discrepancy issues.
- Be wary of a patient requiring revision hip surgery who demonstrates a severe Trendelenburg gait when walking. If possible, plan an approach to the hip joint that avoids violating the abductor mechanism. Warn the

patient that they may still likely be limping with abductor weakness after surgery, especially if the Trendelenburg test is also strongly positive.

Other Impingement Tests

Ischiofemoral impingement (IFI) is an uncommon cause of hip pain caused by abnormal contact between the ischium and the lesser trochanter of the femur. In the **ischiofemoral impingement (HEADER – hip extension, adduction, external rotation) test,** the patient is positioned supine, the ipsilateral knee is flexed to 90° and the hip is then extended, adducted and externally rotated. A positive test elicits pain deep within the groin and/or medial aspect of the buttock.

The **piriformis test** evaluates pathology within the piriformis muscle itself or irritation of the sciatic nerve by the muscle's margin. The patient lies on their side with the affected side uppermost. The hip is then flexed to 45° and the knee to 90°. With one hand, the examiner stabilises the pelvis and with the other adducts the flexed hip. This manoeuvre stretches the piriformis muscle. Localised pain over the piriformis muscle suggests tendonitis, but when the pain is along the course of the sciatic nerve, this may be an indication of entrapment of the sciatic nerve by the piriformis muscle itself.

Snapping Hip

(Internal): Iliopsoas tendon snapping (coxa saltans interna). This is a well-recognised pathological hip condition particularly seen in young athletes such as ballet dancers. On occasion, the iliopsoas tendon can snap over the anterior capsule or iliopectineal ridge during hip movements. This is because the iliopsoas tendon moves from lateral to the iliopectineal ridge in flexion to medial in extension.[10] To identify this, the examiner brings the ipsilateral hip from flexion, abduction and external rotation (similar to FABER) into extension, adduction and internal rotation (opposite of FABER). The test is positive when there is an audible click or clunk, which can sometimes be painful. This usually occurs at 30° to 45° of flexion (Figure 8.26a,b). The diagnosis can be confirmed with a dynamic ultrasound scan. Surgical treatment can be by tenotomy.

(External): Iliotibial band (ITB). This is especially seen in women because of the wider pelvis. The ITB snaps over the greater trochanter. To test for it, the patient lies on the side with the affected side uppermost. The patient actively flexes their hip and then adducts. From this position, it is passively brought by the examiner into extension and abduction. A snap is felt over the greater trochanter (Figure 8.27a,b).

References

1. Byrd JW. Physical examination. In Byrd JW (ed), *Operative Hip Arthroscopy*. New York: Springer, 2005; pp. 36–50.

2. Beals RK. Painful snapping hip in young adults. *West J Med* 1993;159:481–482.

3. Hardcastle P, Nadi S. The significance of the Trendelenburg test. *J Bone Joint Surg* 1985;67 (5):741–746.

4. Thurston A. Assessment of fixed flexion deformity of the hip. *Clin Orthop* 1982;169:186–189.

5. Griffin DR, Dickenson EJ, O'Donnell J, et al. The Warwick Agreement of femoroacetabular impingement syndrome (FAI syndrome): an international consensus statement. *Br J Sports Med* 2016;50(19): 1169–1176.

6. Frangiamore S, Mannava S, Geeslin AG, et al. Comprehensive clinical evaluation of femoroacetabular impingement: part 1, physical examination. *Arthrosc Tech* 2017;6(5):e1993–2001.

(a)

(b)

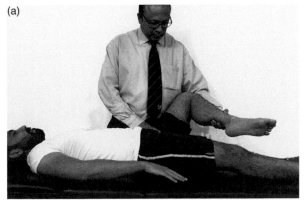
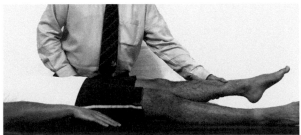

Figure 8.26a,b Internal snapping hip. Iliopsoas tendon snapping. (a) Bring the ipsilateral hip from flexion, abduction and external rotation (Figure-4 position) into (b) extension, adduction and internal rotation. The test is positive when there is an audible click or clunk, which can sometimes be painful. This usually occurs at 30° to 45° of flexion.

(b)

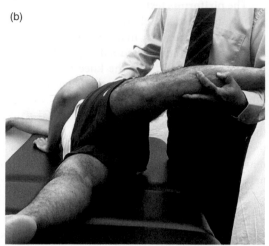

(a)

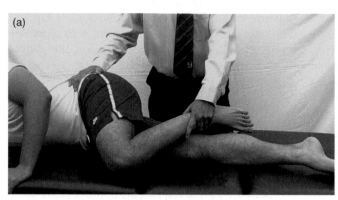

Figure 8.27a,b External snapping hip. Iliotibial band snapping. (a) The patient lies on their side with the affected side uppermost. Patient actively flexes their hip and then adducts. (b) From this position, it is passively brought by the examiner into extension and abduction. A snap is felt over the greater trochanter.

7. Ratzlaff C, Simatovic J, Wong H, et al. Reliability of hip examination tests for femoroacetabular impingement. *Arthritis Care Res (Hoboken)* 2013;65(10):1690–1696.

8. Shanmugaraj A, Shell JR, Horner NS, et al. How useful is the flexion-adduction-internal rotation test for diagnosing femoroacetabular impingement: a systematic review. *Clin J Sport Med* 2018; 30 (1):76–82.

9. Broadhurst N, Bond M. Pain provocation tests for the assessment of sacroiliac joint dysfunction. *J Spine Disorders* 1998; 11:341–345.

10. Via A, Floruzzi A, Randell F. Diagnosis and management of snapping hip syndrome. A comprehensive review of literature. *Rheumatology* 2017;7(4).

Examination of the Knee

Jeevan Chandrasenan, Derek Bickerstaff and Fazal Ali

Steps in Knee Joint Assessment

A. History
B. Clinical Examination

Step 1

Stand the patient and look

Step 2

Walk the patient and look

Step 3

Sit the patient down and look

• Assess patella height, tracking and crepitus

Step 4

Lie the patient down

• Look (quantify quadriceps wasting)
• Feel for effusion and tenderness
• Move

Step 5

Assess ligaments

• Cruciates
• Collaterals

Step 6

Further tests based on the findings above:

• Meniscal stimulation tests
• Other ligaments
• Patellofemoral tests
• Consider rotational profile and Beighton's score
• Examine hip

Stand and Look

On standing the patient, inspect from the front, side, both laterally and medially and the popliteal fossa at the back. Note any scars, wasting, swelling or deformity. It is also important to comment on the Q angle and rotational profile whilst looking from the front.

Walk

Comment particularly on any obvious varus or valgus lurch, as well as foot and patella progression angles.

Sit

Whilst the patient is sitting with the legs hanging over the side of the couch, look at the patella height. Ask them to extend their knee, in particular looking at the patella tracking and the J sign, which may be present in patients with ligamentous laxity with patella instability. Feel for crepitus.

Lie Patient Down

Look, Feel, Move, Then Test the Ligaments

Look

Especially look at the quadriceps and quantify quadriceps wasting by measuring from a fixed point, e.g. anterior superior iliac spine.

Feel

Effusion.

▪ Wipe or bulge test for mild effusion.
▪ Patellar tap for moderate effusion.
▪ Ballottement test for significant effusion.

Continue feeling by resting hands over knee and palpating the popliteal fossa, joint line, tibial tubercle, patella tendon and medial and lateral collateral ligaments in turn.
Palpation is with the knee first in extension (for effusion testing) then 90° flexion.

Move

First, assess extension by asking the patient to straight leg raise and then lifting both heels in the hands and assessing any degree of recurvatum. Flexion is assessed first actively and then passively, comparing both knees.

Ligaments

Cruciate Ligaments

- Flex both knees to 90° with heels together. Observe from the side and look for a posterior sag. If there is a sag, then perform the quadriceps active test.
- In the quadriceps active test, the foot is fixed and the patient is asked to extend their leg. In the presence of a posterior sag, the tibia will be pulled forwards to a neutral position by the contraction of the quadriceps muscle.
- Next, perform the anterior and posterior draw test.
- Then, perform the Lachman's test with the knee flexed to 20°–30°.
- Note that pivot shift test is not usually recommended for the examination or in clinics, as this test is most commonly and reliably performed in the anaesthetic room, as it can be quite painful.

Collateral Ligament

Test the medial collateral ligament (MCL) and the lateral collateral ligament (LCL) in extension and then in 30° of flexion.

Further Tests

The above sequence is carried out in all cases of knee examination. After testing the ligaments, proceed in one of **three** directions depending on the previous findings:

1. If there is the likelihood of meniscal pathology, then meniscal provocation tests may be performed.
2. If there is ligamentous pathology, then assessment of the posterolateral corner should be carried out. The most common test for this is the dial test.
3. If the findings indicate patellofemoral pathology, then other patellofemoral tests can be carried such as patella glide test, patella apprehension test and Clarke's test. In these, patient's rotational profile and/or Beighton's score assessment must also be considered, as they can be associated with patella maltracking.

History

General Questions

Patients usually present with a combination of symptoms relating to pain, swelling, locking,

clicking and giving way. These form the basis of the specific questions asked when taking a history. The diagnostic specificity of each of these symptoms in isolation is poor; rather, they are used in combination to guide the examiner to a differential diagnosis. In addition, the presence and degree of each of these symptoms at presentation and then how they changed with the passage of time are important.

It is then important to ascertain the duration of symptoms, exact details of the mechanism of injury and then the general course of events, including response to any treatment already received.

Other key questions include occupation, sport and lifestyle.

Specific Questions

Pain

The site of pain within the knee is an indication as to the structure damaged but is by no means diagnostic, particularly with traumatic disorders such as meniscal tears. As an example, lateral joint pain from a patellofemoral disorder is frequently mistaken for a lateral meniscal tear. The site of pain following an episode of injury, however, such as an MCL strain, is a clear indication of the possible structures involved. It is useful to obtain a description of the pain at the time of injury or presentation and then how the pain has progressed. Of particular importance is whether the pain is constant and whether it occurs at night. For instance, these symptoms are an indication to recommend arthroplasty in assessing a patient with severe degenerative changes. Constant pain may indicate more sinister pathology such as tumour or infection.

It is then important to relate the pain to the level and type of activity, such as whether the symptom appears after a few steps of walking or only after running. In addition, questions about the pain related to specific actions such as twisting and turning may indicate a problem with the main weightbearing areas of the knee such as a meniscal tear or chondral defect. Bent knee activities such as kneeling, crouching or squatting may indicate a patellofemoral problem, though posterior horn tears of the medial meniscus are aggravated by loaded bent knee activities such as coming up from a squatting position. Patients with patellofemoral problems also have exacerbation of symptoms ascending or descending slopes and stairs.

The examiner should always be aware of the possibility of referred pain from the hip or lumbar spine, particularly when assessing a patient with degenerative symptoms.

Swelling

Swelling can be outside the joint, such as with a lateral meniscal cyst, or inside the joint, such as with a haemarthrosis. The timing of the swelling is important. Immediate swelling or within a few hours is an indication of haemarthrosis. Gradual swelling indicates effusion.

Generalised swelling may be secondary to a haemarthrosis, which is generally defined as swelling appearing within 4 hours of an injury. The main differential diagnosis in a traumatic haemarthrosis is an anterior cruciate ligament (ACL) rupture, an osteochondral fracture (often associated with a patella dislocation) or a peripheral meniscal tear. Indeed, if an athlete gives a history of a twisting injury on the sports field followed by swelling within 4 hours, they have a 70–80% chance of having sustained an ACL rupture.[1] The commonest misdiagnosis in this setting is to confuse an ACL rupture with a lateral patella dislocation. Indeed rarely, both can occur together.[2] Both occur on the slightly flexed weightbearing knee forced into external rotation. This reinforces the need for a skyline radiograph in the acutely injured knee to identify a possible osteochondral fragment from the patellofemoral joint that occurs in patella dislocation.

Haemarthoses are painful due to the degree of tension within the knee. A relatively painless haemarthrosis or diffuse swelling rather than true haemarthosis should alert the examiner to the possibility of a more extensive ligamentous injury with disruption of the capsule. The examiner can be lulled into thinking the injury is less severe than is the case. However, in these cases there is usually bruising extending down the calf, which should alert the surgeon to capsular damage.

Locking

Locking can be subdivided into true locking and pseudo-locking. True locking is relatively rare. It occurs when an intra-articular structure, loose body or meniscal tear, interposes between the femoral condyle and tibial surface. Classically, the patient can lose *terminal extension* but is able to flex the knee (though usually also losing some terminal flexion which is less noticeable). Loose bodies may also be felt by the patient in the suprapatella pouch but more commonly in either the medial or lateral gutter. They are classically elusive and once found immediately move to another area, hence their eponym of 'joint mouse'.

Pseudo-locking is a far more common presentation, and usually occurs in patients with anterior knee pain secondary to some form of patella maltracking. Classically, it is associated with marked pain and there is no movement of the knee.

Giving Way

There are two types of giving way: true giving way, which is usually associated with some form of ligamentous instability, and a buckling type of sensation, which is usually associated with anterior knee pain and the symptom of pseudo-locking previously described.

An example of true giving way is seen in ACL instability. The patient has no problem running in a straight line, but on planting the foot and twisting with the upper body internally rotating, the knee suddenly collapses.

Instability from chronic medial insufficiency usually presents with difficulty performing cutting movements rather than rotation. Isolated posterior cruciate ligament (PCL) rupture does not usually present with instability unless there is associated posterolateral or posteromedial instability. In these situations, the knee again feels unstable with rotatory movements but also on walking downstairs due to the unimpeded anterior displacement of the femur on the tibia.

Buckling of the knee is frequently seen in patients with anterior knee pain. These patients often report their knee buckling without any rotary movement, usually occurring when walking in a straight line or down stairs. The knee buckling is rarely associated with an effusion.

Examination

Examination of the knee should follow the usual orthopaedic routine of inspection, palpation, movement and ligaments. This is sequence is followed for all knee examinations. Following this, specific tests related to the presumed diagnosis should be then addressed – e.g. patellofemoral pathology, meniscal tears or other ligaments.

One must always remember to use the opposite limb for comparison, and to gain the patient's trust, leave any possible painful tests to the end. A tense patient will make any assessment of subtle instabilities impossible.

The examination should start immediately as the patient enters the clinic to assess their gait, walking aids and general mobility. To fully assess the patient, however, they should be undressed from mid-thigh.

Inspect (Look)

Initial inspection should begin with the **patient standing** to assess overall limb alignment and any shortening.

The **Q angle** (quadriceps angle) has an influence on patellofemoral symptoms by affecting the line of pull of the quadriceps muscle on the patella. It is the angle between a line drawn from the anterior superior iliac spine and the midpoint of the patella, with another line drawn from the tibial tubercle through the midpoint of the patella (Figure 9.1). It averages 15°, with females being slightly more and males slightly less because of the width of the pelvis.

Limb alignment includes any femoral or tibial rotational malalignments, which also have a bearing on knee function (Figure 9.1a).

The foot position should be assessed for evidence of any abnormalities such as hyperpronation, which again can affect patellofemoral function. It is easier at this stage to assess the posterior aspect of the knee for scars, swellings or bruising. The anterior aspect can be

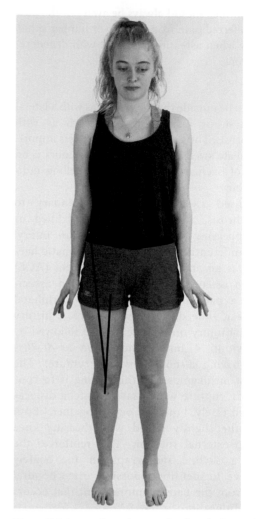

Figure 9.1 Inspect the patient standing from the front, side and back. The 'Q angle' is the angle formed between a line drawn from the anterior superior iliac spine to the midpoint of the patella and a line drawn from the tibial tubercle through the midpoint of the patella.

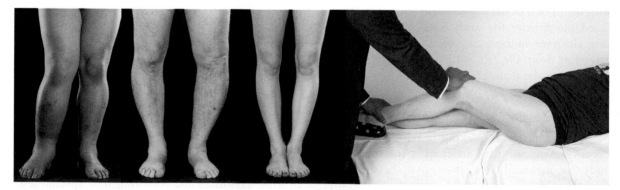

Figure 9.1a From left to right: valgus right knee; bilateral varus knees; young patient with miserable malalignment syndrome with both patellae pointing inwards; fixed flexion deformity of the knee.

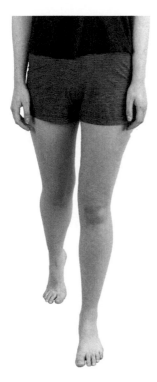

Figure 9.2 When walking, look for rotational abnormalities as well as any varus or valgus lurch.

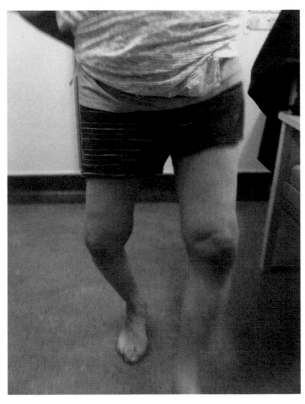

Figure 9.2a Patient walking with a varus lurch as they weightbear on the right leg. This would represent osteoarthritis of the medial compartment or lateral ligament incompetence.

assessed at this stage or later when the patient is supine.

The next step is to observe the gait pattern whilst **walking**. There should be sufficient room to watch the patient walking both towards and away from the examiner (Figure 9.2). As the patient walks, it is important to observe the foot progression angle (angle that the foot makes with an imaginary straight line: normal 10°–15° external) and the patella progression angle (angle that the patella makes with an imaginary straight line: normal 0°). This would indicate rotational malalignment.

A varus or valgus thrust may also be an important sign. A valgus thrust may indicate lateral compartment osteoarthritis or medial ligament laxity. A varus thrust may indicate medial compartment osteoarthritis or lateral ligament laxity or posterolateral corner (PLC) injury (Figure 9.2a). With the PLC injuries, the varus may be combined with recurvatum/hyperextension at the knee joint. It may be helpful to observe whether the patient walks with a foot drop, as 20% of patients with these PLC injuries also have a common peroneal nerve palsy.

Next, have the patient **sit down** with the legs hanging over the side of the couch (Figure 9.3). Patella height is best demonstrated here. Ask the patient to extend and flex the knees to feel crepitus and to observe patella tracking. A J-sign can be observed in some cases. Here the patella moves centrally and then subluxes laterally as the knee comes into extension. This is seen in some cases of patella instability, commonly in tall individuals with generalised laxity. Unless the patient has been examined in this sitting position with the legs hanging over the edge of the couch, this J-sign can be missed.

The patient is now **laid supine** on the examination couch with their head relaxed on a pillow and their hands placed on their chest. A patient straining to watch an examination may increase muscle tone, affecting observations such as knee laxity. As well as inspecting the anterior aspect of the knee for scars, swellings or bruising, any quadriceps or calf wasting

157

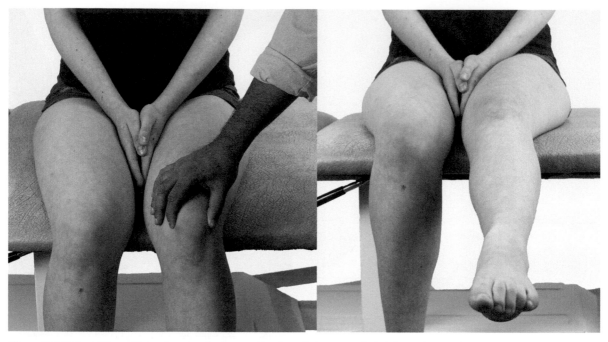

Figure 9.3 Patient sitting with legs hanging freely over side of couch. Assess patella height, tracking and crepitus.

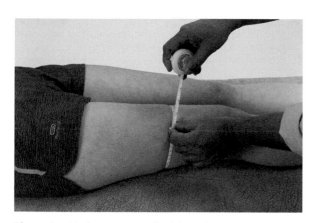

Figure 9.4 Lie the patient comfortably on the couch. Muscle bulk may be assessed by measuring the circumference of the thigh from a fixed point such as the anterior superior iliac spine.

can be observed and measured from a fixed bony point such as the anterior superior iliac spine (Figure 9.4).

Palpate (Feel)

There are three basic tests for the presence of an effusion: the ballottement test, the patellar tap test and the wipe (or bulge) test. The **ballottement test** checks for

a massive effusion and is performed like a fluid thrill test for abdominal ascites. In this test, pressure on one side is transmitted via the fluid to the hand on the other side of the knee. The **patellar tap test** is performed for moderate effusion (Figure 9.5a). A hand is placed over the suprapatellar pouch and pressed on to occlude this space. The patella is then pressed on with the other hand in order to allow the patella to touch the femoral trochlea. In the presence of a moderate effusion, this gives the sensation of a tap. The **wipe/bulge test** is performed for a small effusion (Figure 9.5b). Here the suprapatellar pouch is occluded with one hand. Then the lateral gutter is stroked and the fluid is observed to move across to the medial side with a bulge (or vice versa).

If there is the appearance of swelling in the knee and yet no effusion, one must consider synovial hypertrophy as seen in conditions such as pigmented villonodular synovitis.[3]

The knee joint is largely subcutaneous apart from posteriorly, and as such many structures can be **palpated** directly. The anatomical location of the tenderness is usually a good indicator of the underlying pathology. This is best done with the knee bent up to 90° with the foot firmly planted on the examination couch in a neutral position (Figure 9.6). The fingers can then be

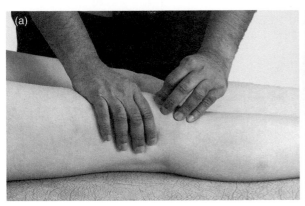
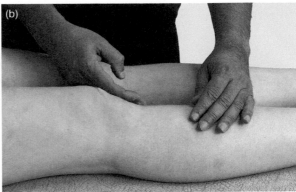

Figure 9.5a,b (a) Patellar tap for moderate effusion. (b) Bulge test for small effusion. If necessary a hand can be placed on the suprapatellar pouch to occlude the space.

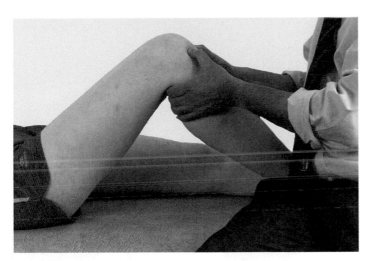
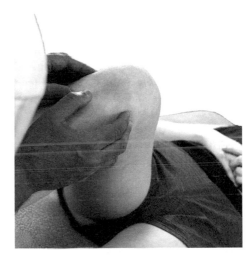

Figure 9.6 Palpation of the knee joint is best done in the flexed knee. Illustration is showing palpation of popliteal fossa and patella tendon followed by palpation of the joint line.

used to palpate along the joint lines starting with the painless side. Tenderness along the joint line, particularly posteromedially, may indicate a meniscal tear. The borders of the femoral and tibial condyles, the patella tendon and medial (MCL) and lateral (LCL) collateral ligaments can also be palpated for tenderness.

The patella tendon should be palpated in full extension and then tensed at 90° of flexion. In chronic patella tendinosis, tenderness in the proximal tendon is more noticeable in extension (**Bassett's sign**) compared to flexion. In flexion, the normal superficial fibres cover the damaged deep fibres, resulting in less pain on palpation.

The posterior aspect of the knee should also be palpated to identify soft tissue masses in the popliteal fossa, which may not have been evident on inspection.

Move

The assessment of movement relates to active and passive movement of the joint (Figure 9.7). The normal range of passive movement is assessed comparing both sides and including hyperextension. The range can be noted as degrees of movement. Alternatively, hyperextension can be

159

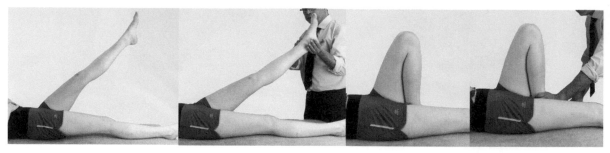

Figure 9.7 Range of movement involves extension and flexion. Here, active straight leg raising demonstrates an intact extensor mechanism. Passive extension performed by allowing the patient to place the weight of their leg in the examiner's hand will demonstrate hyperextension if present. Active flexion should be followed by passive if necessary.

measured as the distance the heel can be lifted off the examination couch and flexion by the heel-to-buttock distance.

The patient should be asked to actively perform a straight leg raise to assess the integrity of the extensor mechanism and flex the knee as far as possible. If a straight leg raise is not performed, then an extensor lag may be missed. This is seen, for example, in patients who previously had a patellectomy or a chronic quadriceps rupture or repair.

After active straight leg raise, hold the leg up by the heel and ask the patient to relax their leg whilst you lift the weight of the leg. This allows the examiner to demonstrate any hyperextension in the joint.

Ligament Testing

ACL and PCL Instability

The first step in assessing anterior cruciate ligament (ACL) or posterior cruciate ligament (PCL) instability involves both knees viewed from the side when flexed to 90° to identify any **posterior sag** indicating PCL injury. The levels of the tibial tubercles are compared (Figures 9.8 and 9.8a). If this is not recognised, anterior movement from an abnormally posteriorly placed tibia may be misinterpreted as anterior instability.

A variation to the posterior sag is to flex the hip to 90° and hold the heels of the leg with the knee bent also to 90° **(Godfrey's test)**. A posterior sag will be evident (Figure 9.8b).

If there is a positive posterior sag, then the **quadriceps active test** can be performed. This test works by contractions of the quadriceps being transmitted to the tibial tubercle via the patella and the patella tendon. It is performed by fixing the foot and asking the patient to

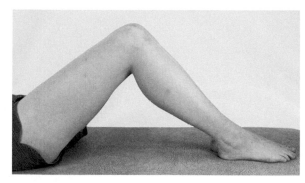

Figure 9.8 Cruciate ligament testing starts with both knees flexed to 90° and observing the level of the tibial tubercles from the side (posterior sag).

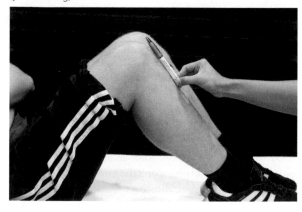

Figure 9.8a A positive posterior sag indicating a ruptured PCL. A pen placed on the surface of the tibial tubercle on both sides will demonstrate the difference.

try to extend the leg (Figure 9.9). If there is a posterior sag, the quadriceps will pull the tibia forwards.

In the **anterior and posterior drawer tests,** the knees are flexed to 90° and the feet are fixed to the couch. Sitting on the patient's foot is described.

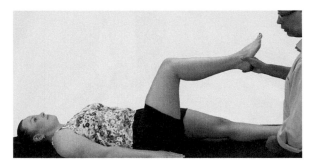

Figure 9.8b Godfrey's test. Another method of demonstrating a posterior sag.

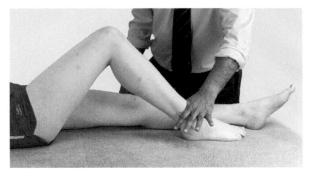

Figure 9.9 Quadriceps active test to confirm the posterior sag. Examiner's hand holds the foot, and the patient is requested to straighten their knee against resistance. The quadriceps contraction will reduce the tibia to a neutral position.

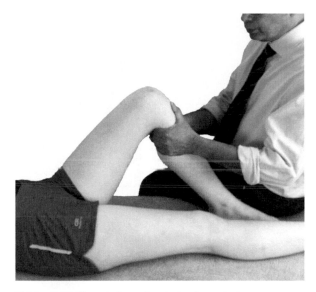

Figure 9.10 The anterior and posterior drawer tests.

However, this is not usually necessary and can be painful. Both hands are used to grasp the upper tibia with the thumbs on the tibial tubercles (Figure 9.10). At this angle of flexion, the anterior tibial condyles should be anterior to the corresponding femoral condyles. From the neutral position, excessive movement forwards indicates a positive anterior drawer sign and excessive movement backwards indicates a positive posterior drawer sign. A positive posterior drawer sign suggests a PCL rupture. A positive anterior drawer sign suggests an ACL rupture. However, because secondary restraints such as the posterior capsule prevent the tibia coming forwards, a positive anterior drawer sign would suggest an

injury not only to the ACL but also to the secondary restraints.[4]

The most reliable test for ACL instability is the **Lachman test**, because at 20° of flexion the ACL is isolated by relaxing the posterior capsule and the other secondary restraints, the collaterals.

With a knee of normal size, the best technique is to grasp the distal femur with one hand holding the femur still while flexing the knee to 20° and then the other hand grasps the proximal tibia and displaces the tibia anteriorly (Figure 9.11a). The amount of anterior displacement is then estimated and can be graded.

Grading is the degree of translation and graded as I (3–5 mm), II (5–10 mm) or III (>10 mm).

The presence or absence of an endpoint is important to note. An endpoint grade A indicates a firm and sudden endpoint to passive anterior translation of tibia on fixed femur, whilst a grade B is given for an absent, ill-defined or softened endpoint and is indicative of a complete rupture.

For patients with large thighs or examiners with small hands, it is better to fix the femur over the examiner's flexed knee whilst displacing the tibia with the other hand (Figure 9.11b).[5]

The other classic test for ACL instability is the **pivot shift test,**[6] which can be performed a number of different ways, though the basic principle is the same. The pivot shift test recreates the anterolateral subluxation of the tibia on the femur, which results in the 'giving way' sensation experienced by the patient when twisting on a planted foot. The pivot shift test measures the rotational component of ACL function, whereas the anterior

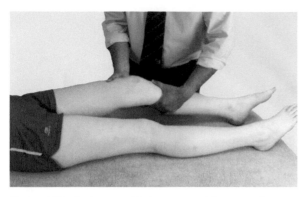

Figure 9.11a Lachman test is the most sensitive test to detect an ACL insufficiency. It is performed with the knee flexed to 20°.

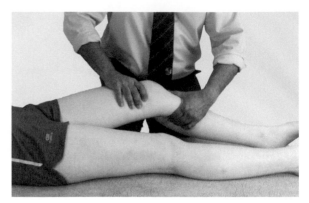

Figure 9.11b In patients with large thighs, the Lachman test may be better performed in the position shown here, with the examiner's thigh under the patient's thigh and one hand clasping the front of the patient's thigh in order to steady it.

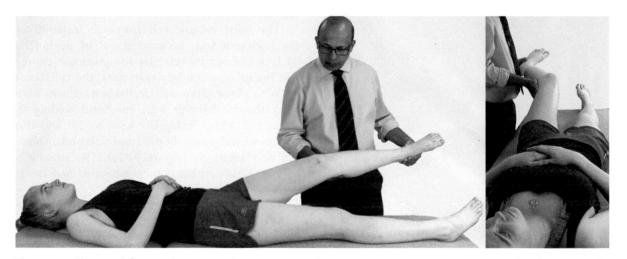

Figure 9.12 The pivot shift test. In the presence of an ACL injury, the tibia is subluxed when an internal rotation and valgus force is applied to the knee. If there is an intact MCL, the ITB reduces the tibia as the knee goes into flexion.

drawer and Lachman tests measure the anteroposterior stability.

In this test, the patient's leg is held in full extension and the lower leg is then internally rotated and a valgus strain applied to the knee via the laterally placed hand. In this position, the tibia is anterolaterally subluxed. The knee is then flexed gently, and at about 20° the tibia suddenly reduces, which can be seen in obvious cases and palpated in more subtle cases (Figure 9.12). This reduction is a result of the iliotibial band (ITB) being tense and pulling the joint back into place.

As such, the degree of instability is increased if the hip is abducted as this decreases tension in the ITB.[7] It is not possible to perform this test with medial instability (MCL rupture), as the medial pivot is lost. The key to this test is obtaining the patient's confidence as if performed too forcibly, it can be distressing for the patient. Sometimes, with the leg securely held by the hands around the knee, the patient feels more confident, which allows this test to be performed gently and quickly. This test is more commonly performed under anaesthetic rather than in clinics or examinations.

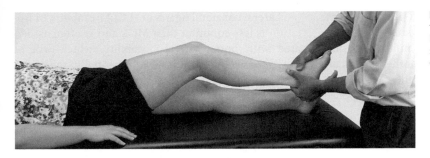

Figure 9.12a Flexion-rotation drawer test. By holding the ankle instead of the knee, this method of performing the pivot shift test may be found to be a bit more comfortable by the patient.

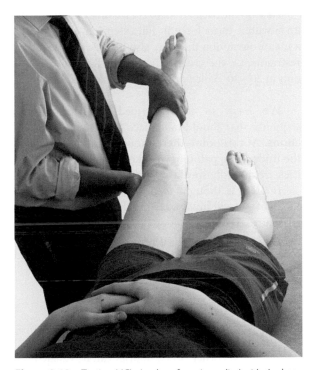

Figure 9.13a Testing MCL. A valgus force is applied with the knee extended then this is repeated with the knee flexed to 20°.

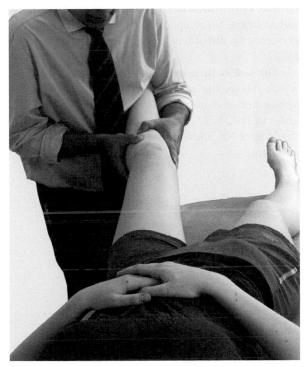

Figure 9.13b Alternative way of holding the leg to test for the collateral ligament.

There are different variations to the pivot shift test, mainly to make it more comfortable. In one, a reverse method is described (**jerk test**) where the knee is first flexed with the tibia in the reduced position and then subluxes as it extends, whilst applying the valgus force and internal rotation.

In another (**flexion-rotation drawer test**), the same manoeuvre as the standard pivot shift is performed, but instead the *ankle* is grasped with both hands and then the flexion, valgus and internal rotation are applied indirectly from the ankle (Figure 9.12a).

MCL and LCL Instability

The medial collateral ligament (MCL) injuries result in the commonest form of knee instability.

The superficial MCL is the main restraint to valgus forces through the knee. The deep MCL (meniscofemoral and meniscotibial ligaments) provide less restraint. The posteromedial capsule also provides an important restraint in extension, but in flexion it is lax and therefore has less of a role in flexion.

To examine the MCL, the leg is held with one hand above and the other hand below the knee

163

(Figure 9.13a). It is first placed in full extension. A valgus force is then applied to the knee by pushing the lower hand away from the midline against the laterally placed upper hand. In another technique, the lower leg is held between the elbow and body and a similar direction of forces applied (Figure 9.13b).

The degree of opening can be assessed, but the most important point is whether there is a soft or hard endpoint. If there is no endpoint with the leg in full extension, this signifies a major disruption of the knee with additional damage to the posteromedial capsule and the cruciate ligaments, which act as secondary stabilisers to valgus strain. Some opening with an endpoint may be present with disruption of only the deep fibres of the MCL.

The test is then performed in 20°–30° of flexion, which relaxes the secondary restraints and allows an assessment of mainly the superficial but also the deep fibres of the MCL. Again, an assessment is made as to the degree of movement and the presence of an endpoint.

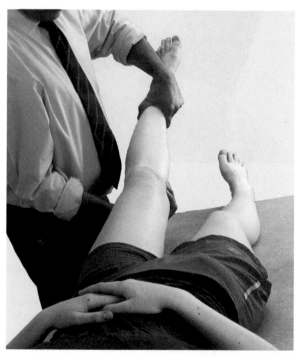

Figure 9.14 Testing LCL. A varus force is applied with the knee extended. It is then repeated with the knee flexed to 20°. Note that from testing the MCL to testing the LCL, the examiner's right hand has moved in such a way that the palm acts as the fulcrum for the MCL and then the fingers act as a fulcrum for the LCL.

Lateral collateral ligament (LCL) instability in isolation is less common than MCL and is often associated with posterolateral instability, which will be described in the next section. Essentially, the test is the same as for the MCL except the forces are exerted in the opposite directions to those described for the MCL. This will mean the position of the examiner's hands have to be adjusted (Figure 9.14). There is normally greater laxity in the lateral structures compared to the medial and thus care should be taken to interpret the findings and so it is best to compare any opening of the joint with the uninjured knee.

As with the MCL, if there is excessive opening of the knee with a varus force in full extension, this signifies a major disruption that may also include the secondary restraints, i.e. the cruciate ligaments. If the opening is only at 20°–30° of flexion, then it is an isolated LCL tear.[8]

We have so far described the examination sequence that should take place for all knee examinations. At this point, there should be an idea of what the underlying pathology is likely to be. The possibilities are, broadly speaking, arthritic or soft tissue.

If there is thought to be ligament damage, then further tests will involve testing the other ligamentous structures. If the pathology is thought to be meniscal, then meniscal stimulation tests should be performed. If patellofemoral, then tests of the patellofemoral joint should be performed.

Further Tests

Posterolateral Instability

Posterolateral corner (PLC) injuries can be isolated but are more commonly associated with PCL and ACL injuries. If this is not recognised, the cruciate ligament reconstructions may fail in the absence of a corrective osteotomy and/or a separate reconstruction of the PLC.

There are many tests described to diagnose posterolateral instability. Some of the more common ones will be described here. The key to the clinical examination features is increased external rotation. These patients may also walk with a pronounced varus/lateral thrust. Always remember to look for any signs of common peroneal nerve injury in these patients.

The **external rotation recurvatum** test involves lifting one or both legs off the couch by grasping the great toes (Figure 9.15). In a positive result, the knee goes into varus and hyperextension (recurvatum) and externally rotates. When positive, this usually

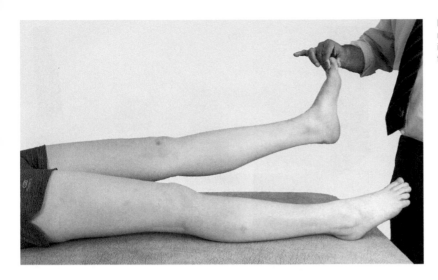

Figure 9.15 The external rotation recurvatum test for posterolateral corner injuries. Both legs can be lifted by the toes for comparison.

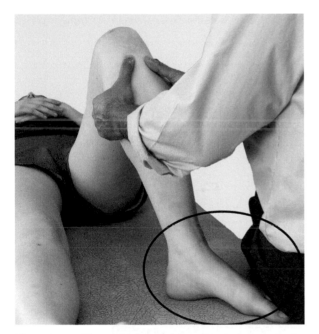

Figure 9.15a The posterolateral drawer sign is demonstrated by performing the posterior drawer test in neutral alignment, internally rotated and externally rotated. An increase in magnitude of the posterior drawer in external rotation indicates a PLC injury.

represents a significant injury with the posterolateral corner including an LCL rupture.

The **posterolateral drawer sign** is demonstrated by performing the posterior drawer test in neutral alignment, with the tibia internally rotated and then with the tibia externally rotated (Figure 9.15a). An

increase in magnitude of the posterior drawer in external rotation indicates a PLC injury.[9]

The **dial test** is passive external rotation of the tibia (relative to the femur), with the knee at 30° and 90° of flexion (Figure 9.16a,b). This is best performed with the patient prone. The knees are kept together in order to prevent rotation at the hips. It is also best to control the rotation of the tibia by grasping above the ankles. The feet indicate the degrees of rotation from neutral. In the rare case of isolated PLC injury, increased external rotation (greater than 10° difference between the two feet) is noted at 30° but less so at 90°. When combined PCL and PLC injuries are present, increased external rotation is noted in both positions (Figure 9.16c).[10]

The dial test utilises the fact that the posterior cruciate ligament is active when the knee is in 90° of flexion but inactive at 30°. The posterolateral corner normally resists the external rotation forces; therefore, the foot will externally rotate more than the contralateral side with a PLC injury. Hence, if the PCL is also ruptured, there will be no restriction at 90°, and the foot will continue to externally rotate, indicating a combined PCL and PLC injury. If the PCL is intact, the increase of external rotation will be less at 90° compared to the external rotation at 30°.

Meniscal Pathology

The diagnosis of a meniscal tear is usually from the history and the presence of joint line tenderness. Meniscal stimulation tests have a wide-ranging sensitivity and specificity (see Chapter 1, Table 1.4).

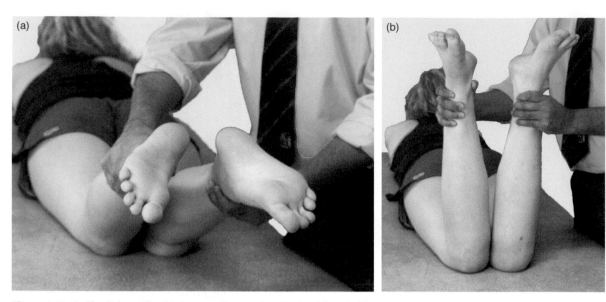

Figure 9.16a,b The dial test. The tibia is externally rotated at (a) 30° and (b) 90° of flexion. Note that the knees are placed together to prevent hip movements and the legs are held above the ankles to prevent movement in the ankles.

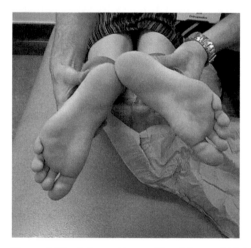

Figure 9.16c Patient with a positive dial test, which indicates a posterolateral corner injury. With a combined PLC and PCL injury, the increased external rotation is present at both 90° and 30°. In an isolated PLC injury, there is increased external rotation at 30° compared to 90°.

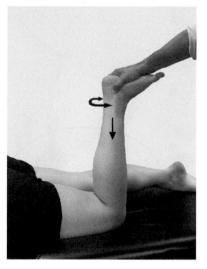

Figure 9.17 Apley grind test. Examiner pushes down the axis of the leg and rotates.

The absence of positive signs does not rule out a meniscal tear.

The following clinical tests are infrequently performed in a clinical setting, but the Thessaly test has the highest accuracy in detecting a meniscal tear with 94% for medial meniscal and 96% for lateral meniscal tears.[11]

The **Apley grind test** is historical and involves forcing the tibiofemoral surfaces together to 'catch' the meniscus. In this test, the patient is prone with the knee flexed to 90° and the examiner pushes downwards on the foot and rotates the leg (Figure 9.17).

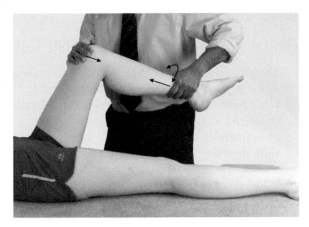

Figure 9.18 McMurray's test is a provocation test for meniscal pathology.

McMurray's test was to recreate displacement of a meniscal tear which is painful and probably not in the patient's best interests. A modification of this is a compression test to produce discomfort along the joint line, which may indicate pathology in the medial or lateral compartment.[12] The patient is supine with the knee flexed. The examiner places one hand on the top of the knee with the fingers and thumbs positioned to palpate the joint line and the other under the heel or holding the ankle (Figure 9.18). The examiner can then compress the joint by pushing down on the top hand while the lower hand controls flexion and can also rotate the leg, thereby stressing each compartment in varying degrees of flexion. This test is most specific for a tear of the posterior horn of the medial meniscus.

Childress' test. Another, less specific test is to ask the patient to fully squat, and if possible, duck walk. This action compresses the posterior horns of the menisci but can also cause patellofemoral pain.

Thessaly test. Here the patient is asked to stand on one leg at a time: first, the unaffected leg as a trial, then the affected leg (Figure 9.19). The examiner holds the patient's hands to prevent them overbalancing. The patient flexes their knee to 5° and then internally rotates and externally rotates their knee and body three times. This is repeated with the knee flexed to 20°. Pain, locking or catching represents a positive result. The test is more sensitive at 20° compared to 5°.

Sometimes when a patient presents with symptoms and signs of a meniscal tear, radiographs or magnetic resonance imaging (MRI) instead show appearance of

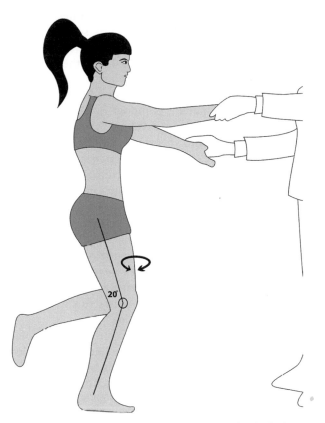

Figure 9.19 Thessaly test. The patient is supported and asked to stand on one leg in turn. The leg to be examined is flexed 5°, and the patient is asked to rotate three times. This is then repeated at 20°.

osteochondritis dissecans. Although not very sensitive, **Wilson's test** may prove the diagnosis. To perform this test, the patient is supine, and both the hip and knee are flexed to 90°. The examiner then passively internally rotates the lower leg and then extends it fully. In a positive test, the patient experiences discomfort at terminal extension as the ACL impinges on the area of osteochondritis on the lateral part of the medial femoral condyle.

Patellofemoral Pathology

The commonest patellofemoral pathologies include maltracking, which manifests in pain, subluxation or frank dislocation and osteoarthritis.

An assessment of this patient will first include looking for *generalised* joint laxity. Following this, the patient is examined *regionally*, whereby the overall alignment of the leg including rotational profile is assessed. Third, a *local* examination of the patellofemoral joint is performed.

167

Examine for lateral retinacula tightness, which one finds with patella tilting such as seen in excessive lateral pressure syndrome. To do this, the patella should be just engaged in the femoral trochlea.

In the **patellar glide test,** the knee is flexed slightly and the patella is moved maximally medially and laterally (Figure 9.20a). If one imagines the patella split into quadrants, the patella should be able to move at least one quadrant medially; any less indicates lateral retinacula tightness. The medial retinaculum is naturally more lax, but movement of greater than two quadrants laterally indicates laxity in the medial retinaculum which one may see in recurrent patella dislocation. With the patella held in this lateral position, the knee is now flexed and the patient's reaction observed (Figure 9.20b). A positive **patellar apprehension test** is seen when the patient resists further flexion for fear of the patella dislocating.

Clarke's test is used to demonstrate patellofemoral pathology such as chondromalacia and patellofemoral arthritis. In performing this test, put a hand over the suprapatellar pouch with gentle pressure on the superior pole of the patella (Figure 9.21). Ask the patient to contract the quadriceps or to attempt straight leg raise. Pain in the patellofemoral joint indicates pathology is present.

Advanced Corner
Clinical Significance of the Pivot Shift Test

- The pivot shift tests for the rotational component of the ACL. A positive pivot shift is believed to result from a tear of the ACL plus the anterolateral ligament (ALL) of the knee. It is currently recommended that if a patient has a positive pivot shift, then the ALL should be reconstructed or an anterolateral tenodesis performed.[13]
- When treating partial tears of the ACL, it is recommended that if the pivot shift test is negative, then conservative treatment can be tried. However, if it is positive, then ACL reconstruction is advised.[14]

Reverse Pivot Shift Test

This is another test for the postcrolateral corner of the knee that is frequently used. It can be painful, so its use is mainly under anaesthesia. It has a low sensitivity of 25% but a high specificity of 95%.[15]

This test is performed as follows (Figure 9.22): The patient is supine. The hip and knee are both flexed to 90°. Allow the foot to rest on the examiner's anterior superior iliac spine so that axial load can be exerted by the examiner's pelvis. The examiner then externally

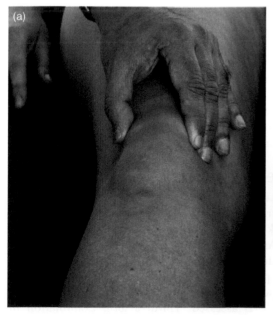
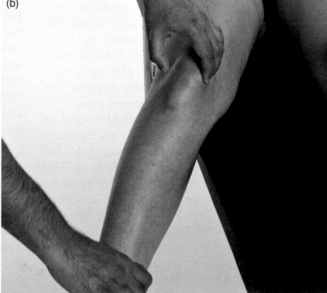

Figure 9.20a,b. Assessing patella stability by (a) patellar glide test (b) patellar apprehension test.

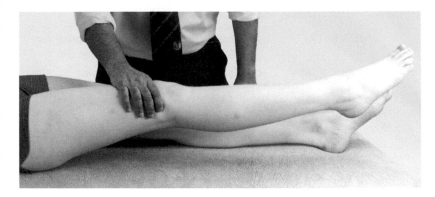

Figure 9.21 Clarke's test for patellofemoral problems. A hand is placed on the superior pole of the patella. The patient is asked to contract the quadriceps by attempting to perform a straight leg raise.

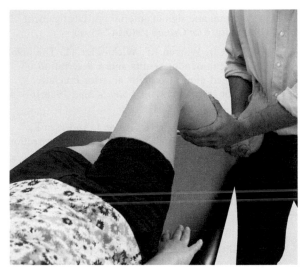

Figure 9.22 Reverse pivot shift test. For posterolateral corner injuries. In this test the tibia is first subluxed in the flexed position. It is then reduced by the ITB as the knee goes into extension.

rotates the leg and provides a valgus force. This subluxes the tibia posterolaterally. The knee is then straightened while the axial load, external rotation and valgus are applied. At about 20°, there is a 'clunk' as the subluxation is reduced. This is because at 20° the ITB changes from a flexion vector to an extension vector and therefore pulls the tibia anteriorly and reduces the subluxation.

Anteromedial Rotatory Instability

Injury to the PMC of the knee (especially the posterior oblique ligament) usually is not isolated and involves other ligaments and is frequently part of a multi-ligament knee injury. The MCL is most commonly involved, but it can be the ACL and also the PCL.

Failure to recognise an injury to the PMC may therefore predispose to failure of reconstructions of the MCL, ACL or PCL.[16]

PMC injuries, especially those associated with MCL injuries, result in anteromedial rotatory instability (AMRI).

To test for AMRI: The patient is supine and the knee flexed to 30° with a valgus force applied to it. At the same time, the foot is externally rotated. Opening of the joint in this position is a sign of AMRI.

Slocum Test

This test is a modification of the anterior drawer test and can be used to test for AMRI and antero-lateral rotatory instability (ALRI) by placing the foot in external rotation or internal rotation, respectively.[17]

The knee is flexed to 90° and the foot is placed in neutral, 15° external rotation and 30° internal rotation, in turn. An anterior drawer is performed. If there is subluxation of the anteromedial tibial plateau on external rotation, then this is suggestive of AMRI. If there is subluxation of the anterolateral tibial plateau on internal rotation, then ALRI is the diagnosis.

Anterolateral rotatory instability is suggestive of ACL rupture together with LCL and/or arcuate ligament.

Clinical Evaluation of the Acutely Injured Knee in the Child

This evaluation is more difficult to make in a child than in an adult. Children are poor historians; hence, information such as mechanism of injury may not be accurate. They may not be able to tolerate a painful clinical examination as well as an adult, and their ligaments are generally more physiologically lax

Table 9.1 Diagnostic accuracy of clinical examination and MRI in children (adapted from Kocher et al)[19]

Diagnosis	Sensitivity (%)		Specificity (%)		Positive predictive value (%)		Negative predictive value (%)	
	Clin Exam	MRI	Clin Exam	MRI	Clin Exam	MRI	Clin Exam	MRI
ACL tear	81.3	75.0	90.6	94.1	49.0	58.6	97.8	97.1
LM tear	62.1	79.3	80.7	92.0	14.5	34.3	97.6	98.8
MM tear	50.0	66.7	89.2	82.8	34.0	30.1	94.1	95.7

compared to adults, making interpretation of ligament rupture more difficult. Therefore, always remember to compare the injured limb with the other side.[18]

In the acutely swollen knee, apart from the usual differential diagnosis of ACL rupture, patella dislocation, peripheral meniscal tear and osteochondral fracture, children can also get sleeve fractures of the patella, epiphysiolysis and tibial eminence fractures. Therefore, a radiograph is essential in the early evaluation of these patients.

Both clinical examination and MRI are not as accurate in children compared to adults. The negative predictive values of clinical examination and MRI for ACL injuries and meniscal tears are higher than the positive predictive values (Table 9.1).

This means that if the clinical examination and MRI are negative for injury, then the chance of a patient having an ACL or meniscal injury is low. However, if the tests are positive, it does not mean that the clinician can always believe that the structures are injured. This contrasts with the adult, where if both are positive it is likely that the patient has sustained the injury (ACL or meniscus).[19]

References

1. Maffuli N, Binfield PM, King JB, Good CJ. Acute haemarthrosis of the knee in athletes. A prospective study of 106 cases. *J Bone Joint Surg Br* 1993;**75**(6):945–949.

2. Simonian PT, Fealy S, Hidaka C, O'Brien SJ, Warren RF. Anterior cruciate ligament injury and patella dislocation: a report of nine cases. *Arthroscopy* 1998;**14**(1):80–84.

3. Flandrey F, Hughston JC, McCann SB, Kurtz DM. Diagnostic features of diffuse pigmented villonodular synovitis of the knee. *Clin Orthop* 1994;**298**:212–220.

4. Torg JS, Conrad W, Kalen V. Clinical diagnosis of anterior cruciate ligament instability in athletes. *Am J Sports Med* 1976;**4**(2):84–93.

5. Draper DO, Schulthies SS. Examiner proficiency in performing the anterior draw and Lachman tests. *J Orthop Sports Phys Ther* 1995;**22**(6):263–266.

6. Galway HR, MacIntosh DL. The lateral pivot shift: a symptom and sign of anterior cruciate ligament instability. *Clin Orthop* 1980;**147**:45–50.

7. Bach BR Jr, Warren RF, Wickiewicz TL. The pivot shift phenomenon: results and a description of a modified clinical test for anterior cruciate ligament instability. *Am J Sports Med* 1988;**16**(6):571–576.

8. Nielsen S, Rasmusson O, Oveson J, Andersen K. Rotatory instability of cadaver knees after transection of collateral ligaments and capsule. *Arch Orthop Trauma Surg* 1984;**103**(3):165–169.

9. Reider B. *The Orthopaedic Physical Exam*, 2nd ed. Philadelphia: Elsevier Saunders, 2005.

10. Bae JH, Choi IC, Suh SW, et al. Evaluation of the reliability of the Dial test for posterolateral rotator instability: a cadaveric study using an isotonic rotation machine. *Arthroscopy* 2008 May;**24**(5):593–598.

11. Karachalios T, Hantes M, Zibis AH, et al. Diagnostic accuracy of a new clinical test (the Thessaly test) for early detection of meniscal tears. *J Bone Joint Surg* 2005;**87A**(5):955–962.

12. Solomon L, Warwick D, Nayagam S. *Apley's System of Orthopaedics and Fractures*, 8th ed. London: Arnold, 2001.

13. Dodds AL, Halewood C Gupte CM, Williams A, Amis AA. The anterolateral ligament: anatomy, length changes and association with the Segond fracture. *Bone Joint J* 2014;**56-B**:325–331.

14. DeFranco MJ, Bach BR. Current concepts review. A comprehensive review of partial anterior cruciate ligament tears. *J Bone Joint Surg Am* 2009;**91**:198–208.

15. Rubenstein RA, Shelbourne KD, McCarroll JR, VanMeter CD, Rettig AC. The accuracy of the clinical examination in the setting of posterior cruciate ligament injuries. *Am J Sports Med* 1994;**22**(4):550–557.

16. Dold AP, Swensen S, Straus E, Alaia M. The posteromedial corner of the knee: anatomy, pathology and management strategies. *J Am Acad Orthop Surg* 2017 Nov;**25**(11):752–761.

17. Larson RL. Physical examination in the diagnosis of rotatory instability. *Clin Orthop Relat Res* 1983;172:38–44.

18. Ardern CL, Ekås GR, Grindem H, et al. 2018 International Olympic Committee consensus statement on prevention, diagnosis and management of paediatric anterior cruciate ligament (ACL) injuries. *Br J Sports Med* 2018;**52** (7):422–438.

19. Kocher MS, DiCanzio J, Zurakowski D, et al. Diagnostic performance of clinical examination and selective magnetic resonance imaging in the evaluation of intraarticular knee disorders in children and adolescents. *Am J Sport Med* 2001;**29**:292–296.

Examination of the Foot and Ankle

Jimmy Ng, Yulanda Myint and Nick Harris

Assessment of the Foot and Ankle

A. History
B. Clinical Examination

Step 1
Stand the patient and look

Step 2
Walk the patient and look
Ask the patient to tiptoe

Step 3
Think – Special tests?
(Consider doing a single leg tiptoe test or a Coleman block test at this stage if the diagnosis is obvious)

Step 4
Sit the patient and look
Look at the sole of the foot, between the toes, shoes and walking aids

Step 5
Move

Step 6
Feel

Step 7
Other special tests

The above sequence of **look, move, feel, special tests** flows best. Palpation takes a long time to perform, and, in most cases, a provisional diagnosis can be made following inspection, walking and assessment of the joint movements.

Stand
When standing the patient, first look from the front, side and back and note any deformities or scars. Whilst looking from the back, it is important to observe the position of the heel and to look for any 'too many toes

sign', indicating tibialis posterior dysfunction. Always consider looking at the spine, as many foot and ankle problems are a manifestation of a neurological condition. Looking at the hands may give a clue to Charcot–Marie–Tooth in patients with pes cavus. In patients with flat feet, remember to look for underlying hyperlaxity (confirm by Beighton's scoring system).

Walk
Walking will give clues to the diagnosis. Foot and ankle pathology will almost always affect gait. Ask the patient to go onto tiptoes as a quick screen.
Before sitting the patient down, the examiner may prefer to do relevant special tests here rather than later on, e.g. the single leg tiptoe test if the patient has pes planus or the Coleman block test if the patient has a pes cavus.

Sit Patient Down
Sit the patient down and inspect the sole of the foot. Inspection of the foot is not complete without observing the sole and between the toes. This should now be a cue for looking at the shoes and walking aids.

Move
Depending on the underlying pathology, consider examining the joints from proximal to distal or distal to proximal. If the patient has possible ankle arthritis, then examine the ankle joint first. If the patient has a forefoot problem such as hallux valgus, then it may be more sensible to examine the distal joints first.

Feel
The foot and ankle joints are superficial, and therefore tenderness in a particular area would mean pathology in that underlying structure. It would also lead the clinical examination on to the relevant special test, e.g. tenderness in the third web space will lead on to Mulder's test, tenderness behind the medial malleolus would lead on to the tiptoe test.

Coleman Block Test

A patient with a cavovarus foot would have a plantarflexed first ray. In order to assess the flexibility of the hindfoot, a block is placed beneath the foot such that the first ray is not supported. If the heel is mobile, then it should adopt a valgus position. If it remains in varus, then it is a fixed deformity. This test is described in more detail later in the chapter.

Single Leg Tiptoe Test

Ask the patient to hold on to a stable support or put their hands on the wall so that they do not overbalance. Ask them to stand on tiptoes on both legs. Then ask them to repeat the manoeuvre on one leg. In the presence of a tibialis posterior tendon rupture, the patient will have difficulty doing this on one leg.

History

General

Age, sex, occupation and problems with shoewear must be elicited from patients with foot and ankle problems. Patients usually present with pain, swelling, stiffness, deformity, instability and paraesthesia. It is important to establish how their symptoms affect their activities of daily living, gait, hobbies and work.

There are several medical conditions that are relevant in managing patients with foot and ankle problems. Systemic conditions such as diabetes mellitus, inflammatory arthritis including rheumatoid arthritis, crystal arthropathies and vasculitis can cause pain, stiffness, swelling and/or deformity of the foot and ankle. They are usually bilateral, and management strategies will differ from degenerative conditions. Pitting oedema of the lower legs may represent underlying cardiac, renal or liver disease.

Painless unilateral swelling in a diabetic patient must be investigated for peripheral neuropathy and Charcot foot.

Neuromuscular conditions and spinal lesions such as a cerebral palsy, poliomyelitis, prolapsed intervertebral disc, spina bifida and spinal stenosis may also affect the foot.

History of smoking and alcohol consumption must be established. Smoking increases the risk of wound problems and non-union in fusion surgery, and excess alcohol consumption can lead to peripheral neuropathy.

Specific

Pain

The most important symptom in foot and ankle pathology is pain. Localised pain often directs the clinician to the diagnosis. Referred pain is uncommon except in entrapment neuropathies such as tarsal tunnel syndrome.

Ankle pain is often felt anteriorly especially in degenerate disease with impingement. Rheumatoid involvement in the ankle is less common than in the other joints of the foot and usually manifests as a tenosynovitis.

Pain in the subtalar joint is often localised below and behind the malleoli and also in the sinus tarsi. Vainio[1] stated that 60–70% of patients with rheumatoid arthritis will have involvement of the subtalar and midtarsal joints. The resulting deformity is one of valgus, with patients complaining that the foot is gradually 'going over'. Tibialis posterior tenosynovitis may exacerbate this.

Heel pain may be localised to either side of the calcaneus, especially in conditions such as insufficiency fractures of the calcaneus and Paget's disease. Pain at the insertion of the Achilles tendon, and plantar fascia is associated with systemic conditions such as gout, pseudogout and seronegative arthropathies especially when bilateral. Burning pain anterior to the medial calcaneal tuberosity on the plantar aspect of the foot worse with the first few steps in the morning is typical of plantar fasciitis. The presence of a plantar heel spur on plain radiograph neither confirms nor refutes the existence of plantar fasciitis. Pain located at the insertion of the Achilles tendon made worse with resisted plantarflexion activities is typical of Achilles tendinitis.

Pain and swelling *posterior to the medial malleolus* along the course of the posterior tibial tendon often reflects posterior tibial tendinitis. Any loss of the normal medial longitudinal arch as in acquired pes planus might also suggest attenuation or rupture of the posterior tibial tendon.

Posteromedial pain might also represent flexor hallucis longus tendinitis. Pain of this origin is typically made worse by movement of the hallux. In severe cases, triggering of the hallux can occur due to flexor hallucis longus tendon stenosis between the medial and lateral tubercles of the talus. Lateral ankle pain can be caused by peroneal tendinitis and instability.

Midfoot pain is less common than hindfoot and forefoot pain. Post-traumatic, degenerative and inflammatory arthritic conditions can all lead to

Table 10.1 Differential diagnosis of forefoot pain

Metatarsalgia		
Callosity	**No callosity**	
	Neuritic symptoms	*No neuritic symptoms*
Hallux valgus	Morton's neuroma	MTP instability
Bunionette	Tarsal tunnel syndrome	MTP joint capsulitis
Claw, hammer, mallet toes	PID	Stress fracture
IPK		

IPK, intractable plantar keratosis; MTP, metatarsophalangeal; PID, prolapsed intervertebral disc

Table 10.2 Acquired cavovarus foot

Differential diagnosis of acquired cavovarus foot	
Neuromuscular	• Cerebral palsy
	• Spinal dysraphism
	• Spinal cord tumour
	• Poliomyelitis
	• Hereditary motor and sensory neuropathy (Charcot–Marie–Tooth disease)
	• Muscular dystrophy
Structural	• Trauma

midfoot pain. In the diabetic patient swelling of the midfoot with or without pain is typical of Charcot neuroarthopathy of the midtarsal joint if there is no evidence of infection. Navicular stress fractures are also a cause of midfoot pain especially in athletes.

Forefoot pain or metatarsalgia has many causes. It is simplified by initially establishing whether the patient has an associated callosity, and second whether the patient has neuritic symptoms.[2] Table 10.1 outlines a simple algorithm to help in diagnosis. Patients with hallux valgus and lesser toe deformities complain of pain with shoewear and cosmesis.

Intractable plantar keratosis (IPK) usually occurs under the second or third metatarsals and is the result of either a transfer lesion because of medial column insufficiency (for example in hallux valgus) or because of problems with the ray itself such as metatarsal overlength.

Nerve compression or irritation can occur at many levels. An accurate history will help localise the pathology. Local lesions can cause narrowing of the tarsal tunnel such as a ganglion, schwannoma or lipoma. Patients with tarsal tunnel syndrome complain of vague diffuse burning pain and tingling over the plantar aspect of the foot, which is often worse with exercise. Occasionally, patients complain of pain radiating up the medial aspect of the leg (Valleix phenomenon).

In contrast, patients with a Morton's neuroma complain of a burning plantar pain well localised between the metatarsal heads. The pain often radiates to the toes of the involved interspace, usually the third and fourth. Atypical neuritic symptoms should alert the physician to more proximal lesions such as a prolapsed intervertebral disc and mononeuritis of diabetes.

Instability

Ankle instability presents in two ways, either recurrent sprains or a feeling of looseness when walking on uneven ground or wearing high-heeled shoes. Pain is an uncommon feature unless there is an associated talar lesion. Tarsal coalition may present with ankle instability.

Deformity

Acquired foot deformity in the adult typically presents with pain associated with overloading. The acquired cavovarus foot has either a neuromuscular or traumatic aetiology (Table 10.2). Patients with a cavovarus deformity often complain of pain under the metatarsal heads together with lateral instability. They also complain of uneven shoewear in the early stages. The acquired flat foot deformity in the adult often results from posterior tibial tendon dysfunction, rheumatoid disease, trauma, infection or tumour (classically osteoid osteoma). Pain is often felt medially over the prominent talar head and laterally due to impingement of the lateral talar process in the angle of Gissane. Tarsal coalition usually presents in childhood but can present in adults with a fixed planus deformity and ankle instability.

Examination

Inspection (Look)

The patient is first examined **standing**. The position of the heel in relation to the floor is best assessed from the back, as is any asymmetry of the calves. Swelling of the Achilles tendon or posteromedial or posterolateral aspects of the ankle is also best assessed from behind. In this position, the relationship between the long axis of

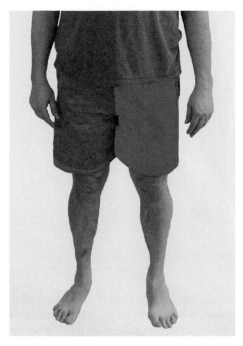

Figure 10.1a Stand the patient and look from the front, side and back. Pay particular attention to any deformity, the arches and the hindfoot. Remember to look at the spine.

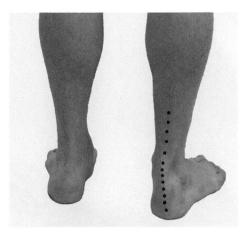

Figure 10.1b The tibiocalcaneal angle – usually 5° of valgus.

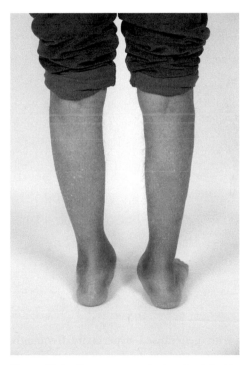

Figure 10.1c 'Too many toes sign' on the right. Up to 1.5 toes visible is normal. Three toes visible here signifies possible tibialis posterior rupture.

the tibia and the long axis of the os calcis should be commented on. This represents the tibiocalcaneal angle and is usually 5° of valgus (Figures 10.1a and 10.1b).

From behind the patient, it is also possible to comment on the amount of the forefoot visible. This has important implications in patients with posterior tibial tendon disruption, e.g. the 'too many toes sign' (Figure 10.1c). Normally, about one and a half toes are visible when looking from behind. More than this or asymmetry between the two sides indicates that the arch has dropped.

From the front, the examiner should start with the ankle, commenting on any swelling that might represent synovitis, an effusion or osteophytes (Figure 10.1d). Moving to the side, the examiner then comments on the medial longitudinal arch. The arch may be flatter than expected (planus) or higher than expected (cavus). There may also be deformity of the midfoot.

The forefoot can have many different deformities in the same foot. It is important to describe the deformities in a logical fashion, starting with the hallux and moving laterally. Skin and nail changes must be sought, especially in diabetic patients where ulceration is common and in patients with psoriasis where pitting of the nails can be found.

Many foot and ankle deformities have a neurological basis; therefore, it is important to inspect the lumbar spine for signs suggestive of spinal dysraphism such as a hairy patch, naevus, lipoma, dimple or sinus.

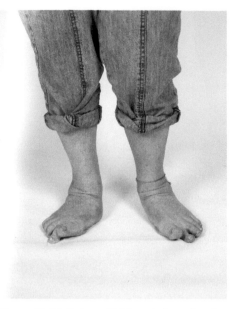

Figure 10.1d Patient with bilateral planovalgus feet as evident from the front.

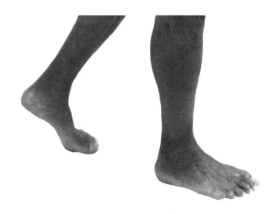

Figure 10.2 Walk the patient looking at the gait and the rockers.

Patients with generalised hyperlaxity frequently have foot problems such as flat feet. Beighton's scoring (Chapter 1) may confirm this.

Walking the patient may be regarded as part of inspection (Figure10.2). Walking can reveal disability, pain or stiffness. Patients with an arthritic ankle may have difficulty moving through the second rocker of gait. They may externally rotate the leg through the hip to compensate during gait in order to avoid the second rocker. Patients with an arthritic first metatarsophalangeal (MTP) joint will have difficulty with toe-off.

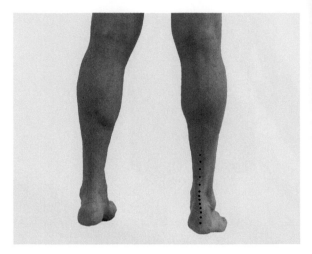

Figure 10.3 Ask the patient to tiptoe, observing the arches.

At the end of walking the patient is then asked to **rise onto tiptoes**. This serves as a useful screen and confirms that the gastrosoleus complex is functioning. If both heels adopt a varus position during this manoeuvre, this suggests that both tibialis posterior tendons are functioning (Figure 10.3).

At this point of the examination process, the examiner must decide if they would perform special tests if relevant to the underlying pathology. In postgraduate exams, this may look better as usually the provisional diagnosis is obvious from performing the previous steps (look, walk and tiptoe).

Therefore, if the patient has a flat foot, then perform the single leg tiptoe test. If the patient has a pes cavus, then consider performing a 'Coleman block test' at this stage. Both of these tests are described in more detail below.

Ask the **patient to sit**. Then **inspect the plantar aspect** of the foot and between the toes for evidence of plantar keratoses or ulcers. Diabetic ulcers are typically found under the first metatarsal head, the pulp of the hallux and beneath the second and third metatarsal heads (Figure 10.4). Do not forget to look at shoes and walking aids, as these will give an indication of any pressure points in the foot and any degree of disability.

Movement (Move)

Terminology

There still exists a considerable ambiguity in the use of terms concerning the joints of the human foot and

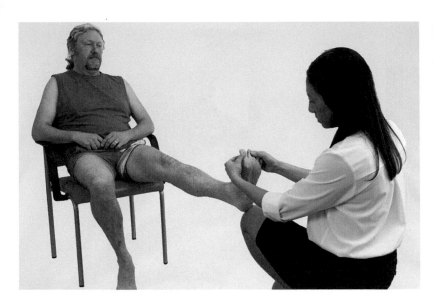

Figure 10.4 Sit the patient down and look at the sole of the foot and between the toes. Use this as a cue to also look at the shoes and walking aids.

their motions despite the efforts toward standardising these by anatomists and clinicians.[3]

There are several reasons for this. The first is an embryological one. The foot is initially aligned with the leg but rotates through 90° during development. This causes two of the axes of motion of the foot to do the same. Position and movement of hindfoot are usually described with reference to the axes of motion of the leg whilst the mid- and forefoot (distal to Chopart's joint) are described relative to their embryological axes. If internal and external rotation of the mid- and forefoot are replaced with pronation and supination, there become obvious similarities with upper limb movements.

Another reason for the confusion is that movements of the foot and ankle rarely occur in one plane. Combination patterns of movement have been described as early as 1889 by Farabeuf.[4] Inversion refers to plantarflexion, adduction and supination of the mid- and forefoot together with plantarflexion, adduction and internal rotation of the hindfoot. Eversion is the opposite with dorsiflexion, pronation and abduction of the mid- and forefoot together with dorsiflexion, abduction and external rotation of the hindfoot.

Active and passive ankle movement is assessed with the patient seated, both with the knee flexed and extended. Ideally, it is best to have the legs hanging over the side of the couch. The usual range of ankle movement is 20° of dorsiflexion and 50° of plantarflexion. An ankle that cannot plantarflex to neutral is described as being in *calcaneus*. An ankle that cannot dorsiflex to neutral is described as being in *equinus*.

Passive movement must be assessed with the forefoot in supination to exclude dorsiflexion at Chopart's and the midtarsal joints. Inversion of the heel to lock the subtalar joint will further ensure that the passive movement is isolated to the ankle joint.

To examine, put one hand on the heel and invert it to lock the subtalar joint. Use the same forearm to support the foot (Figure 10.5). The other hand supports the tibia. Dorsiflex the ankle by lifting the forearm under the foot. Plantarflex by bringing it downwards. Alternatively, the heel can be inverted to lock the subtalar joint and the forefoot supinated to lock the midfoot.

Causes of reduced ankle dorsiflexion include:

- Primary problems within the joint such as ankle arthritis.
- Obstruction from the front either by soft tissue or osteophytes (impingement) usually seen in footballers, ballet dancers and other sports persons.
- Contracture or tightness of the gastrocnemius (assessed by Silfverskiöld's test described below).
- Scarring of the tibiofibular syndesmosis. The widest part of the talus is anterior; therefore, to achieve full dorsiflexion the syndesmosis has to separate slightly. If it is damaged or scarred, e.g. following ankle sprains or fractures, this separation does not occur, and the dorsiflexion is reduced.

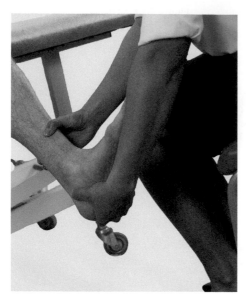

Figure 10.5 Ankle movements. The knee is flexed, the heel is inverted to lock the subtalar joint and forefoot is supinated slightly by resting it on the forearm.

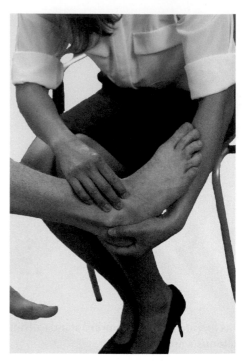

Figure 10.6 Subtalar movements. The talus is felt between the index finger and thumb of one hand. The other hand grasps the patient's heel and inverts/everts it.

Subtalar movement can be assessed with the foot hanging over the side of the couch or can be examined with the patient prone. Giannestras[5] stated that in the plantigrade position there is only 5° of valgus and 5° of varus movement in the subtalar joint.

To examine the subtalar joint, hold the calcaneus with one hand and the talar head/neck with the thumb and index finger of the other hand. Apply a varus and valgus stress with the hand that is holding the calcaneus and at the same time feel for movement of the talus with the other hand. Holding the talus isolates subtalar from ankle motion (Figure 10.6).

Inversion and eversion are assessed with the foot in a relaxed position of slight plantarflexion to assess inversion, and a neutral position to assess eversion, remembering that these movements reflect movement not just at the subtalar joint but also at Chopart's and the midtarsal joints (Figure 10.7). Whilst performing these movements passively, it is possible to assess whether movement is occurring at the subtalar joint or elsewhere in the foot. The amount of inversion is generally twice that of eversion, approximately 20° of inversion and 10° of eversion.

By fixing the hindfoot, the amount of passive pronation and supination occurring at Chopart's and the midtarsal joints can be assessed and their contribution to overall inversion and eversion can

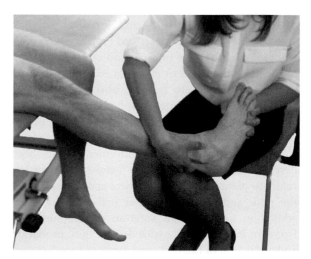

Figure 10.7 Inversion is a combined movement of subtalar joint and midfoot that is best assessed with the ankle slightly plantarflexed.

then be calculated. Similarly, by fixing the hindfoot (holding the calcaneum in neutral position with one hand) **abduction and adduction** of the mid tarsal

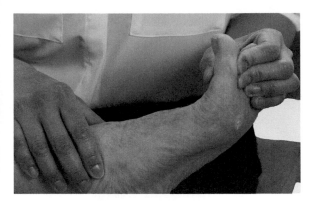

Figure 10.8 Dorsiflexion of the first MTP joint of the big toe.

joints can be assessed. This movement is minimal (about 5°). Whilst examining the midfoot, pay particular attention to the mobility of the **first tarsometatarsal joint**, which may be a contributing factor in hallux valgus and may need to be addressed by a Lapidus fusion. To assess this joint, use one hand to fix the tarsal bones and the other to grasp the first metatarsal and to move it in a dorsal and plantar direction.

Active and passive **movement of the hallux** is then assessed. The usual range is 70° of dorsiflexion and 40° of plantarflexion relative to the long axis of the first metatarsal. In hallux rigidus active and passive movement will be restricted and painful. During passive movement, it is often easy to demonstrate impingement between the base of the proximal phalanx and the prominent cheilus on the dorsal aspect of the neck of the first metatarsal (Figure 10.8). A **grind test** has been described to support a diagnosis of hallux rigidus. The great toe is grasped, loaded and then rotated in the coronal plane. This reproduces the patient's symptoms if there is complete joint involvement rather than isolated impingement.

Palpation (Feel)

This must again follow a systematic approach starting with the ankle and moving distally. It is important to know the anatomy of the underlying structures (Figure 10.9a,b,c,d). *Palpation may reveal an area of tenderness that may make the examiner suspicious of a particular diagnosis. It is useful at this point of the clinical examination to then perform a special test that may help to confirm the diagnosis.*

Medially, the examiner assesses the ankle for swelling or tenderness that might reflect synovitis or rupture of the posterior tibial tendon, irritation or compression of the posterior tibial nerve or snapping of the flexor hallucis longus.

Moving anteriorly in a clockwise fashion, ankle synovitis or an effusion can be felt in the notch of Harty, which is the space medial to the tibialis anterior. Crepitus might also be felt here with passive movement.

Moving laterally, the tibialis anterior, long extensors and peroneus tertius can be palpated. As the examiner moves further lateral, the anterolateral aspect of the ankle joint can be palpated. Again synovitis, an effusion and crepitus can be detected here.

Thumb pressure applied over the anterolateral gutter with the foot in plantarflexion will push any hypertrophic synovium into the joint causing pain. If the foot is then moved into dorsiflexion the pain intensifies which is positive for synovial impingement. This is the **anterolateral impingement test**[6] (Figure 10.10a,b).

From this position, the examiner can move superiorly over the inferior tibiofibular syndesmosis. Tenderness here may reflect injury to this structure. Further tests to support this are the **squeeze test,** in which the examiner squeezes the calf at midcalf level, compressing the fibula and tibia in the coronal plane[7] (Figure 10.11). External rotation of the foot with the leg stabilised anteriorly is also a *provocation test* for syndesmosis injuries.

Moving distal to the joint line, the examiner can palpate the anterior talofibular ligament that runs at an angle of approximately 70° to the long axis of the fibula from the anterodistal aspect of the fibula to the talus. Further anteriorly, the sinus tarsi can be palpated. Tenderness here may reflect irritation of the subtalar joint.

Moving posteriorly, the examiner can palpate the peroneal tendons. The calcaneofibular ligament runs deep to the peroneal tendons, creating an angle of approximately 100° with the anterior talofibular ligament. Tenderness in this region may reflect injury to the peroneal tendons, the superior peroneal retinaculum or the calcaneofibular ligament.

Continuing in a clockwise direction, the examiner then moves on to the Achilles tendon. Tenderness, thickening and nodules can be detected as well as any bony swelling such as in a Haglund's deformity. To distinguish between thickenings of the tendon or tendon sheath, passive dorsiflexion and plantarflexion are performed. A thickening of the tendon will move

(a)

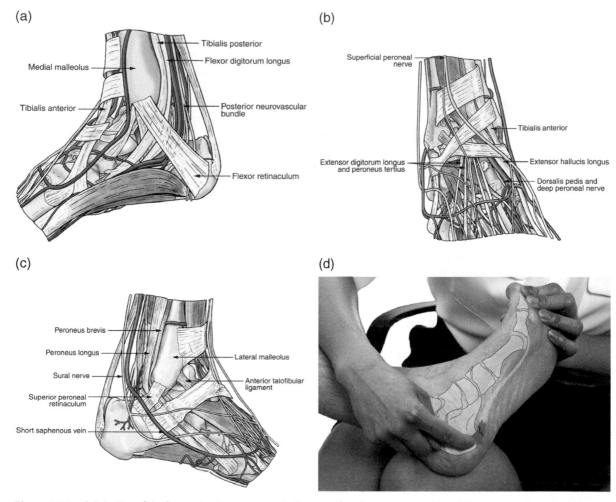

Medial malleolus

Tibialis anterior

Tibialis posterior

Flexor digitorum longus

Posterior neurovascular bundle

Flexor retinaculum

(b)

Superficial peroneal nerve

Extensor digitorum longus and peroneus tertius

Tibialis anterior

Extensor hallucis longus

Dorsalis pedis and deep peroneal nerve

(c)

Peroneus brevis

Peroneus longus

Sural nerve

Superior peroneal retinaculum

Short saphenous vein

Lateral malleolus

Anterior talofibular ligament

(d)

Figure 10.9a–d Palpation of the foot and ankle systematically. The area of tenderness gives an idea of the pathology based on the underlying anatomical structures.
(a) The anatomy of the medial aspect of the ankle
(b) The anatomy of the anterior aspect of the ankle
(c) The anatomy of the lateral aspect of the ankle
(d) The site of maximum tenderness in a patient with plantar fasciitis

with movement of the tendon, whilst a thickening of the sheath will remain fixed.

Having palpated the ankle, the examiner then moves more distally. The calcaneus is the site of origin of the plantar fascia from the anteromedial tuberosity. Tenderness here is indicative of plantar fasciitis. The plantar fascia should also be palpated for plantar fibromatoses. Side-to-side compression of the calcaneus is helpful in identifying patients with structural abnormalities of the heel, e.g. stress fractures.

Maximally dorsiflexing the great toe tenses the plantar fascia and may provoke further discomfort. This manoeuvre also recreates the medial longitudinal arch in a patient with a mobile pes planus deformity, the so-called windlass effect (Figure 10.12).

Moving distally, the examiner then palpates Chopart's joint (talonavicular and calcaneocuboid) for evidence of tenderness and/or crepitus. Between the two joints is the sinus tarsi; tenderness here is often suggestive of irritation of the subtalar joint. The midtarsal joints should be assessed in a similar way.

Moving on to the forefoot, the examiner starts with the hallux. Tenderness and swelling dorsally at the level of the metatarsophalangeal joint is suggestive of a cheilus associated with hallux

(a)

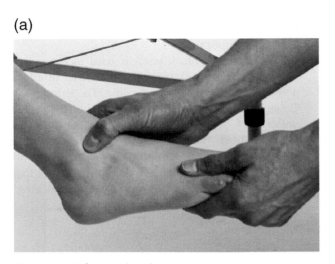

(b)

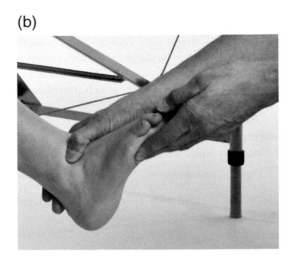

Figure 10.10a,b Anterolateral impingement test.
(a) Apply thumb pressure over the anterolateral gutter with the foot in plantarflexion. This causes pain.
(b) If the foot is then moved into dorsiflexion, the pain intensifies, which is positive for synovial impingement.

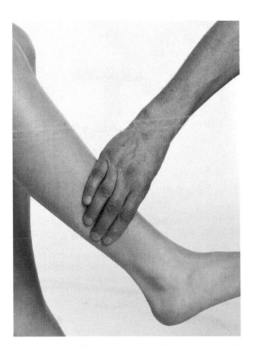

Figure 10.11 The 'squeeze test'. For assessment of the distal tibiofibular syndesmosis.

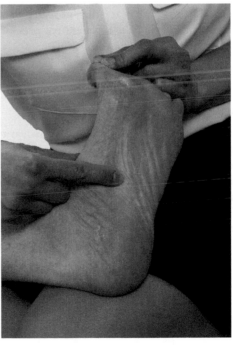

Figure 10.12 The 'windlass effect'. The great toe is maximally dorsiflexed, which tightens the plantar fascia and helps to reform the medial arch.

rigidus. Tenderness and swelling along the shaft of a metatarsal, especially the second, might reflect a stress fracture.

Tenderness and swelling of a lesser metatarsophalangeal joint might reflect a synovitis, such as that associated with Freiberg's disease, which typically

affects the second metatarsal head. Isolated metatarsophalangeal joint synovitis can be detected by passively plantarflexing the toes. This manoeuvre is painful in the presence of synovitis. Swelling and tenderness of all the metatarsophalangeal joints is typical of rheumatoid or psoriatic arthritis. In this case, there may be evidence of the *'daylight sign'*. Due to the synovitis the toes are pushed apart so daylight can be seen between each. The *'squeeze test'* reinforces this. The toes are squeezed in a medial-lateral direction, which provokes discomfort if a synovitis is present.

Palpation of the plantar aspect of the forefoot attempts to identify specific areas of tenderness often related to plantar keratoses beneath prominent metatarsal heads.

Tenderness between the metatarsal heads, especially in the third web space and if associated with burning pain and paraesthesia radiating to the toe, is typical of a Morton's neuroma. Reproduction of the pain when squeezing the toes in a mediolateral direction and the production of a click by applying dorsally directed pressure from beneath the affected web space further support the diagnosis and is described as *Mulder's sign*[8] (Figure 10.13).

Pain beneath the first metatarsophalangeal joint should alert the examiner to the possibility of a sesamoiditis, the result of a degenerative process, stress fracture or avascular necrosis (AVN).

Special Tests

Coleman Block Test

This is performed in a cavovarus foot. A cavovarus foot can be forefoot driven or hindfoot driven.[9]

Forefoot-driven deformities are usually due to neuromuscular causes such as Charcot–Marie–Tooth disease or spinal dysraphism. In forefoot-driven deformity, the first ray is plantarflexed due to sparing of peroneus longus. As the foot works as a tripod (formed by first metatarsal head, calcaneum and fifth metatarsal head), a plantarflexed first ray will cause the hindfoot to go into varus on weightbearing.[9]

Hindfoot driven deformities are due to trauma, such as varus malunion in previous talus fracture causing hindfoot varus.[9]

The Coleman block test[10] is used to determine whether the hindfoot varus is forefoot or hindfoot driven and if it is fixed or flexible. To perform the Coleman clock test, a 2.5 cm block or book is placed under the foot such that the first ray is unsupported (Figure 10.14). We recommend the examiner place the block next to the foot and ask the patient to lift up the foot. The examiner then holds the patient's foot and positions it accurately onto the block to avoid unclear instructions.

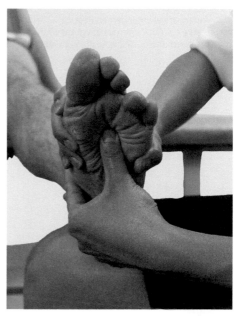

Figure 10.13 Mulder's test. The forefoot is being squeezed in a medial-lateral direction whilst at the same time pressure is applied from the plantar aspect of the foot under the affected web space. A click may be felt, and the patient feels pain.

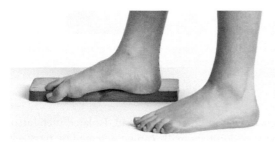 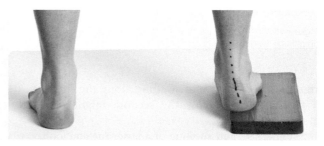

Figure 10.14 The Coleman block test. The first ray and the great toe are placed off the edge of the block, allowing the heel to move back into a valgus position if there is no fixed deformity.

Hindfoot varus that corrects with Coleman block test suggests that it is forefoot driven and the hindfoot is flexible. On the other hand, hindfoot varus that does not correct on Coleman block test suggests that the deformity is hindfoot driven or the hindfoot is rigid (likely degenerative change in subtalar joint due to long-standing deformity causing limited subtalar motion).

Single Leg Tiptoe Test

This is performed in planovalgus deformity. Take the patient to a wall so that they can lean on it to support themselves. Normally, when a patient goes onto their tiptoes, the heel will go into varus and the medial longitudinal arch will be elevated (Figure 10.15). This is because of the 'windlass effect' whereby forced dorsiflexion of the MTP joint of the big toe tightens the plantar fascia and results in the medial arch raising and the heel going into varus.[11,12]

When a normal patient is asked to tiptoe on both legs and then one leg, they are able to do so. In the presence of a tibialis posterior tendon rupture, when the patient is asked to perform a double heel rise, the affected foot remains in valgus rather than shifting into varus. When asked to perform a single heel rise, the patient is unable to do this (Figure 10.15a,b).

Testing the Muscles around the Ankle

It is important to test the muscles around the ankle, particularly in planovalgus (to assess the function of tibialis posterior) and cavovarus foot (to confirm muscle imbalance and assess power of the muscle that may be used in tendon transfer).

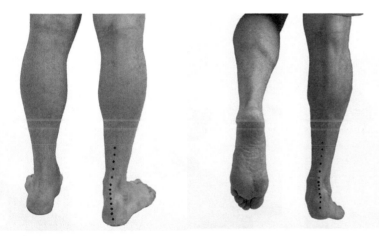

Figure 10.15 Tiptoe test. Normally, as the patient goes on to tiptoes, the medial arch will elevate and the heel will go into varus.

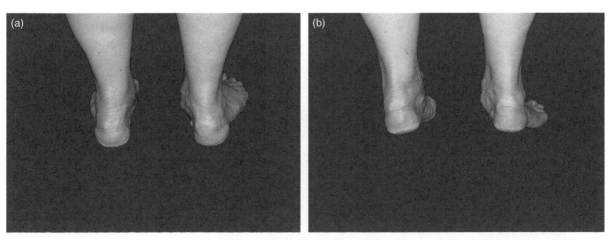

(a) (b)

Figure 10.15a,b This patient has a tibialis posterior rupture on the right side. (a) The heel is in valgus when standing. (b) When on tiptoes, note that the heel remains in valgus. This patient is unable to perform a single leg tiptoe test.

Tibialis posterior: To test tibialis posterior function, the foot is plantarflexed. From this position, resisted inversion is undertaken that stresses the tibialis posterior (Figure 10.16). Palpate the tendon behind the medial malleolus.

Tibialis anterior: Place the patient's ankle in maximum dorsiflexion and some inversion. Ask them to resist your attempt to plantarflex. Palpate the tendon at the front of the ankle (Figure 10.17).

Peroneus longus: To test for peroneus longus, place the patient's ankle in plantarflexion and with the foot everted (the opposite of tibialis anterior). Ask the patient to maintain this position as the examiner

pushes inwards (Figure 10.18). Feel the tendon behind the lateral malleolus.

Peroneus brevis: To distinguish between peroneus brevis and longus, the foot is placed in the neutral position and resisted eversion performed

Silfverskiöld's Test

This test is performed to determine whether gastrocnemius or soleus is the cause of reduced dorsiflexion of the ankle. Maximally dorsiflex the ankle first with the knee extended then with the knee flexed to 90° (Figure 10.19a,b). It is important to also lock the subtalar joint to prevent valgus escape.

Because the gastrocnemius originates from above the knee, it tightens when the knee is extended and relaxes when the knee is flexed. If the loss of dorsiflexion is due to gastrocnemius tightness alone, then there

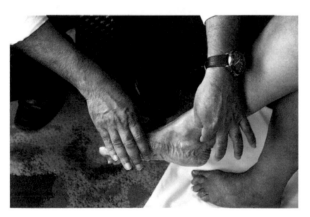

Figure 10.16 Testing for tibialis posterior. Resisted plantarflexion and inversion. Palpate the tendon behind the medial malleolus.

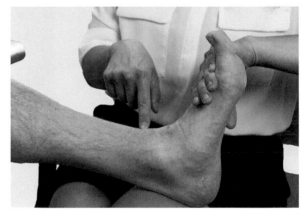

Figure 10.17 Testing for tibialis anterior. Resisted dorsiflexion and inversion. Palpate the tendon.

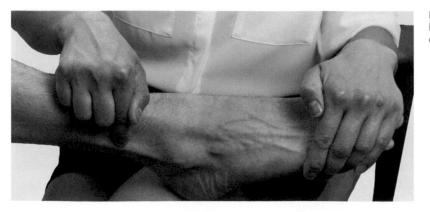

Figure 10.18 Testing for peroneus longus. Resisted plantarflexion and eversion. Palpate the tendon.

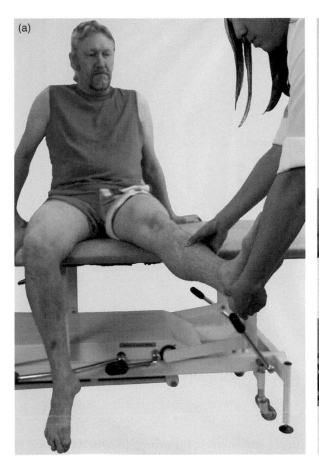

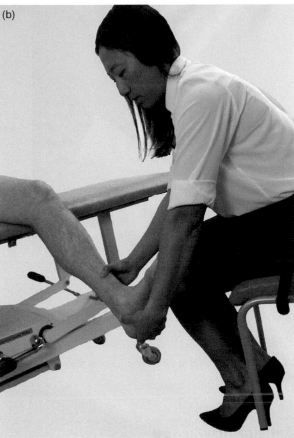

(a)

(b)

Figure 10.19a,b Silfverskiöld's test. This test is performed to determine whether gastrocnemius is the cause of reduced dorsiflexion of the ankle. (a) Maximally dorsiflex the ankle first with the knee extended, (b) then with the knee flexed to nearly 90°.

will be reduced dorsiflexion with the knee extended. If there is no change of ankle dorsiflexion with knee flexion or extension, then the contracture is in both gastrocnemius and soleus.

Thompson's Test

This is a test (also known as Simmonds test) to determine if there is a rupture of the Achilles tendon. The patient lies prone on the couch with both ankles freely dangling over the end of the couch (Figure 10.20). Normally, the resting tone of the gastrocnemius results in slight plantarflexion of the ankle. If there is a rupture of the Achilles tendon, the position of the ankle is more neutral. Squeeze the calf. In the presence of an intact tendon (sometimes also with a partial tear), there will be passive plantarflexion at the ankle. If there is a complete tear, then there will be no response to the calf squeeze.[13]

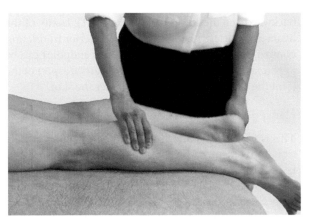

Figure 10.20 Thompson's calf squeeze test. Squeeze the calf with the patient in the prone position. Loss of passive plantarflexion of the ankle results from a compete rupture of the Achilles tendon.

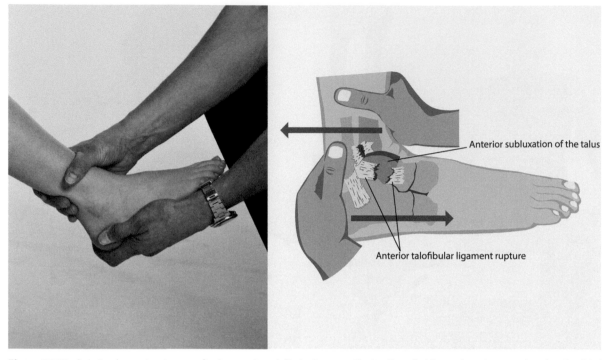

Figure 10.21 Anterior drawer test to assess for the anterior talofibular ligament. The heel is pulled forwards at the same time that the tibia is pushed backwards.

Anterior Drawer Test

This test is used to assess the anterior talofibular ligament of the lateral ligament complex. The patient is seated with the legs hanging over the side of the couch. The examiner grasps the heel with one hand and with the other hand holds on to the lower part of the leg. The examiner then pulls forwards on the heel and pushes backwards on the lower leg (Figure 10.21). Laxity of the ligament is determined by increased anterior translation compared to the uninjured side. A soft endpoint can be appreciated. Sometimes, in the anterolateral aspect of the joint the dome of the talus tents under the skin.

Neurovascular Assessment

This is undertaken after the three basic steps of inspection, movement and palpation have been completed. It is important to emphasise that many foot and ankle deformities result from neurological conditions. Inspection of the lumbar spine is therefore an integral part of the examination of the foot and ankle. Similarly, in anyone complaining of neurological symptoms in the foot, it is also important to exclude lumbar nerve root tension. Assessment for clonus will distinguish between upper and lower motor neuron lesions. Assessment of sensation will help identify patients at risk for ulceration and will also distinguish between conditions such as poliomyelitis (which has normal sensation) and spina bifida, both of which are lower motor neuron lesions. The use of 5.07 Semmes–Weinstein monofilament test is recommended to test for peripheral neuropathy.[14] Motor testing should initially assess myotomal function and then concentrate on specific muscle groups as directed by the history and examination.

Assessment of the pulses concludes the initial general examination (Figure 10.22).

Specific Pathological Conditions

Lesser Toe Deformities

Lesser toe deformities are varied. When describing these deformities, there are specific differences that need to be appreciated:

Mallet toe – A flexion deformity of the distal interphalangeal joint (DIPJ).

Hammer toe – A flexion deformity of the proximal interphalangeal joint (PIPJ).

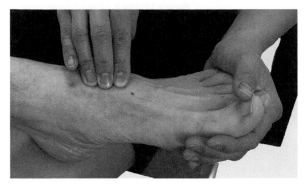

Figure 10.22 The final stage of the foot and ankle examination is to perform a neurovascular assessment.

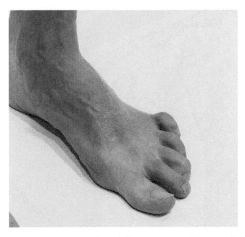

Figure 10.23 Forefoot deformities. The third toe shows a mallet deformity (flexed DIPJ), the fourth shows a hammer toe deformity (flexed PIPJ) and the fifth toe shows a claw deformity (MTPJ extension and PIPJ flexion).

Claw toe – An extension deformity of the metatarsophalangeal joint (MTPJ) and a flexion deformity of the PIPJ or DIPJ (Figure 10.23).

In assessing a hammer toe deformity, it is important to be able to differentiate between a fixed deformity at the PIP joint and a flexible deformity because the treatment is influenced by the degree of stiffness. To do this, the PIP joint movements need to be examined with the long flexors of the toes relaxed. This can be accomplished by either plantarflexing the ankles or exerting upward pressure on the metatarsal heads (Figure 10.24).

Cavovarus Foot Deformities

The commonest cause in the adult is Charcot–Marie–Tooth disease (hereditary motor and sensory neuropathy type I). It is autosomal dominant inherited and typically presents in the second decade with symmetrical deformities. Asymmetrical cavovarus deformities are more typical of spinal dysraphism. Patients with Charcot–Marie–Tooth develop hindfoot varus, pes cavus, clawing of the toes and hands and plantarflexion of the first ray (Figure 10.25a,b). The Coleman block test will help to determine whether the hindfoot varus is fixed or flexible.

Posterior Tibial Tendon Disruption

This results from progressive degenerative change within the tendon. Symptoms range from pain and swelling along the medial aspect of the ankle to postural changes with loss of the medial longitudinal arch and hindfoot valgus (planovalgus foot). In patients with complete disruption of the tendon, more toes

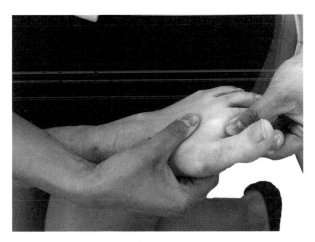

Figure 10.24 To assess the flexibility of the PIP joints, the long flexors to the toes need to be relaxed. This is achieved by elevating the metatarsal heads. Alternatively, the ankle can be plantarflexed.

are visible when viewing the patient from behind, the so called too many toes sign[15] due to increased abduction of the forefoot (Figure 10.26). This patient is unable to perform a tiptoe test on the affected side. There may also be talonavicular uncoverage with the talar head palpable medially. It is important to assess whether the hindfoot is fixed in valgus or corrects into varus and whether any compensatory forefoot position is fixed or flexible, as this affects the treatment options.

(a)

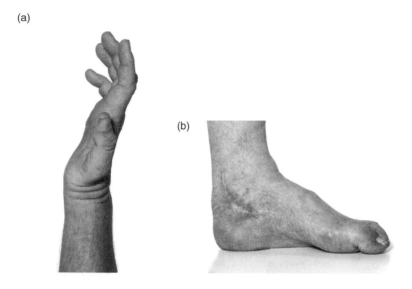

(b)

Figure 10.25a,b Charcot–Marie–Tooth disease. (a) Wasting of the intrinsic muscles and clawing of the hand. (b) Pes cavus and hindfoot varus

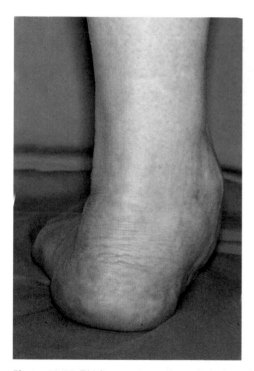

Figure 10.26 Tibialis posterior tendon rupture. Note the flattened medial arch, hindfoot valgus and 'too many toes'.

Rheumatoid Foot

This condition has a characteristic pattern of involvement. Symmetrical clawing of the lesser toes and deformity of the hallux are typical of the rheumatoid forefoot. The synovitis causes extension of the metatarsophalangeal joints with subsequent rupture of the volar plate leading to clawing of the toes. The clawed toes pull the plantar fat pad distally and expose the metatarsal heads. On the plantar aspect of the foot, there are callosities over the prominent metatarsal heads. Patients describe a feeling of 'walking on pebbles'.

The hindfoot is often in valgus due to involvement of the subtalar joint and also the posterior tibial tendon. The midfoot is abducted with loss of the medial longitudinal arch (Figure 10.27).

Tarsal Coalition

This condition usually presents in children when the fibrocartilaginous bar, which represents a failure of segmentation of the tarsal bones, ossifies. Patients complain of foot fatigue and hindfoot pain. In adults, recurrent ankle sprains may be a presenting feature. Tenderness is detected in the sinus tarsi with a calcaneonavicular bar and medially around the sustentaculum tali with a talocalcaneal bar. The classical description of presentation with a tarsal coalition is one of a 'peroneal spastic flatfoot'. The hindfoot is fixed in valgus with no inversion of the foot permitted. Not all patients with a coalition, however, have a fixed valgus deformity; some have neutral alignment and some a varus deformity.

The differential diagnosis of a fixed flatfoot deformity in an adult includes septic arthritis, osteoid osteoma, inflammatory arthropathy, trauma and posterior tibial tendon disruption.

Achilles Tendon Disruption

The patient often describes being struck at the back of the leg. They are unable to perform a heel raise;

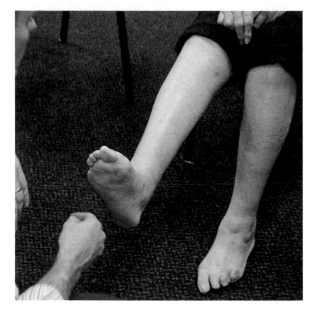

Figure 10.27 Rheumatoid foot. Note that the callosity is picked up only by deliberate inspection of the sole of the foot.

a palpable gap is felt and when placed supine. The patient may still be able to actively plantarflex their ankle because the long toe flexors are intact. However, squeezing the calf does not produce plantarflexion (Thompson's test).[13]

Peroneal Tendon Dislocation

This results from disruption of the superior peroneal retinaculum. It recurs in more than 50% of cases. In the chronic setting, the patient describes a popping or snapping sensation lateral to the ankle. Movement of the foot and ankle from full plantarflexion and inversion to full dorsiflexion and eversion will often reproduce the dislocation. Pain and tenderness over the tendons are suggestive of a concomitant tear of the tendons.

Ankle Instability

This can only be diagnosed with certainty using stress radiographs. Chronic instability is usually of the lateral ligaments (anterior talofibular ligament and the calcaneofibular ligament).

To test the calcaneofibular ligament, an *inversion stress test (varus stress test)* is performed. With one hand, hold the ankle dorsiflexed to lock it. With the other hand, hold the calcaneus and invert it (Figure 10.28). Opening of the joint indicates laxity.

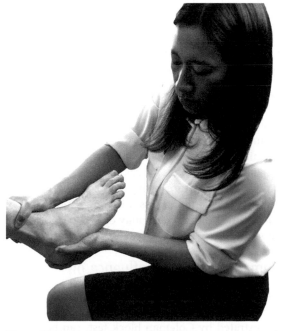

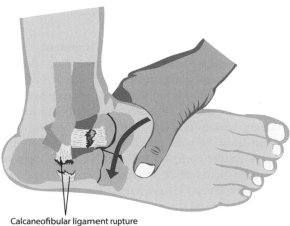

Calcaneofibular ligament rupture

Figure 10.28 Test for the calcaneofibular ligament. An inversion stress is applied to the foot to demonstrate the tear in the ligament

Comparison with the other side may reveal a difference, but radiographs are needed to define whether the instability is occurring in the ankle, subtalar or both joints. The anterior drawer test (as described above) assesses the anterior talofibular ligament. In severe cases, a suction sign develops just anterior to the lateral malleolus. Again, though, radiographs are required to confirm that the instability is occurring in the ankle.

Entrapment Neuropathies

Although it is always important to consider the possibility of distant neurological disease affecting the foot and ankle, there are certain entrapment neuropathies around the foot and ankle that can be responsible for numbness, paraesthesia and wasting.

Tarsal tunnel syndrome results from compression of the posterior tibial nerve in the tarsal canal. It is characterised by diffuse plantar pain associated with paraesthesia and numbness. Percussion over the area of the entrapment may reproduce the symptoms, and palpation along the course of the nerve may reveal local causes such a lipoma, ganglion or exostosis. Physical findings must be supported with electrodiagnostic studies especially if surgery is planned.

Deep peroneal nerve entrapment occurs most frequently beneath the inferior extensor retinaculum. It is often associated with trauma such as repeated ankle sprains. Patients complain of pain in the dorsum of the foot with radiation into the first web space. Examination may reveal reduced sensation in the first web space and wasting of the extensor digitorum brevis.

Superficial peroneal nerve entrapment results from impingement of the nerve on the deep fascia as it exits the lateral compartment approximately 10 cm proximal to the ankle joint. Patients complain of pain in the lateral distal calf often associated with numbness and paraesthesia on the dorsum of the foot. Examination reveals point tenderness where the nerve exits the compartment. Where either deep or superficial peroneal nerve entrapment is suspected, the examiner must always palpate the common peroneal nerve around the neck of the fibula.

Other entrapment neuropathies have been described such as sural nerve entrapment and entrapment of the first branch of the lateral plantar nerve. These must be considered once more common lesions have been excluded.

Charcot Foot

A Charcot foot is a systemic pathological process that results in fractures, dislocations and progressive deformity of the foot and ankle. If left untreated it results in a deformed, unstable foot (typically rocker bottom deformity) which causes limited mobility, recurrent ulceration, deep infection and has a 15% major amputation rate.[16]

Patients will typically present with a red, hot and swollen foot that is often indistinguishable from infection. They may or may not have pain. Patients with a Charcot foot will have peripheral neuropathy and background of an underlying systemic disease (most commonly diabetes mellitus). The temperature of the foot will also be about 3.5°C higher on the affected side. Presence or history of ulceration significantly increases the odds of a diagnosis of infection over Charcot's.[16,17]

Elevation test: A useful clinical test to distinguish infection from a Charcot foot is elevation of the foot above the level of the heart for at least 1 minute. In a Charcot foot, the erythema will decrease with foot elevation, but it remains in infection.[16,17]

Advanced Corner

First Metatarsal Rise Sign

Another simple but sensitive test to detect early posterior tibial tendon dysfunction is the first metatarsal rise sign as described by Hintermann and Gächter.[18] The authors described externally rotating the tibia with the foot plantigrade on the ground. If the posterior tibial tendon is dysfunctional, the first metatarsal head will lift off the ground.

Silfverskiöld's Test: Influence on Treatment

Consider performing this test routinely for all hindfoot deformities, including planovalgus and cavovarus deformities. The Achilles tendon is at a shorter length when the calcaneum is in a varus or valgus position. This can result in contracture in long-standing deformity. It is therefore important to assess this pre-operatively when planning any hindfoot deformity correction as Achilles tendon lengthening may be required.[15]

Coleman Block Test: Influence on Treatment

A forefoot-driven deformity with flexible hindfoot, as demonstrated by Coleman block test, can be treated

Table 10.3 Surgical treatment options for cavovarus foot

Forefoot driven/ flexible hindfoot	• First metatarsal osteotomy + tendon transfers
	• Jones transfer (hallux PIPJ fusion + extensor hallucis longus transfer to first metatarsal shaft)
Fixed hindfoot/ hindfoot driven	• Lateral closing wedge osteotomy of calcaneum or lateral calcaneal displacement osteotomy

Table 10.4 Surgical treatment options for planovalgus foot

Flexible	Medial calcaneal displacement osteotomy, flexible digitorum longus transfer +/– spring ligament reconstruction +/– Achilles tendon lengthening
	+ Lateral column lengthening (if evidence of forefoot abduction/talonavicular uncoverage)
	+ Medial cuneiform opening wedge (Cotton) osteotomy (if fixed forefoot varus/supination after other reconstructive procedures performed)
Fixed	Triple arthrodesis +/– Achilles tendon lengthening
	+ Deltoid ligament reconstruction (if correctable talar tilt)
	Pantalar fusion (in fixed talar tilt)

with a corrective orthotic (with lateral posting and first metatarsal cut out). If surgery is required, forefoot procedures with tendon transfers are usually sufficient. A hindfoot-driven or fixed-hindfoot deformity will require bony reconstructive procedures of the hindfoot (Table 10.3).[11]

Tiptoe Test: Influence on Treatment

The single leg tiptoe test will help distinguish between a flexible and fixed hindfoot (Figure 10.29). A flexible planovalgus foot will respond to a corrective orthotic, whereas a fixed deformity will not. A typical orthotic used in flexible planovalgus foot is medial heel wedge with medial longitudinal arch support.

Surgical treatment for flexible and fixed deformity also varies. Flexible deformity can be reconstructed, whereas fixed deformity requires fusion (Table 10.4).[11,12,19,20]

Lesser Toe Deformity Treatment

There are a vast number of surgical treatments available for lesser toe deformities and these options vary significantly between clinicians. Plantarflexing the ankle or elevating the metatarsal heads will help differentiate between fixed and flexible lesser toe PIP joints by relaxing the long flexors.

In general, flexible deformities can be treated with mainly soft tissue procedures (but sometimes bony) to rebalance the forces creating the deformity. Fixed deformities often require fusion of the affected joint(s).

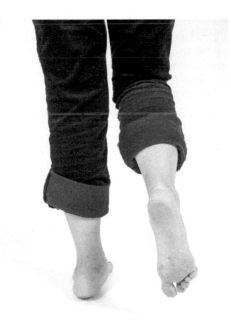

Figure 10.29 Single leg tiptoe test. This patient is unable to adequately lift the heel on the left. The heel stays in valgus, indicating a fixed deformity.

References

1. Vainio K. The rheumatoid foot; a clinical study with pathological and roentgenological comments. *Ann Chir Gynaecol Fenn Suppl* 1956;**45**(1):1–107.

2. Coughlin MJ. Common causes of pain in the forefoot in adults. *J Bone Joint Surg Br* 2000 Aug;82 (6):781–790.

3. Sarrafian SK. *Anatomy of the Foot and Ankle*, 2nd ed. Philadelphia: Lippincott,1993.

4. Farabeuf L. *Précis de manuel operatoire*. Paris: Masson, 1889; pp. 816–847.

5. Giannestras N. *Foot Disorders: Medical and Surgical Management*, 2nd ed. Philadelphia: Lea & Febiger, 1970.

6. Molloy S, Solan MC, Bendall SP. Synovial impingement in the ankle. A new physical sign. *J Bone Joint Surg Br* 2003 Apr;**85**(3):330–333.

7. Hopkinson WJ, St Pierre P, Ryan JB, Wheeler JH. Syndesmosis sprains of the ankle. *Foot Ankle* 1990 Jun;**10**(6):325–330.

8. Mulder JD. The causative mechanism in Morton's metatarsalgia. *J Bone Joint Surg Br* 1951 Feb;**33-B**(1):94–95.

9. Krähenbühl N, Weinberg MW. Anatomy and biomechanics of cavovarus deformity. *Foot Ankle Clin* 2019 Jun 1;**24**(2):173–181.

10. Coleman SS, Chesnut WJ. A simple test for hindfoot flexibility in the cavovarus foot. *Clin Orthop Relat Res* 1977 Apr;(123):60–62.

11. Johnson KA, Strom DE. Tibialis posterior tendon dysfunction. *Clin Orthop Relat Res* 1989 Feb;(239):196–206.

12. Myerson MS. Adult acquired flatfoot deformity: treatment of dysfunction of the posterior tibial tendon. *Instr Course Lect* 1997;**46**:393–405.

13. Thompson TC, Doherty JH. Spontaneous rupture of tendon of Achilles: a new clinical diagnostic test. *J Trauma* 1962 Mar;2:126–129.

14. Feng Y, Schlösser FJ, Sumpio BE. The Semmes Weinstein monofilament examination is a significant predictor of the risk of foot ulceration and amputation in patients with diabetes mellitus. *J Vasc Surg* 2011 Jan 1;**53**(1):220–226.e5.

15. Yao K, Yang TX, Yew WP. Posterior tibialis tendon dysfunction: overview of evaluation and management. *Orthopedics* 2015 Jun;**38**(6):385–391.

16. Dodd A, Daniels TR. Charcot neuroarthropathy of the foot and ankle. *J Bone Joint Surg* 2018;**100**(8):696–711.

17. Yousaf S, Dawe EJC, Saleh A, Gill IR, Wee A. The acute Charcot foot in diabetics. *EFORT Open Rev* 2018 Oct 1;**3**(10):568–573.

18. Hintermann B, Gächter A. The first metatarsal rise sign: a simple, sensitive sign of tibialis posterior tendon dysfunction. *Foot Ankle Int* 1996 Apr;**17**(4):236–241.

19. Chadwick C, Whitehouse SL, Saxby TS. Long-term follow-up of flexor digitorum longus transfer and calcaneal osteotomy for stage II posterior tibial tendon dysfunction. *Bone Joint J* 2015 Mar 1;**97-B**(3):346–352.

20. Chan JY, Greenfield ST, Soukup DS, Do HT, Deland JT, Ellis SJ. Contribution of lateral column lengthening to correction of forefoot abduction in stage iib adult acquired flatfoot deformity reconstruction. *Foot Ankle Int* 2015 Dec 1;**36**(12):1400–1411.

11

Examination of the Brachial Plexus

Fazal Ali, Joe Garcia, Armughan Azhar and Simon Kay

Full understanding of this topic is only achieved if the reader has knowledge of:

- Examination of the rotator cuff and muscles around the shoulder girdle – see Chapter 2
- Examination of the peripheral nerves of the upper limb – see Chapter 6
- Examination of the dermatomes and myotomes of the upper limb – see Chapter 7
- Anatomy of the brachial plexus – see below

Assessment of the Brachial Plexus

A. History
B. Clinical Examination

Step 1
Stand the patient and look:

- Can the patient actually stand?
- Look at the position in which the arm is held
- Look for wasting, scars (including axilla)
- Look for presence of Horner's syndrome

Step 2
Feel

- Over bony areas
- Sweating and pulse
- Sensation- dermatomes and peripheral nerves

Step 3
Move
Motor testing is performed in the anatomical sequence of the brachial plexus.

- Assess the myotomes of the upper limb (roots)
- Assess the muscles supplied by the nerves off the roots of the brachial plexus
- Assess the muscles supplied by the nerves arising from the trunks
- Assess the muscles supplied by the nerves arising from the cords
- Assess the muscles supplied by the terminal branches of the brachial plexus

The aims of clinical examination of the brachial plexus are to:

1. Determine the **level** of the lesion (supraclavicular or infraclavicular).
2. Determine the **extent** of the injury (sensory and motor deficit).
3. Determine the presence of **any poor prognostic signs** (including preganglionic injuries).

To examine competently for the level and extent of a brachial plexus lesion, the examiner should have sound knowledge of the following aspects of the clinical examination.

Sensory Testing

- Dermatomes of the upper limb
- Cutaneous nerve supply to the upper limb such as area supplied by radial nerve, median nerve, ulnar nerve and musculocutaneous nerve, etc.

Motor Testing

- Myotomes to the upper limb
- Demonstrate power in the muscles of the shoulder girdle
- Demonstrate muscles of the rotator cuff
- To be able to examine terminal branches of the brachial plexus including radial nerve, ulnar nerve, median nerve, axillary nerve and musculocutaneous nerve

Once the examiner is proficient in doing the above, then assessment of the brachial plexus injury is much easier. The system for the examination is *look, feel, move.*

Look

- On standing, look at the position in which the patient holds the arm. It may be adducted and internally rotated, as in upper trunk lesions (Erb's palsy) with the 'waiter's tip' position. There may be a clawed hand, as in lower trunk lesions (Klumpke's palsy)

- Look for scars, including in the axilla. These may be surgical scars or scars related to a penetrating injury. Look for wasting of the muscles of the shoulder girdle in the upper limb.
- Look for Horner's syndrome, which includes ptosis, myosis, anhydrosis and enophthalmos. Horner's syndrome is damage to the sympathetic chain, which is in proximity to the nerve roots and signifies the possibility of a preganglionic lesion.
- If the patient cannot stand, then the long tracts of the spinal cord may be damaged, as these are close to the roots of the brachial plexus.

Feel

- Feel over bony prominences for previous fractures, especially clavicle and scapular fractures.
- It is important also to feel the pulse in the upper limb, as the brachial plexus is closely related to the subclavian and axillary arteries.
- Feeling for sweating on the affected limb is an important sign, as this sign may be preserved in the presence of a neuropraxia.
- Test the dermatomes and the area supplied by the peripheral nerves. A dermatomal pattern of loss of sensation may indicate root or trunk injuries, whereas a peripheral nerve pattern of sensory loss may indicate lesions of the cord or the terminal branches of the brachial plexus.

Move

Examine the following muscle groups in the anatomical sequence of the brachial plexus:

- Myotomes, i.e. C5/6/7/8 and T1 of the upper limb
- Muscles supplied by nerves arising off the roots:
  - Dorsal scapular nerve (C5) – rhomboids
  - Long thoracic nerve (C5, 6, 7) – serratus anterior
- Muscles supplied by nerves arising from the trunks:
  - Suprascapular nerve (C5/6) upper trunk – supraspinatus and infraspinatus
  - Trapezius can be tested to indicate trunk lesions because the eleventh cranial nerve (spinal accessory) lies in the posterior triangle of the neck near to the trunks.
- Muscles supplied by nerves arising from the cords:
  - Medial and lateral pectoral nerve (medial and lateral cord) – pectoralis major
  - Thoracodorsal nerve (posterior cord) – latissimus dorsi
  - Upper and lower subscapular nerve (posterior cord) – subscapularis

- Muscles supplied by the terminal branches of the brachial plexus:
  - Radial nerve, median nerve, ulnar nerve, axillary nerve and musculocutaneous nerve.

Anatomy

It is impossible to learn to examine the brachial plexus without knowing the anatomy (Figure 11.1) and (Table 11.1).

The brachial plexus is formed by the ventral primary rami of C5, C6, C7, C8 and T1. It originates in the neck, and emerges in the interscalene space and passes laterally and inferiorly between the central part of the clavicle and the first rib. It then passes deep to the muscles attached to the coracoid process before entering the axilla and the upper arm from behind the lateral border of pectoralis major.

The brachial plexus consists of roots, trunks, division, cords and branches.

- Five roots (C5–T1): between anterior and middle scalene muscles and lie superior and posterior to subclavian artery.
- Three trunks: upper, middle, lower, in the posterior triangle of the neck.
- Six divisions: behind the clavicle, two from each trunk, no peripheral nerves originate directly from the divisions.
- Three cords: named because of their anatomical relationship to axillary artery, posterior, lateral and medial.[1]
- Terminal branches: The posterior cord terminates as the radial nerve and the axillary nerve. The medial cord terminates as the ulnar nerve but gives a branch to the median nerve. The lateral cord also contributes to the median nerve and has another terminal branch, the musculocutaneous nerve.

Anatomical Relationships

The **skeletal** relationships are most easily understood. The spinal column lies medial to the plexus and may lie in the same zone of trauma. The clavicle and first rib may each be fractured, and fracture of the first rib is associated with the dissipation of large amounts of kinetic energy. In exceptional circumstances, fracture of the scapula and clavicle may indicate that the arm has suffered a near avulsion injury; a brachiothoracic

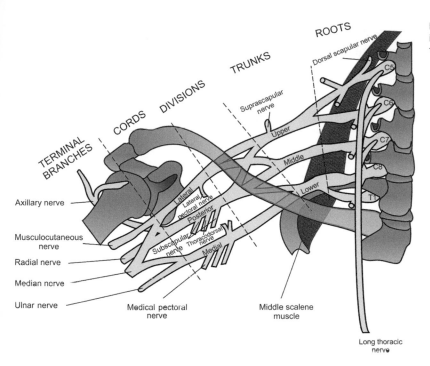

Figure 11.1 Brachial plexus with division into roots, trunks, divisions and cords together with branches.

dissociation and the integrity of the skin envelope disguises substantial deep trauma.

Two important **neural** associations with the brachial plexus are the sympathetic nerves and the phrenic nerve. The sympathetic rami for the arm and face emerge from the T1 root immediately after it exits the cervical foramen. Avulsion of this root therefore carries a high incidence of Horner's syndrome (Table 11.2).

The phrenic nerve arises from the C5 root as it lies on the medial scalene muscle and receives its main additional contribution from C4. Phrenic nerve palsy is therefore most likely to indicate avulsion of the C5 root with or without avulsion of the C4 root. In the latter case, other signs of cervical plexus palsy may include numbness over the lateral neck and ear, or, rarely, trapezius palsy from involvement of the closely associated spinal accessory nerve.

The **vascular** relationships of the brachial plexus are important, for not only do they provide evidence of collateral damage in cases of brachial plexus palsy, but that damage may itself be of great importance. The T1 spinal nerve arches cephalad and lateral to join C8 at the first rib and so form the lower trunk. The subclavian artery also crosses the first rib immediately anterior to the plexus and is intimately associated with the brachial plexus for the remainder of its course.

The artery is therefore susceptible to injury in the same manner as the T1 nerve root, and penetrating or avulsion injuries of the plexus are often associated with vascular damage. Arterial injury is of greater significance than injury to the subclavian vein.

History

In the history, the first point to determine is whether there is a history of trauma. If no recent trauma, then was it from birth (obstetric brachial plexus palsy)? Was there no trauma at all? If so, then consider a Parsonage–Turner syndrome.

If there has been trauma following sport such as American football or rugby and the symptoms and signs are resolving after only a brief period, then consider a diagnosis of 'burner' or 'stinger'. All of these diagnoses will be considered further in the 'Advanced Corner' of this chapter.

Age and co-morbidities are important prognostic indicators. The older the patient is, then the worse the prognosis will be. Both of these factors will have a bearing on the decision for any surgery. Hand dominance, to some degree, will also have a bearing on the decision for surgery.

If there is a history of trauma, then the energy of injury and the mechanism of injury must be

195

Table 11.1 Branches of the brachial plexus

Branches	Spinal segment	Function & nerve supply
Roots		
Dorsal scapular nerve	C5	Function: Motor Rhomboid major & minor
Long thoracic nerve	C5, C6, C7	Function: Motor Serratus anterior
Trunks (upper)		
Suprascapular nerve	C5, C6	Function: Motor Supraspinatus, infraspinatus
Nerve to subclavius	C5, C6	Function: Motor Subclavius
Cords		
Lateral cord		
Lateral pectoral nerve	C5, C6, C7	Function: Motor Pectoralis major (clavicular head)
Musculocutaneous Nerve (terminal branch)	C5, C6, C7	Function: Motor All muscles in the anterior compartment of the arm
Medial cord		
Medial pectoral nerve	C8, T1	Function: Motor Pectoralis major (sternal head), pectoralis minor
Medial cutaneous nerve of arm	C8, T1	Function: Sensory Skin on medial side of distal one-third of arm
Medial cutaneous nerve of forearm	C8, T1	Function: Sensory Skin on medial side of forearm
Ulnar nerve (terminal branch)	C7, C8, T1	Function: Motor All intrinsic muscles of the hand (except three thenar muscles and two lateral lumbricals); also FCU and medial half of FDP in the forearm Function: Sensory Skin over the palmer surface of the medial 1½ digits and associate palm and wrist, skin over the dorsal surface of the medial 1½ digits
Posterior cord		
Upper subscapular nerve	C5, C6	Function: Motor Subscapularis
Thoracodorsal nerve	C6, C7, C8	Function: Motor Latissimus dorsi
Lower subscapular nerve	C5, C6	Function: motor Subscapularis, teres major
Axillary nerve (terminal branch)	C5, C6	Function: motor Deltoid, teres minor Function: Sensory Skin over upper lateral part of arm – 'regimental badge'
Radial nerve (terminal branch)	C5, C6, C7, C8 & T1	Function: motor All muscles in the posterior compartments of arm and forearm Function: sensory Skin on the posterior aspects of the arm and forearm; the lower lateral surface of the arm, and the dorsal lateral surface of the hand
Medial & lateral cords		
Median nerve (terminal branch)	C5, C6, C7, C8, T1	Function: motor All muscles in the anterior compartment of the forearm (expect FCU and medial half of FDP), three thenar muscles and two lateral lumbrical muscles Function: sensory Skin over the palmer surface of the radial 3½ digits FCU, flexor carpi ulnaris; FDP, flexor digitorum profundus

Table 11.2 Clinical signs of Horner's syndrome

Meiosis	Constricted pupil in the absence of sympathetic tone
Anhydrosis	Unilateral loss of sweating in the face
Ptosis	Drooping of the upper eyelid resulting from loss of sympathetic tone in Müller's muscle
Enophthalmos	Relative atrophy of orbital contents – eye appears sunken (late stages)

determined. Low-energy injuries will most likely cause a neurapraxia, e.g. following an anterior dislocation of the shoulder. High-energy injuries will signify worse prognosis and could be associated with other injuries such as shoulder girdle fractures and thoracic trauma. These patients will not uncommonly have other major trauma such as head injuries and long bone fractures, which take priority in management, and the brachial plexus injury is secondary at this point.

The mechanism of injury may help to determine the type of brachial plexus lesion. Common mechanisms include cervical extension, rotation or lateral bending. Depression of the shoulder, like falling onto the shoulder, can result in upper brachial plexus injuries. Hyperabduction of the shoulder, like grabbing on to something whilst falling, can result in a lower brachial plexus injury.

The common symptoms that a patient presents with are pain, paresthesia, dysaesthesia, numbness and weakness. Severe pain with an anaesthetic limb indicates root avulsions and has a poor prognosis for recovery.

Examination

Brachial Plexus Injury Following Major Trauma

With significant trauma, it is important to be alert to injury to the adjacent structures, e.g. the cervical spine or the great vessels and the thoracic cavity and contents. Having excluded life-threatening injury, the examiner should note the extent of the paralysis and sensory loss and chart this accurately where possible. Often pain and distress will make this examination incomplete, but data should be recorded for future comparison. The examiner must be aware of the possibility of a Horner's syndrome in lower trunk injury, in which case the pupil inequality may be mistaken for a sign of cerebral injury. The vascular status of the limb should also be established and recorded, and evidence of subclavian artery rupture may include expanding supraclavicular haematoma.[2]

Routine investigation for all patients at this early stage should include a trauma computed tomography (CT). In cases with extensive sensory loss in the arm, unappreciated fractures should be sought, especially of the wrist and forearm, where relatively subtle injuries can determine final outcome if undetected and untreated. The development of CT angiography has superseded contrast angiography in many units, and bony injury may be defined simultaneously where appropriate CT scanning protocols are employed.

After appropriate care has been given to the urgent treatment of bony, visceral or vascular injuries, the patient may then be assessed in more detail. This is the first opportunity to detect and record important data that will have bearing in the days to come when deciding whether clinical signs are evolving. The use of a standard brachial plexus chart for recording the findings is useful but not essential. A simple scheme is to record sensory findings on a sketch of the limb and to record motor findings by muscle group or by movement.

The Aims of Clinical Examination of the Brachial Plexus

Regarding how to approach a brachial plexus examination, one must first understand the aims of this examination. There are three main aims:

- Determine the level of the lesion.
- Determine the extent of the injury.
- Determine the presence of any poor prognostic signs.

Regarding the **level** of the lesion, first determine whether the injury is supraclavicular or infraclavicular.

- In supraclavicular lesions – roots and trunks are affected.
- In infraclavicular lesions – cords and branches affected.

Involvement of nerves arising from the roots of the brachial plexus such as the dorsal scapular nerve to the rhomboids and the long thoracic nerve to serratus anterior muscles are suggestive of a supraclavicular lesion. Involvement of the only nerve that arises from a trunk, the suprascapular nerve from the upper trunk, is also suggestive of a supraclavicular lesion.

For supraclavicular injuries, it is important to decide whether the injury is preganglionic or postganglionic. Preganglionic means the lesion is proximal to the dorsal root ganglion on the sensory side and at the level of the rootlets from the anterior horn cells on the motor side.

To examine the **extent** of the brachial plexus lesion competently, the examiner should have sound knowledge of the sensory and motor examination of the upper limb as described below.

The accuracy of identifying the structures injured (i.e. level and extent) in brachial plexus trauma by clinical examination is about 60%.

The **poor prognostic signs** include:

- High-energy injury
- Older age
- Flaccid limb
- Painful anaesthetic limb
- Signs of preganglionic injuries

Signs of preganglionic injuries include Horner's syndrome (Table 11.2) and signs that the rhomboids or serratus anterior muscles are affected. Preganglionic lesions may also be associated with long tract injuries to the spinal cord.

The sympathetic chain is not part of the brachial plexus. However, the ganglion lies just adjacent to the root. Therefore, any injury of the root (especially T1) can result in damage to the sympathetic system, resulting in Horner's syndrome (Figure 11.2).

The reason why preganglionic injuries have a poor prognosis is that they are not repairable and therefore may require later nerve grafts or muscle transfers.

With postganglionic injuries, there may be a chance of early repair.

Examination System for the Brachial Plexus

Inspection (Look)

Where possible, the initial examination is facilitated with the patient is standing. If the patient is unable to stand, the reason should be determined, bearing in mind that avulsion of the roots of the plexus may be associated with long tract signs that result in unsteadiness. The examiner should also stand and should begin by observation, inspecting the anterior and posterior aspects of the patient, noting posture, symmetry and signs of other injuries, as well as trophic changes and evidence of surgical scars. Look into the axilla, as some surgical approaches are via the axilla (Figure 11.3).

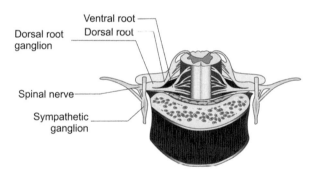

Figure 11.2 Relationship of the sympathetic chain to the dorsal root ganglion and the roots showing that, because of the intimate relationship, if these structures are damaged, then the sympathetic chain is also likely to be damaged.

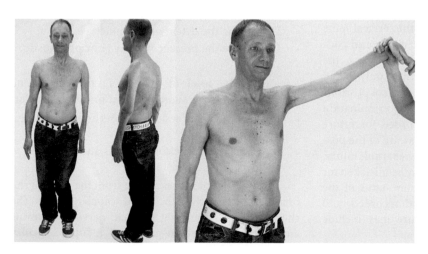

Figure 11.3 This patient has a long-standing brachial plexus injury. Note the gross wasting, clawing of the hand, supination of the forearm and Horner's syndrome. When looking from the side, wasting of the supraspinatus and infraspinatus is seen. Remember to look into the axilla, especially for any scars from previous surgery.

Look at the general attitude of the upper limb. It may be completely flail, indicating preganglionic injury. There are some characteristic appearances that that indicate the roots involved, e.g. an Erb's palsy or Klumpke's palsy.

Erb's palsy results from injuries to the upper part of the brachial plexus (C5, C6). This can be the result of a difficult delivery at birth but can also occur after trauma to the head and shoulder where the two are stretched apart.[3,4] Pressure on the upper brachial plexus from a shoulder dislocation can result in an Erb's palsy. The classical features are loss of sensation in the arm and weakness of the deltoid, biceps and brachialis, resulting in an arm that hangs by the side internally rotated at the shoulder and with the forearm extended and pronated. This is referred to as the 'waiter's tip' position (Figure 11.4).

Klumpke's palsy is a condition in which the lower brachial plexus is injured (C8, T1).[4] It may be the result of a difficult vaginal delivery or trauma in which there is forceful abduction of the shoulder such as hanging from a tree branch. The classic 'claw hand' shows the forearm supinated and the wrist and fingers flexed (Figure 11.5). In this palsy, sensation may be lost in the ulnar forearm and hand.

Horner's syndrome should be sought (Figure 11.6). Horner's syndrome indicates an injury to the sympathetic chain, which is located near to the T1 root immediately after exiting from the foramen, and is usually associated with avulsion of this root.

Feel

First, palpate the bony areas of the shoulder girdle for any areas of tenderness or fracture callus (Figure 11.7).

Then feel for sweating. Autonomic function is often preserved in first-degree injury but is lost acutely in all other degrees.

Because of the possibility of vascular damage, and because the cords are in intimate relation to the axillary artery, the pulse should also be palpated (Figure 11.8).

The sensory examination for different modalities is important, but in the first instance the initial assessment is seeking areas of gross sensory loss, and the most expedient way to undertake this is with a paperclip or pinwheel (pain or nociception) (Figures 11.9a and 11.9b). This offers a measure of threshold assessment, and this may be supplemented by light touch using the examiner's own fingertips. In each case, the perception of each stimulus should be compared to the uninjured side (if such exists), and

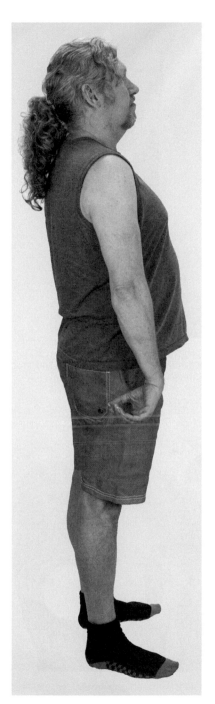

Figure 11.4 Erb's palsy (upper brachial plexus lesion C5, C6) is demonstrated here with the shoulder internally rotated and with the elbow extended and pronated, resulting in the 'waiter's tip position'.

the patient asked to comment on difference and similarity. Such examination may sometimes be usefully supplemented by examining other sensory modalities

199

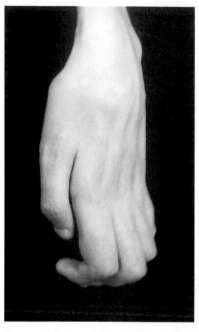

Figure 11.5 Klumpke's palsy (lower brachial plexus lesion C8, T1) is manifested mainly in the hand with flexion of the fingers and wrist (claw hand). In addition, there is supination of the forearm.

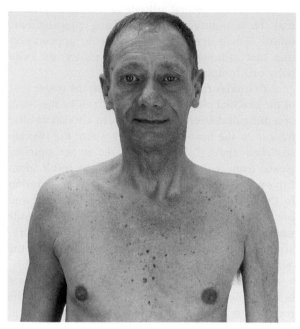

Figure 11.6 Horner's syndrome. This patient has ptosis, meiosis and enophthalmos of his left eye. Anhydrosis completes the classic features of this syndrome.

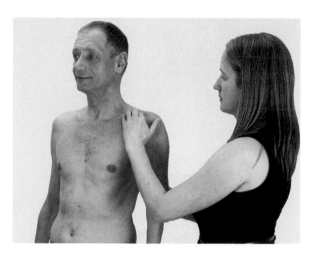

Figure 11.7 Palpation starts with feeling for areas of tenderness or bony prominences such as fracture callus.

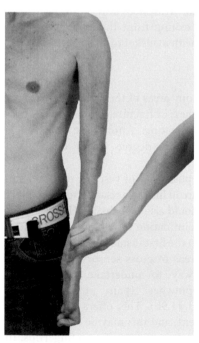

if a neurapraxia or conduction block is suspected, for in these injuries some fibres are preferentially affected, leading to an unpredictable loss of one modality before another.

Figure 11.8 Palpation should include feeling for the pulse, as brachial plexus injuries may be associated with trauma to the subclavian or axillary vessels.

Because of the anatomical arrangement of the brachial plexus, traction (the commonest cause of damage) often produces a mixture of degrees of nerve injury. It is important to distinguish those nerves that have suffered a first-degree injury (neurapraxia), since recovery can be expected without intervention. In these cases, certain characteristics are seen in the sensory loss. First, it may change rapidly, and the densest loss may be only transient, placing great importance on accurate recording of the signs from the first examination. Second, some modalities are more likely to be lost and are slower to recover, especially proprioception and light touch. Nociception, on the other hand, may be preserved, and this finding, in conjunction with the apparent preservation of sensibility in the presence of dense motor loss, should alert the examining surgeon to the likelihood of a first-degree nerve injury.

The sensory loss will then be plotted and will usually be found to correspond to the distribution of a root (dermatome) or branch (off the cords or terminal branch). This allows assessment of the level of injury anatomically (Figure 11.10a–d).

The sensory recovery may be graded using the Medical Research Council (MRC) system (Table 11.3) or, more usefully, with a descriptive system such as:

- No sensibility (i.e. anaesthetic)
- Pinprick sensibility recovered
- Moving touch felt
- Moving two-point discrimination of mm
- Static two-point discrimination of mm.

When assessing nerve injuries, a useful sign is **Tinel's phenomenon**. The principle underlying this sign is that the injured axon and the new growth cones of the regenerating nerve depolarise on mechanical stimulation. Percussion at the site of a significant

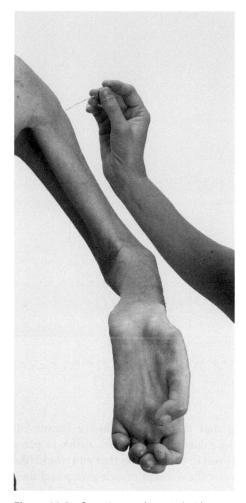

Figure 11.9a Sensation can be tested with a paper clip.

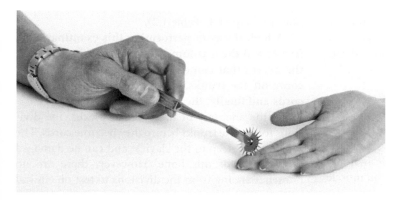

Figure 11.9b The use of a pinwheel to assess sensation. A wide area of assessment can be covered relatively quickly.

201

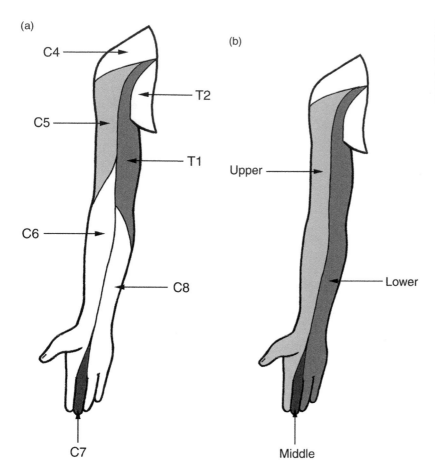

(a)

C4

T2

C5

T1

C6

C8

C7

(b)

Upper

Lower

Middle

Figure 11.10a–d Systematically examine the upper limb for sensory deficit. Plot the areas of deficit on a simple line drawing to determine whether the lesion is at the level of roots, trunks, cords or terminal branches. (a) Roots – dermatomes (b) Trunks

nerve injury results in the patient perceiving tingling distal to the injury in the distribution of that nerve (whether motor or sensory). This is a reliable localising sign of nerve injury, but it should be remembered that this sign may also be present at the site of distal regeneration. Tinel's sign is not quantitative, and the presence of a migrating Tinel's phenomenon indicates that some fibres are regenerating. Its position tells how advanced that process is but does not indicate the eventual extent of recovery (Figure 11.11). The absence of a positive Tinel's sign may also indicate a preganglionic injury.

Motor Examination (Move)

Examination of the motor system should then be undertaken. This is best conducted in a systematic manner from proximal to distal based on the anatomy of the brachial plexus. Initially, this focuses on muscle groups and their power.

Providing that there is still passive movement possible in the joint, it is sometimes easier to **place the patient's joint in the position that you would like it to be in** to test the relevant muscle group and then ask the patient to resist your attempts to straighten it.

In some muscle groups, grading of power is useful, whilst other groups require more descriptive approaches. Use the MRC grading system for motor power (Chapter 1, Table 1.2).

A logical way of performing this examination is first to test the myotomes (roots), then in sequence, the nerves that come off the roots, the nerves that come off the trunks, the nerves that come off the cords and finally, the terminal branches.

In the anatomy of the brachial plexus, the divisions follow the trunks before they become cords. The divisions lie deep to the clavicle and can be damaged in fractures of this bone. However, there are no branches arising from the divisions to test on clinical examination.

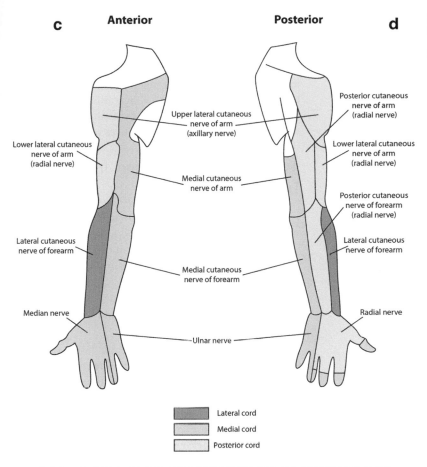

c   **Anterior**   **Posterior**   **d**

Upper lateral cutaneous nerve of arm (axillary nerve)

Lower lateral cutaneous nerve of arm (radial nerve)

Medial cutaneous nerve of arm

Lateral cutaneous nerve of forearm

Medial cutaneous nerve of forearm

Median nerve

Ulnar nerve

Posterior cutaneous nerve of arm (radial nerve)

Lower lateral cutaneous nerve of arm (radial nerve)

Posterior cutaneous nerve of forearm (radial nerve)

Lateral cutaneous nerve of forearm

Radial nerve

Lateral cord
Medial cord
Posterior cord

Figure 11.10a–d (cont.)
(c) Cords and cutaneous branches – anterior view
(d) Cords and cutaneous branches – posterior view

CORDS AND CUTANEOUS NERVES OF UPPER LIMB

Assess the Roots

- **C5** – elbow flexion; **C6** – wrist extension; **C7** – elbow extension; **C8** – finger flexion; **T1** – finger abduction.

The method of assessing the roots are similar to the American Spinal Cord Injury Association (ASIA) system described in Chapter 7 and shown in (Figure 11.12a–e).

In practice, some patterns of injury are common and can easily be recognised. In isolated C5 root lesions, the main loss is abduction of the arm and elbow flexion (which may be weak rather than absent) and some sensory loss over the lateral aspect of the deltoid muscle. This contrasts with an isolated axillary nerve palsy by the presence in the latter case of some activity in supraspinatus.

In C5, C6 root lesions, a classic pattern with three components is seen and, once seen, is easily recognised. Here the shoulder abductors, the external

rotators and the elbow flexors are paralysed. The arm is held internally rotated and cannot be flexed at the elbow or abducted.

Combined C5, C6 and C7 root lesions are as above but with weak elbow extension and weak or absent wrist flexion and extension. Isolated or combined C7, C8, T1 root lesions have good proximal limb muscles but clawing in all digits of the hand with weak flexion and extension of the fingers.

Assess the Nerves Arising from the Roots

- **Dorsal scapular nerve.** To test the rhomboid muscles, ask the patient to shrug the shoulders backwards against resistance (Figure 11.13a).
- **Long thoracic nerve.** To test for serratus anterior, the patient pushes against a wall with outstretched arms, the fingers and palm pointing downwards on the wall (Figure 11.13b).

Table 11.3 The MRC grading of sensation

S0	No sensation
S1	Pain sensation
S2	Pain and some touch sensation
S3	Pain and touch with no overreaction
S3+	Some two-point discrimination
S4	Complete recovery

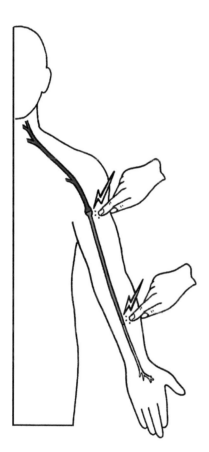

Figure 11.11 The principle of Tinel's phenomenon. Percussion over the site of nerve injury results in tingling or electric shock sensation passing distally in the distribution of the nerve. A similar 'migrating Tinel's phenomenon' is found when percussing over the site of the advancing growth cones of regeneration.

The long thoracic nerve (serratus anterior) and the dorsal scapular nerve (rhomboids) come off the roots and should be assessed just after assessing the myotomes as they may be injured together. Injury to these nerves indicates a preganglionic lesion.

Scapular stability is provided by a large number of muscles, prime amongst which are the rhomboids, serratus anterior and the trapezius. Paralysis of any of these three main muscles may result in an appearance of winging, which is therefore not always caused by long thoracic nerve palsy. Serratus anterior palsy results in the more common presentation of medial winging. Trapezius weakness causes lateral winging.

Assess the Nerves Arising from the Trunks

- **Suprascapular nerve.** This is assessed by testing supraspinatus (shoulder abduction in the scapular plane with the shoulders internally rotated) and infraspinatus (shoulder external rotation) (Figure 11.14a).
- **Spinal accessory.** Trapezius is tested by shrugging the shoulder; the trapezius should be palpated to isolate it (Figure 11.14b).

The muscles to be tested for trunk lesions are the trapezius and those supplied by the suprascapular nerve. The trapezius is supplied by the eleventh cranial nerve (spinal accessory), which is not part of the brachial plexus but lies in the posterior triangle of the neck and is therefore in proximity to the trunks and so can be injured together.

The spinal accessory nerve is commonly injured in the posterior triangle in the course of a node biopsy. The injury is often unappreciated despite the complaint of the patient. In part, this is because the belief exists that trapezius is the primary shrugger of the shoulders. In fact, that action is largely performed by levator scapulae, which can be felt contracting at the medial margin of the superior border of the scapula. Trapezius paralysis results in an inability to sustain abduction of the arm at 90°.

The suprascapular nerve, which supplies the supraspinatus and infraspinatus, comes off the upper trunk.

Distinguishing between weakness of supraspinatus and deltoid can be difficult. Supraspinatus can initiate abduction, whereas deltoid alone cannot. Conversely, supraspinatus can sustain abduction, as can deltoid. In 90° of abduction, the most powerful extender of the glenohumeral joint is deltoid (posterior fibres). Weakness of supraspinatus may be distinguished from a rotator cuff tear with difficulty. External rotation is compromised and, if no contraction of supraspinatus can be felt, imaging of the joint or direct inspection may be required.

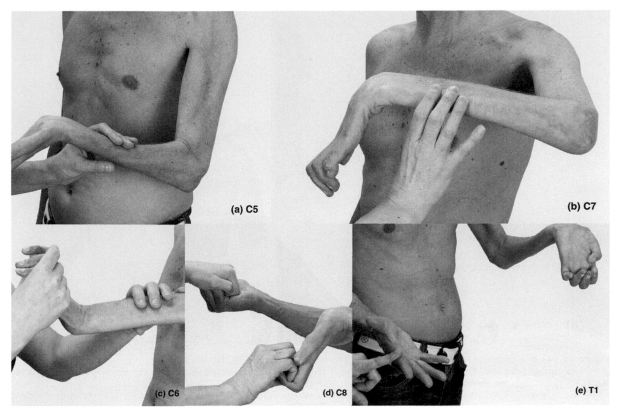

Figure 11.12a–e Assessing the roots of the brachial plexus by testing the myotomes.
(a) C5 – Flexion of the elbow
(b) C7 – Extension of the elbow
(c) C6 – Extension of the wrist
(d) C8 – Flexion of IP joints of the fingers
(e) T1 – Intrinsic muscles of the hand. First dorsal interosseous muscle of right hand is being demonstrated here.

IP, interphalangeal

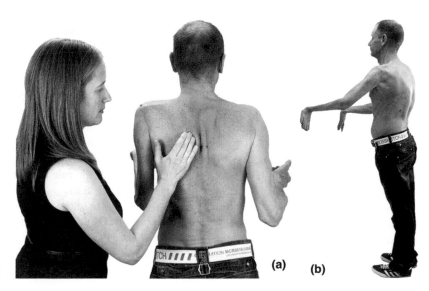

Figure 11.13a,b Assessing the muscles that are supplied by nerves coming off the roots of the brachial plexus.
(a) Testing the rhomboids (dorsal scapular nerve, C5). Push the elbows backwards and towards the midline against resistance and palpate the muscle. Also, the medial border of the scapula should move closer to the midline. Asymmetry between sides is suggestive of weakness.
(b) Testing serratus anterior (long thoracic nerve, C5,6,7). The patient pushes against the wall with outstretched arms, the fingers and palm pointing downwards on the wall. Look for scapular winging.

205

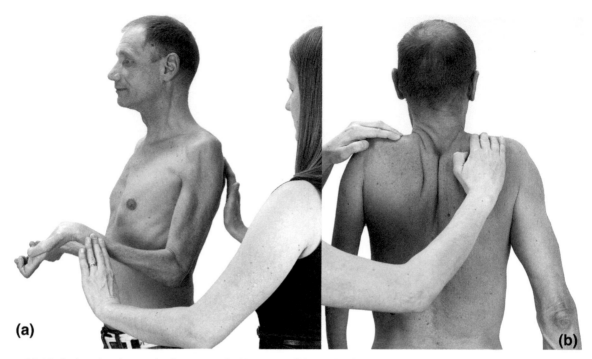

(a)

(b)

Figure 11.14a,b Assessing the muscles that are supplied by nerves off the trunks of the brachial plexus.
(a) Test for supraspinatus and infraspinatus (suprascapular nerve off the upper trunk). Infraspinatus is shown here – elbow to the side and flexed 90°. (i) Ask patient to externally rotate and resist this movement. (ii) Feel the muscle.
(b) Testing trapezius. This muscle is supplied by the eleventh cranial nerve (spinal accessory), but this nerve is located in the posterior triangle of the neck which can therefore be injured together with the trunks. To test, shrug the shoulders against resistance and palpate the muscle.

Assess the Nerves Arising from the Cords

- **Upper and lower subscapular nerve** (posterior cord). 'Gerber's lift-off test'. The hand is placed behind the back of the patient at the level of the lumbar spine, and the patient is asked to maintain the position. If subscapularis is weak, then the patient is unable to maintain the position of elevation off the back (Figure 11.15a).
- **Thoracodorsal nerve** (posterior cord). The patient is asked to apply downward pressure on the examiners shoulder. Feel the latissimus dorsi muscle contract (Figure 11.15b).
- **Medial and lateral pectoral nerve** (medial and lateral cords). The patient is requested to press into their own waist with their hands. Palpate the pectoralis major muscle (Figure 11.15c).

The muscles to be tested for lesions involving the cords are the subscapularis (upper and lower subscapular nerves off the posterior cord), the latissimus dorsi (thoracodorsal nerve off the posterior cord) and the pectoralis major muscle (medial and lateral pectoral nerves off the medial and lateral cords).

Subscapularis is an internal rotator of the shoulder and is tested by Gerber's lift-off test. Shoulder adduction is achieved mainly with two large muscles (pectoralis major and latissimus dorsi) that derive their innervation from several roots each, and so offers little localising information in terms of root involvement, but preservation of these muscles suggests involvement of the plexus distally, since the pectoral nerves emerge from the plexus early and the thoracodorsal nerve emerges from the posterior cord. A qualitative appreciation of latissimus dorsi function can be obtained by grasping the anterior free borders of both muscles and asking the patient to cough, exploiting the role of this muscle as an accessory muscle of respiration.

To determine whether the weakness of the pectoralis major is due to the lateral pectoral nerve, palpate the clavicular head of the muscle that it supplies. Palpating the sternal head tests the medial pectoral nerve.

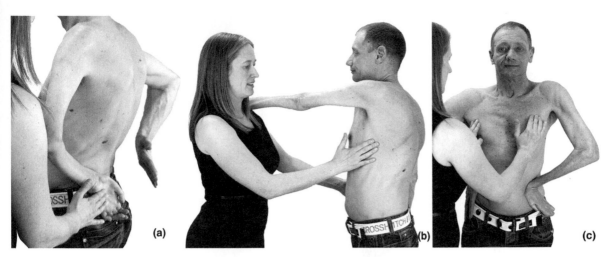

Figure 11.15a,b,c Assessing the muscles supplied by nerves arising from the cords of the brachial plexus.

(a) Testing for subscapularis (upper and lower subscapular nerves, posterior cord). Gerber's lift-off test. The arm is placed behind the back, and the hand is passively positioned away from the body. Patients with subscapularis injuries are unable to maintain this position (lag sign). Power can be assessed by the examiner pushing against the patient's hand.

(b) Testing for latissimus dorsi (thoracodorsal nerve, posterior cord). Downward/backward pressure of the arm against resistance, as though climbing a ladder. Palpate muscle. This force may be exerted on the shoulder of the examiner, as shown here.

(c) Testing for pectoralis major (medial and lateral pectoral nerves, medial and lateral cords respectively). Hands on waist and squeeze inwards. Palpate the muscle.

Assess the Terminal Branches

Axillary nerve (posterior cord). Deltoid is tested by shoulder abduction at 90°.

Musculocutaneous nerve (lateral cord). Biceps brachii is tested by resisted elbow flexion or resisted supination.

Radial nerve (posterior cord). Ask patient to point their index finger.

Ulnar nerve (medial cord). Ask patient to cross their fingers (middle over index).

Median nerve (medial and lateral cords). Ask patient to make an OK sign.

The terminal branches of the cords are assessed in sequence (Figure 11.16a–e).

They are described in more detail in Chapter 6. It may be difficult to separate the loss of movements as a result of terminal branch injuries from that of root (myotome) injuries.

Axillary nerve: Loss of abduction could be because of C5 root lesions or injuries to the axillary nerve (terminal branch of the posterior cord) where the deltoid is affected. To test for the axillary nerve, passively abduct the shoulder to 90°, then extend it. Ask the patient to resist as you push downwards on the arm. Feel the deltoid. This tests the posterior deltoid. The central and anterior fibres of the deltoid can be tested by placing the abducted arm in neutral and flexed positions, respectively. Deltoid function should be differentiated from supraspinatus (suprascapular nerve), especially in the position of forward flexion. The way to do this is to internally rotate the shoulder, thereby defunctioning the deltoid and isolating the supraspinatus.

The axillary nerve also supplies the teres minor muscle. This can be tested by looking for hornblower's sign, as described in Chapter 2.

Musculocutaneous nerve: Elbow flexion (C5, C6). The biceps brachii is innervated by the musculocutaneous nerve (lateral cord), as is the brachialis (predominantly musculocutaneous but some radial nerve laterally), whilst the brachioradialis is innervated by the radial nerve (posterior cord). Elbow flexion should initially be tested without the effect of gravity. Further assessment should record range of elbow flexion and weight lifted or resistance.

Radial nerve: Elbow extension (C7, C8) is predominantly triceps, from the radial nerve (posterior cord), and should be tested in a similar fashion to biceps. Wrist extension is also predominantly C7 via the radial nerve (posterior cord). Finger and thumb

207

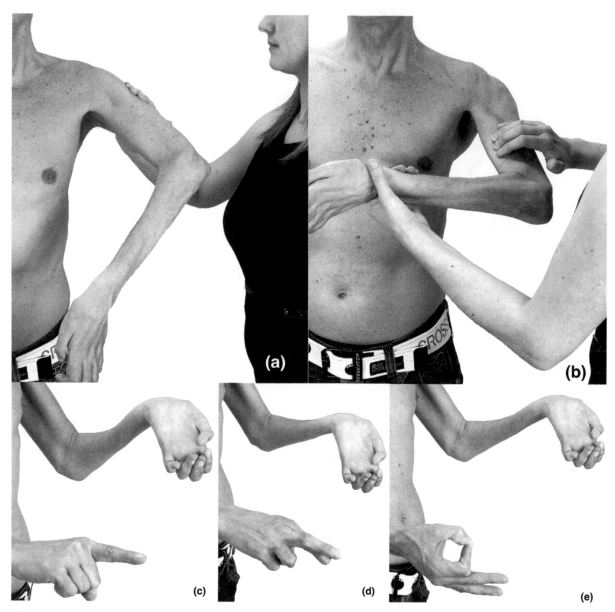

Figure 11.16a–e Assessing the terminal branches of the cords of the brachial plexus.
(a) **Shoulder** –Axillary nerve (terminal branch of the posterior cord). Tested by abducting the shoulder against resistance to test the deltoid.
(b) **Elbow** – Musculocutaneous nerve (terminal branch of the lateral cord). Test the biceps brachii by asking the patient to flex the elbow against resistance. Palpate the muscle. To eliminate gravity, the shoulder is abducted to 90° and the biceps is tested by flexing the elbow in this position.
(c) **Hand** – Radial nerve (terminal branch of posterior cord). Extension of metacarpophalangeal joint assessing extrinsic extensors. Quick screen 'point your finger'.
(d) **Hand** – Ulnar nerve (terminal branch of medial cord). Interosseous muscles of the hand. Quick screen 'cross your fingers'.
(e) **Hand** – Median nerve (from terminal branches of medial and lateral cords). Flexion of the DIP joint of index finger (FDP) and IP joint of thumb (FPL). Quick screen 'OK sign'.

DIP, distal interphalangeal; FDP, flexor digitorum profundus; FPL, flexor pollicis longus; IP, interphalangeal

extension at the metacarpophalangeal (MCP) joints is predominantly C7, 8 (radial nerve).

Ulnar nerve: This nerve supplies the intrinsic muscles which are essentially T1 roots. To separate a T1 lesion from an ulnar nerve lesion, as it branches from the cords of the brachial plexus, test the FDP to the little finger that will be affected in an ulnar nerve lesion and not a T1.

Median nerve: Flexion of the interphalangeal (IP) joint of the thumb, distal interphalangeal (DIP) joint of the index and middle fingers (via flexor pollicis longus (FPL) and flexor digitorum profundus (FDP)) is from the median nerve.

Advanced Corner

Treatment Principles of a Brachial Plexus Injury

The key question at the early stage (assuming that other injuries permit) is whether or not surgery is immediately indicated. Opinions vary on the precise indications for surgery, but some observations may be made.[5]

First, an important reason for performing surgery is to help with diagnosis. No clinical inference or imaging study will substitute for a direct examination of the plexus from foramina to axilla by an experienced surgeon. This is, however, a considerable undertaking and should be done only in the expectation of finding pathology that can then be immediately treated. Thus, the examination aims to predict such pathology and to shape a plan for treatment that can be discussed prior to surgery and completed at surgery.

Faced with a patient many months after injury, the surgeon will have to answer different questions. The results of exploration and repair are poorer after 6 months and, in general, not worthwhile for restoration of motor function in adults after 1 year, although some improvement in sensibility may occur. At this stage, the surgeon will be examining the patient with a view to secondary reconstruction, and the options here are numerous.

In general, they consist of osteotomy, arthrodesis, tendon transfers and, in some cases, nerve transfers to power free-functioning muscle transfers. For these reasons, the surgeon will need to evaluate the degree of recovery and determine whether further recovery is taking place. They will be interested in the function of the hand and its supporting structures and in determining whether the injury is primarily upper root or lower root. In upper root palsy, the hand may function very well

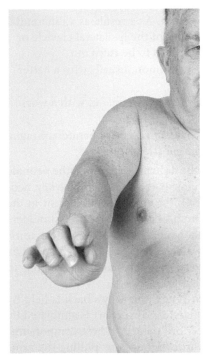

Figure 11.17 A patient with a right brachial plexus palsy. In planning treatment, their age and hand dominance should be noted, as well as duration from the time of injury. It can be seen in this photograph that the patient's shoulder function seems impaired but their hand looks relatively normal, implying an upper brachial plexus injury.

but the patient may lack the vital positioning qualities of a stable shoulder, together with external rotation and elbow flexion (Figure 11.17). In the converse situation, absent lower root function may leave good shoulder or elbow function with little hand use, raising doubts about the value of complex proximal reconstruction.[6]

Obstetric (Birth) Brachial Plexus Injury

This occurs in about 1:1 000 live births. Its incidence is becoming less because of improvements in obstetric care. Associated factors include macrosomia, prolonged labour, breech delivery, forceps delivery and shoulder dystocia.

It was thought that spontaneous recovery would occur in 90% of cases. However, recent data suggest that this is less, leading to a trend for more early surgical intervention.[7]

Presenting features:

- Mostly right-sided, possibly due to occipitoposterior presentation of the baby.

- Child holds arm limply at the side with a lack of any active movement. As a result, as a differential diagnosis, a fracture of the ipsilateral clavicle or proximal humerus has to be ruled out.
- Erb's palsy most common, usually with a better prognosis.
- Klumpke's palsy less common. but with a worse prognosis.
- Horner's syndrome and elevated hemidiaphragm are also poor prognostic features.

Diagnosis may be difficult to make, as the neonate will not be compliant. It is useful to utilise key neonatal reflexes to see if the child has movement in the suspected upper limb. The Moro reflex (shoulders especially but also hands), the asymmetrical tonic neck reflex (elbows especially) and the grasp reflex (hands) should cover the screening movements in the upper limb (Figure 11.18).

With the **Moro reflex**, the baby's back is held by the examiner. Sudden loss of support is simulated by the examiner. The Moro reflex has three components: Abduction of the arms followed by pulling the arms inwards (adduction) and (usually) crying. In the Moro reflex, the neonate also spreads their fingers apart. This reflex disappears by 6 months.

The Moro reflex must not be confused with the **parachute reflex,** which occurs after 6 months of age and lasts forever. In this reflex, the child is held in ventral suspension and then is suddenly lowered. The child extends their arms in a defensive reaction as though they are protecting themselves in a fall.

Asymmetrical tonic neck reflex is present up until about 4 months. If the child's face is turned to one side, the ipsilateral elbows and knees go into extension. The contralateral elbows and knees flex. This is also called the 'fencing reflex', as the position resembles that of a classical fencer.

Grasp (palmar) **reflex** lasts until the baby is about 6 months old. When the palm of the hand is stroked or an object, such as the examiner's finger, is placed in it, the baby will close the fingers of the hand.

'Burners' or 'Stingers'

These refer to a traumatic brachial plexus neurapraxia. Another term for this is 'dead arm syndrome'.

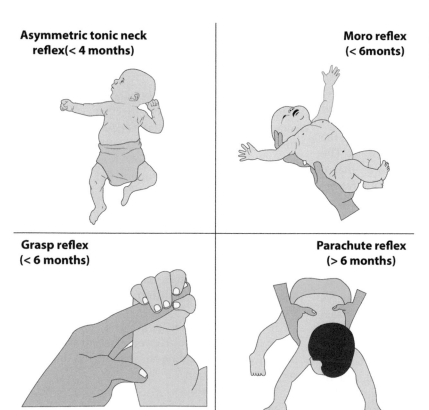

Asymmetric tonic neck reflex(< 4 months)

Moro reflex (< 6monts)

Grasp reflex (< 6 months)

Parachute reflex (> 6 months)

Figure 11.18 Illustration showing three neonatal reflexes: asymmetrical tonic neck reflex; Moro reflex; grasp reflex. Also shown is the parachute reflex, which starts at about 6 months.

These are descriptions of the symptoms that occur following injury.

This injury is most commonly a traction injury following a fall (in sport such as American football or rugby), where there is a traction force on the brachial plexus with simultaneous downward displacement of the arm and forced lateral flexion of the head in the opposite direction (Figure 11.19). It can also be caused by compressive forces or a direct blow to Erb's point (2–3 cm above the clavicle and just posterior to the sternomastoid).

Symptoms and signs only last a few minutes, but in a small proportion of patients they can persist for a few weeks. If bilateral, suspect spinal cord involvement and request a magnetic resonance imaging (MRI) scan.

Burners and Stingers mostly affects the C5, C6 roots or upper trunk. Hence, the biceps, deltoid and rotator cuff muscles will be weak. Serratus anterior and rhomboids will also be affected.

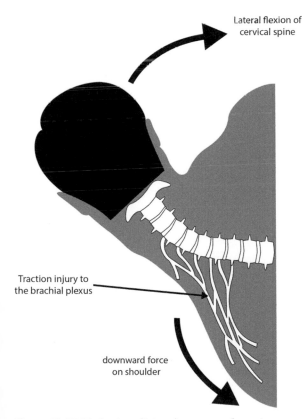

Lateral flexion of cervical spine

Traction injury to the brachial plexus

downward force on shoulder

Figure 11.19 Mechanism of injury that causes a 'burner' or 'stinger'.

Parsonage–Turner syndrome

This is referred to as idiopathic brachial plexopathy, brachial neuritis or neuralgic amyotrophy. The underlying cause is an inflammatory response involving the brachial plexus. Any branch of the brachial plexus can be involved, but the most common branches are the suprascapular nerve, long thoracic nerve and the axillary nerve (essentially the upper brachial plexus).

The patient usually presents following no specific precipitating cause, but Parsonage–Turner syndrome is most commonly seen post-operative, post-traumatic, post-infectious or post-vaccination. They present with severe unilateral shoulder pain. After a period of 24 hours to a few weeks, it becomes a more painless weakness in the affected muscle group. Recovery is the rule. About 90% are recovered by 3 years.[8]

Differential diagnoses include rotator cuff pathology, frozen shoulder, cervical disc disease, entrapment neuropathy (e.g. suprascapular nerve). Clinically it may be most difficult to differentiate from frozen shoulder but in Parsonage–Turner syndrome there is usually full passive range of movement.

Terrible Triad

Groh and Rockwood (1995) described an association between anterior shoulder dislocation, rotator cuff tear and brachial plexus injury.[9] The literature shows that up to 18% of younger patients and up to 32% of patients over the age of 50 years have this triad. In older patients, these can be greater tuberosity fractures rather than rotator cuff tears. Usually, the brachial plexus injury is infraclavicular, especially the posterior cord. The axillary nerve is the most common branch injured and is usually a neuropraxia.[10]

Following an anterior shoulder dislocation, the axillary nerve injury must therefore be specifically looked for. If this is seen, then clinical examination should focus on detecting a rotator cuff tear. This is usually difficult because both abduction (deltoid) and external rotation (teres minor) will be affected by the axillary nerve injury. Early ultrasound or MRI of the rotator cuff is therefore advised.

References

1. Drake RL, Vogal AW, Mitchell AWM. *Gray's Anatomy for Students*, 2nd ed. London: Churchill Livingstone Elsevier, 2010.

2. Midha, R. Epidemiology of brachial plexus injuries in a multitrauma population. *Neurosurgery* 1997;**40** (6):1182–1189.

3. Peleg D, Hasnin J, Shalev E. Fractured clavicle and Erb's palsy unrelated to birth trauma. *Am J Obstet Gynecol* 1997;**177**(5):1038–1040.

4. Shoja MM, Tubbs RS. Augusta Déjerine-Klumpke: the first female neuroanatomist. *Clin Anat* 2007;**20** (6):585–587.

5. Mukund R. Thatte, Sonali Babhulkar, Amita Hiremath. Brachial plexus injury in adults: Diagnosis and surgical treatment strategies, *Ann Indian Acad Neurol* 2013 Jan-Mar;**16**(1):26–33.

6. Martin E, Senders JT, DiRisio AC, et al. Timing of surgery in traumatic brachial plexus injury: a systematic review. *J Neurosurg* 2018 Jun;**1**:1–13.

7. Bahm J, Ocampo-Pavez C, Disselhorst-Klug C, Sellhaus B, Weis J. Obstetric brachial plexus palsy: treatment strategy, long-term results, and prognosis. *Dtsch Arztebl Int* 2009 Feb;**106**(6):83–90. doi: 10.3238/arztebl.2009.0083.

8. Feinberg JH, Radecki J. Parsonage–Turner syndrome. *HSS J* 2010 Sep;**6**(2):199–205. doi: 10.1007/s11420-010-9176-x. Epub 2010 Jul 30

9. Groh GI, Rockwood CA Jr. The terrible triad: anterior dislocation of the shoulder associated with rupture of the rotator cuff and injury to the brachial plexus. *J Shoulder Elb Surg* 1995;**4**(1 pt1):51–53.

10. Gutkovska O, Martynkiewicz J, Urban M, Gosk J. Brachial plexus injury after shoulder dislocation: a literature review. *Neurosurg Rev* 2020;**43** (2):407–423.

Chapter 12

Orthopaedic Examination Techniques in Children

James A. Fernandes

Summary of Orthopaedic Assessment in Children

A. History

B. Clinical Examination

There are certain differences in the way the examiner should approach the child in the examination process as opposed to the adult.

- Remember to communicate with the child as well as the parent.
- Examination of the small child does not necessarily need to be on the couch. They can sit on the parent's lap or even the floor.
- Respect the child's modesty and undress in stages if necessary.

Before examining a paediatric patient for abnormalities, it is important to know the variations within normal development.

Developmental Milestones

3 months	Lifts head when prone
6 months	Sits with some support; 9 months sits without support
9–12 months	Pulls self to stand
15 months	Walks unsupported
2 years	Runs
3 years	Jumps
5 years	Hops
6 years	Skips

Normal Variants

Hip anteversion: 40° at birth; 20° at 9 years; 15° at skeletal maturity.

Knees: 10°–15°varus at birth; Straight at 18 months; 10°–15° valgus at 3 years; 7° valgus from 7 years onwards.

Feet: Feet flat at birth; medial arch develops by 7 years.

Lower limb rotational profile (thigh–foot angle): –7° at birth; +7° at 5 years; +10° to +15° at 10 years onwards.

Based on what observations are made, the subsequent examination is tailored.

Assessment of Rotational Profile

Step 1

Look at the patient standing then walk the patient.

- Foot progression angle
- Patellar progression angle

Step 2

Sit the patient

- Check transmalleolar axis. This indicates tibial torsion. Normally the fibula is 20° posterior to the medial malleolus. In internal tibial torsion, the fibula may be at the same level or in front.

Step 3

Lie patient prone

- Check for metatarsus adductus (can also check whilst sitting).
- Thigh–foot angle. Measures tibial torsion (normal 10°–15° external).

Step 4

- Assess external and internal rotation of the hip.

Step 5

- Gage's test (Craig's test)

Note: There is increased internal rotation of the hip with increased femoral anteversion.
Please refer to Figure 12.15d.

Assessment of Leg Length Discrepancy

Step 1

Stand the patient and look (may be standing with pelvic tilt, FFD of hip or knee)

213

- Look modestly under the underwear.
- Expose spine and look for scoliosis or increased lumbar lordosis.

Step 2
Walk the patient – may see a short-limb gait

Step 3
Trendelenburg test – shortening of neck may result in positive test.

Step 4
- Lie patient down
- Square pelvis
- Thomas test and both hips range of movement (ROM) (because to measure 'true length' both legs have to be placed in similar degree of deformity)
- Tape measure test for leg length – anterior superior iliac spine (ASIS) to medial malleolus

If there is a difference, then proceed to next steps:

Step 5
Galeazzi test – Is shortening from above or below the knee?

- Child supine. Flex hips and knees to 90° with heels together and look from base of bed and from the side.

If shortening is from femoral side, then is it from above or below the greater trochanter?

Step 6
- Use Bryant's triangle: From the ASIS draw a line downwards. Measure the distance from this line to the tip of the greater trochanter. Compare the two sides.
- Can also use Nelaton's line: Draw a line from ASIS to ischial tuberosity. Tip of greater trochanter should be on or just below this line.

Step 7
- Block test: Performed by asking the patient to stand on blocks of increasing heights until the pelvis is level and the patient verbally confirms this. It is the most sensitive test of leg length measurement as the tape measure does not take into consideration shortening arising from below the medial malleolus.

Introduction
Paediatric orthopaedic examination is an art, and the success of the consultation relies on the surgeon's ability to communicate with the parents and the child. Most children who are referred do not require surgery, and time is spent on reassuring the anxious parents or guardian of the normal variations in the development of the child. Quite often, observing the child during the consultation with the parents and a thorough general examination give the clues in making a clinical diagnosis.

The paediatric consulting area should be child friendly, with toys and ample space for the child to play and for the surgeon to observe. Gaining the confidence of the child is crucial, as well as being warm and patient with the parents who are anxious and concerned. Neonates are generally seen in the neonatal wards and therefore the examiner needs to warm their hands before commencing. The initial interview should include introductions, as it is important to know the accompanying adults apart from the parents.

History should be gained from the parents as well as the older child, for, not infrequently, it could be conflicting. Clinical history skilfully obtained is the key to diagnosis, and a methodical examination of the child depending on the symptoms and age confirms your initial impression.[1]

History

General
The history usually starts with asking for demographic data, followed by the presenting complaint. Common complaints are of deformity, limp, gait abnormalities, weakness (generalised or localised), pain, swelling or stiffness of joints.

It is worthwhile asking the older child about their symptoms. The chronological order of the mode of onset of pain, time period, severity, disability and aggravating and relieving factors should be noted. History of trauma should be investigated thoroughly for its aetiological significance as non-accidental injury should always be at the back of your mind especially in a child below the age of 2. Since many of the symptoms arise from the musculoskeletal system that is concerned with support and locomotion, questions should be directed to establishing a relationship of symptoms to physical activity.

Prenatal history is of paramount importance. History of unusual incidents, vaginal bleeding and infections such as toxoplasmosis, rubella cytomegalovirus, herpes simplex and HIV(TORCH) in the first trimester give clues in the congenital afflictions. Maternal history of diabetes mellitus, toxaemia and

Table 12.1 Important developmental milestones

Age	Motor	Language
3 months	Lifts head up when prone	Vocalises without crying
6 months	Head steady when sitting	Smiles and laughs
9 months	Pulls self to stand	Non-specific words (da-da, ma-ma)
1 year	Walks with one hand support	Two or more words
14 months	Walks without support	
2 years	Runs forwards	Three-word sentence
3 years	Jumps in place	Knows whether girl or boy
4 years	Balances on one foot	Counts three objects correctly
5 years	Hops on one foot	Names four colours
6 years	Skips	

syphilis are associated with abnormalities at birth. Fetal movements in later pregnancy can be reduced in arthrogryposis multiplex congenita and Werdnig–Hoffman disease. In the birth history, the type of presentation, birth weight and Apgar score should be sought. Further perinatal-related questions, including jaundice, should be described.

Developmental history for physical and mental milestones should be sought (Table 12.1). Upper limb developmental functions and handedness is important with all children being ambidextrous until age 2. Information about school performance and physical activities give further insight. This is usually followed by a systemic review, including unusual bruising, easy bleeding and allergies. Past illnesses, hospitalisations and family history of significance completes the orthopaedic history. History of consanguinity becomes important whenever dealing with syndromic and/or skeletal dysplasias.

Specific

Limp and Gait Disturbances

Did the child start limping with complaints of pain? How was the onset? Acute transient synovitis of the hip is usually associated with a history of upper respiratory tract infection 7–14 days before the episode. The pain could be in the knee, thigh or hip because of the peculiarity of the same nerve supply. Was there any history of trauma? Post-traumatic avulsions of apophyses around the hip in adolescence produce a painful limp. Where is the pain? Adolescent children developing slipped capital femoral epiphyses more commonly present with aching pain, more often in the knee than the groin, hip or thigh. This may be associated with an abnormal out-toeing gait, especially with chronic slips. In the acute slip, there may be sudden severe pain with difficulty in weightbearing.

Children in the age group of 4–8 years are more likely to have the initial presentation of Perthes' disease.[2] Painful limp and difficulty weightbearing with constitutional and systemic symptoms should be urgently assessed for septic infection of joints, commonly the hip or in bone.

Was the limp noticed from walking age? Painless limp with short leg can be seen in late presentation of a dislocated hip or DDH, and painful limp at the end of the day could be a symptom of adolescent acetabular dysplasia or developmental coxa vara. Abnormal asymmetrical gait could be a feature of a neurological presentation. Abnormal posturing and gait abnormalities might be the only symptoms in rare spinal cord tumours and even in lumbar discitis.

Deformities

Flexible flat feet are usually familial with some family history of ligamentous laxity. Is there a progressive deformity of toes and feet? Pes cavus warrants a family history to rule out hereditary sensorimotor neuropathy (HSMN), Friedreich's ataxia, spinal dysraphism or other disorders. Painful flat feet in adolescence could be the first presentation of tarsal coalitions or inflammatory arthropathies. The former can also present with frequent ankle sprains due to a rigid hindfoot.

In-toeing gait is one of the common complaints (Figure 12.1). If present from walking age and bilateral, usually the common causes are metatarsus adductus, persistent excessive femoral anteversion or internal tibial torsion, with the latter two remodelling 95% of the time by age 7–9 years.

Any unilateral in-toeing or out-toeing needs to be further assessed and if rapidly progressive,

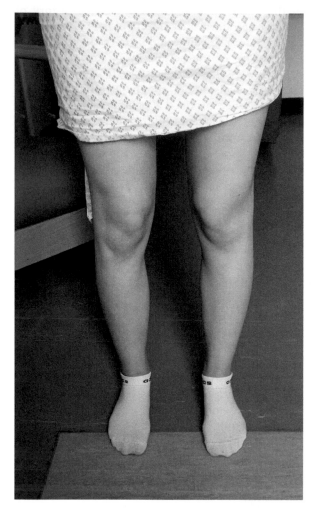

Figure 12.1 This child has patellae pointing inwards. She will walk with an in-toeing gait or a neutral foot progression angle if there is compensatory external tibial torsion (as in miserable malalignment syndrome).

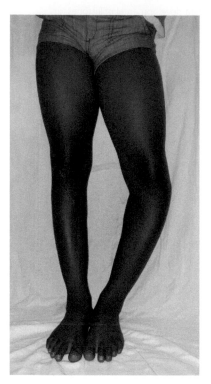

Figure 12.2 A clinical example for Blount's disease. As this is unilateral, it is more likely to be adolescent onset.

pathological conditions such as neurological, tumour, infection and congenital causes should be considered.

Bow legs and knock-knees are common deformities for which parents ask for consultation. Ask about the progression of these deformities. Quite often, they are physiological and, if severe, need to be investigated further.[3] Nutritional rickets is one of the commonest causes in the developing world, whereas questions relating to renal and familial rickets should be asked when such deformities are seen in the developed world. Any asymmetrical deformity could have an underlying cause. Consider Blount's disease in an Afro-Caribbean child with proximal tibial varus (Figure 12.2).

Limb Length Discrepancy

Limb length discrepancy, with or without associated deformities, could have various causes.[4] When was it first noticed? Was it noticed at birth and is it progressing? Is one shoe size smaller than the other? Was it noticed with a unilateral tiptoeing gait at walking age, suggesting a possibility of a late presentation of developmental dysplasia of the hip (DDH) (Figure 12.3). Is the child using a shoe raise? Does the child complain of any backache? Is one limb larger in length and girth as in hemihypertrophy or hypoplastic as in hemiatrophy? Is there a family history of neurofibromatosis? Was there any history of trauma or injury to the growth plates? Was there any history of infection of a joint or bone? These could cause discrepancy with deformity. A positive family history for deformity may indicate a syndrome or some indication for skeletal dysplasias.

Weakness

Localised weakness in the lower or upper limbs is rare and could be due to neuropraxias after injury or to any

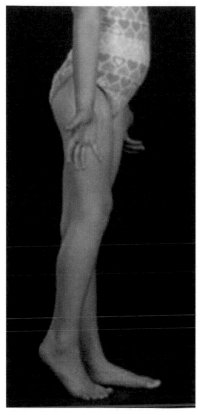

Figure 12.3 Late presentation of developmental dysplasia of the hip with unilateral tiptoe gait and a leg length discrepancy.

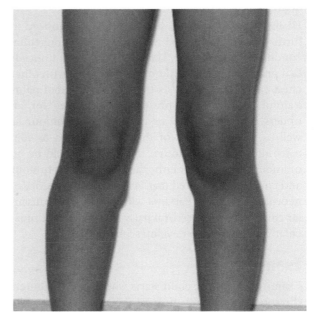

Figure 12.4 Exostoses on the proximal medial aspects of the tibiae in a patient with hereditary multiple exostoses (HME).

bony lumps pressing on nerve structures, as in hereditary multiple exostoses (HME). Adolescents may occasionally present with back pain, sciatica and weakness of toe dorsiflexors with acute disc protrusion.

Generalised weakness could be a feature of metabolic bone disorders. Those who complain of being easily tired and who are toe walkers should be investigated for muscular dystrophy with a simple blood test for creatine phosphokinase. Neuromuscular conditions like myopathies and others may present with floppy baby syndrome, slow developmental milestones, awkward gait and weakness. Space-occupying lesions in the base of the skull or spinal cord may have unusual presentations of weakness with abnormal gait and posturing.

Obstetric birth palsies can present with deformities, abnormal posture and partial or total loss of movements of the upper limb. Was there a large head or breech presentation? Was there a history of difficult labour? When was it first noticed and is there any progress in recovery of movements?

Swelling

When did the swelling appear and is it getting larger? Is there pain and has it progressed in size rapidly? These could be localised swellings or generalised around joints. Soft tissue swellings are usually slow growing and benign like ganglia and are usually pain free. Any swelling associated with pain should be evaluated for soft tissue sarcomas. Does the swelling fluctuate in size? Haemangiomas, which are common around the knee, give a history of fluctuation in size as well as the semi-membranosus bursa at the back of the knee. Bony lumps are usually in the metaphyseal regions of the long bones and could be multiple, as in HME (Figure 12.4). The practitioner should ask about any associated pain, functional loss or compromise in joint movement.

Swelling of joints with associated joint stiffness needs further questioning regarding the onset, periodicity and whether there was a rash or erythematous reaction. Small joint swellings of the fingers and toes are usually suggestive of seronegative arthropathy as the first presentation otherwise called 'sausage toes'. Family history of inflammatory conditions should be part of the history taking. Single joint affections need to be further explored for any foci of infection and systemic symptoms like pyrexia.

217

Scoliosis

History should include whether this was noticed at birth or was associated with any other congenital condition or syndrome. If later, when was it noticed? Is it progressing rapidly and is it associated with other chest cage deformities? Is there any associated pain? Painful scoliosis is a presenting syndrome for an underlying spinal cord or cauda equina tumour as well as bony tumours of the spine such as osteoid osteoma or osteoblastoma.[5] Night pain could be an ominous symptom for either an infection or a tumour and considered as a red flag. Ask for family history of neurofibromatosis. Patients with other neuromuscular conditions like cerebral palsy and Duchenne muscular dystrophy also develop scoliosis.

Examination

Examination of the child starts when the child enters the room and observation takes place while the history is being taken. Many clinical signs can be picked up from the parents giving clues in the genetically inherited conditions like neurofibromatosis, flat feet and scoliosis. The child should be undressed appropriately and in stages if required. Babies below the age of 6 months can be examined on the couch, whereas the toddler and infant can remain on the parent's knee until confidence is gained. Respecting the older child's modesty is vital and request for the presence of a chaperone. Examining the orthoses, shoewear, walking aids and presence of a wheelchair may give further information.

Sometimes the orthopaedic surgeon is called upon to assess a neonate. This is usually because of deformity that is noticed or suspected developmental dysplasia of the hip. Sometimes it is to investigate a possible neurological problem, e.g. an obstetric brachial plexus palsy or the baby is not using their legs.

Because the neonate will obviously not follow commands, it is helpful to know the neonatal reflexes that can be utilised to carry out a neurological assessment. In the upper limb, the Moro reflex, the grasp reflex and the asymmetrical tonic neck reflex can be used (described in more detail in the 'Advanced Corner' in Chapter 11). In the lower limb, the stepping reflex and also the grasp reflex and asymmetrical neck reflex will help with an assessment.

- **Moro reflex:** Sudden loss of support results in abduction followed by adduction of the arms and usually crying.

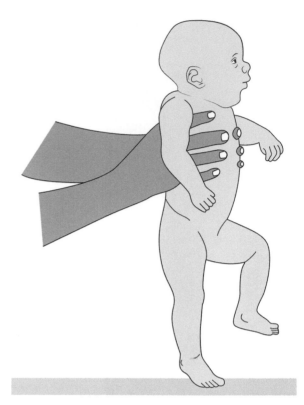

Figure 12.5 Stepping reflex in a neonate. On contact with the surface of the floor, the baby makes an attempt to step. This reflex disappears at around 3 months.

- **Asymmetrical tonic neck reflex:** Turn baby's neck to one side. There is ipsilateral extension of the elbow and knee and flexion of those joints on the contralateral side. Also called 'fencing' reflex because of the resulting position of the limbs.
- **Grasp reflex:** On stroking the palm of hand or sole of foot, the digits flex and grasp the examiner's finger.
- **Stepping reflex:** Suspend the neonate upright and place their feet on the floor. The baby makes an attempt to take a step once one foot is touching the floor. Also called 'walking' or 'dancing' reflex. It disappears at around 3–4 months of age and reappears just before the baby starts to walk at 12–13 months (Figure 12.5).

General

Inspection of the facies may give valuable clues in syndromic conditions and other skeletal dysplasias. When noted, dysmorphic features need to be of significance; looking at the parents' facies may also help. Blue sclerae can clinch the diagnosis of osteogenesis

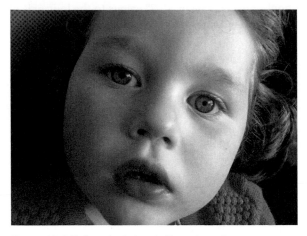

Figure 12.6 Unilateral miosis as in Horner's syndrome

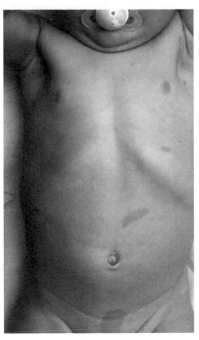

Figure 12.7 'Coast of California' smooth-edged café-au-lait spot of neurofibromatosis.

imperfecta, mongoloid features for Down syndrome and the classic face in achondroplasia with deep-set midface. Asymmetrical sizes of pupils, i.e. miosis, with or without ptosis, are a sign of Horner's syndrome (Figure 12.6).

The height of the child should be recorded both standing and sitting as well as the heights of the parents. The latter can be used in final height prediction of the child as well as using the modern-day height apps. Final height is one of the important decision makers in the choice of limb length equalisation, especially for the consideration of epiphysiodesis of the longer leg.

Metabolic disorders or skeletal dysplasias should be considered where there is short stature associated with lower limb deformities.[6] Short stature is defined as a height that is less than the third percentile for the chronologic age. Anthropometric measurements should include head and chest circumference, span, segmental lengths and ratios of the different segments (see the 'Advanced Corner' in this chapter). Any asymmetry in the body proportions of each side, including the tongue, should be sought, especially in hemihypertrophy. Hemiatrophy with history of low birth weight/low blood sugars may instigate an investigation for Russell–Silver syndrome.

Standing Examination in General

Examine from the front, side and the back; assess the standing posture and the normal curves of the spine. Look at the level of the shoulders and contour, level of the ASIS and symmetry. A plumb line held at the centre of the occiput should pass through the natal cleft. Frontal and sagittal balance should be assessed. Look for external spinal markers of dysraphism such as a dimple, a tuft of hair, naevus or a lipoma. In neurofibromatosis, look for café-au-lait spots (Figure 12.7), axillary or inguinal freckling and neurofibromas as well as in polysototic fibrous dysplasia.

Are there any vascular markings, as in Klippel–Trenaunay syndrome, or other blemishes? Note whether there are any defects of the limbs. If the creases of the limbs are not matching and the pelvis is not square, use blocks to lift the shorter side and level the iliac crests.

The general alignment of the lower limbs is then assessed for genu varum or genu valgum (Figure 12.8a,b), and this can be quantified with graduated wooden triangles at the intercondylar or intermalleolar levels. The reference is the knee, and the child should be made to stand with the patellae facing straight forward, medial malleoli touching each other when varus and the medial femoral condyles touching each other when valgus. The standing mechanical axis views for deformity planning are based on this clinical positioning, which is of paramount importance.[7]

The feet should be assessed for any cavus, flat footedness and hindfoot alignment. Standing on tip-toes should lead to the formation of a robust medial longitudinal arch (Figure 12.9a) and the heels should go into neutral or varus (Figure 12.9b). The hindfoot should normally be in 6°–7° valgus to the long axis of the calf when standing.

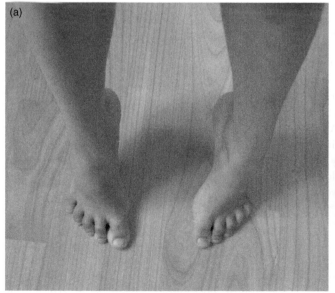

Figure 12.8a Bilateral genu varum in X-linked hypophosphataemic rickets.

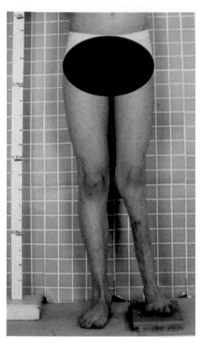

Figure 12.8b Congenital longitudinal deficiency with predominant fibular hemimelia, short limb and ipsilateral valgus deformity.

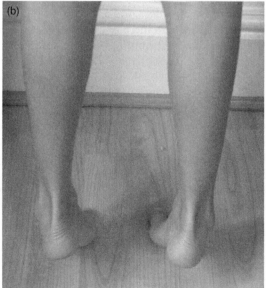

Figure 12.9a,b The medial longitudinal arch forms on standing on tiptoes when flexible and the heels invert into varus with creation of the arch.

Gait

Next, ask the child to walk in a straight line and look for any abnormal upper limb movements suggesting hemiplegia, athetoid or spastic movements. Look at the foot progression and knee progression angles, which give the degree of in-toeing or out-toeing, and the level at which they arise as well as being dynamic vector assessments, these help in surgical planning in de-rotation osteotomies. Look at the way the foot strikes the ground and whether a normal heel-to-toe type of gait is present. Assess knee extension on heel strike and flexion in swing. Look at the pelvis in all three planes.

Limp

Limp can be described as any asymmetrical movement of the lower limbs. A limp can be due to pain where it is called 'antalgic' or result from limb length discrepancy, instability at the hip or neurological causes.

In an **antalgic gait**, the stance phase of the affected limb is hurried with a quick swing phase of the opposite limb. It can result from any painful cause, from the sole of the foot to the pelvis. One can therefore broadly classify any gait as antalgic or non-antalgic gait and then specify.

In a **short-limbed gait**, the shoulder dips down on the shorter side on stance phase, as seen in children with longitudinal deficiencies such as congenital short femur, fibular hemimelia and with a reasonable functional hip.

The **Trendelenburg gait** is due to failure of the abductor mechanism on the affected side to hold the pelvis level in the stance phase, with a compensatory sway of the ipsilateral shoulder, classically called the 'lurch', thereby shifting the center of gravity to the midline. This produces a characteristic waddling or swaying, which becomes very dramatic in bilateral conditions, e.g. bilateral neglected congenital dislocation of the hip (DDH), bilateral coxa vara and in bilateral severe genu varum.

High stepping gait is seen with a foot drop when the dorsiflexors are ineffective at the ankle in achieving foot clearance; this produces the slapping foot. This is seen in paralytic neurological disorders of the lower motor neuron for example after common peroneal nerve injuries and hereditary sensorimotor neuropathy. This abnormality is seen in the swing phase.

In **toe walking** or **tiptoe gait,** the child's initial contact is with the forefoot and the contralateral foot follows the same.[8] This is seen in habitual tiptoe walkers with or without a tight heel cord and could be the earliest presentation of Duchenne muscular dystrophy. It is good practice to routinely request for creatine phosphokinase in males who are habitual tiptoe walkers so that early diagnosis is made and counsel the family. Any increase in tone of the limbs should suggest features of cerebral diplegia.

When the triceps surae is weak, a **calcaneus gait** is seen with lack of push-off and, when severe, is called the **'peg' gait**, as the stance phase remains on the heel throughout. This is often seen in lower motor neuron paralytic conditions and in overcorrected clubfeet after radical surgery.

The stiff knee produces a limp, and the pelvis is either hiked to clear the foot or the patient can circumduct the leg.

When the quadriceps is weak, patients compensate by 'back kneeing' to prevent the knee from collapsing, and fixed equinus helps to achieve this. Some children with paralytic conditions will use the hand to push the front of the thigh backwards to achieve back kneeing, otherwise called the **'quadriceps'** or **'hand-to-knee' gait**, to stabilise themselves in their gait.

Neurological gaits are of various types and can be combinations. **Spastic gait** is of equinus at the ankle, flexion at the knee and hips, with adduction and internal rotation of the lower limbs, producing dragging or scraping characteristics and, when static, has the 'jump' posture. Scissoring of the lower limbs can be seen when there are adduction and internal rotation deformities driven by these vectors from the hips.

In **crouch gait**, the triceps is weak and the gait lacks push-off with the ankles dorsiflexed in stance with knee and hip in flexion. This is quite often an iatrogenic condition caused by lengthening the tendoachilles in spastic conditions.

Ataxic gait is associated with a broad base and, when severe, the feet are thrown out, producing the double tapping stamping type of gait. Cerebellar ataxia also has a broad-based gait, irregular and unsteady, with or without eyes open, and the child is unable to do tandem walking.

Children with myopathies have a **penguin type of gait** and 'Gower's sign' is positive – the child uses the hands to climb upon themselves to stand up from sitting posture which is timed. The hypertrophied or bulky calves are seen in these children, with wasting of the thigh musculature.

Spine

Any head tilt with the chin rotated to the opposite side suggests torticollis or wry neck of the side to which it tilts. In babies one can feel a lump in the sternomastoid which may be the cause and, if not, one should seek other causes such as congenital cervical spinal anomalies. In the older child consider rotary instability of C1–C2 secondary to trauma or para- pharyngeal infections (otherwise called Grisel's syndrome). Rarely, head tilt can result from ophthalmological causes.

Assess the primary and secondary curves of the spine from the side. From the back the spine should be straight, and any lateral curvature seen is called scoliosis (see Chapter 13). Any list of the upper body and flank creases should be sought. Feel the spine for alignment, tenderness or a step at the lower lumbar spine as in spondylolisthesis.

Forward bending will reveal a structural scoliosis with the development of an asymmetrical rib or lumbar prominence (Figure 12.10). Postural or non-structural scoliosis does not show this and can be caused by leg length discrepancy or pain from nerve root entrapment. Scoliosis resulting from leg length inequality can be corrected by using appropriate blocks and making the pelvis level. Structural scoliosis should be assessed for the type of curve and the level of the curve. The usual curve patterns of single right thoracic, single left thoracolumbar or lumbar are those generally seen in adolescent idiopathic scoliosis.

The flexibility of the curve should then be assessed by side bending and whether part of the curve is correctable can be determined. Decompensation signs of the curve should be assessed by using the plumb line as well as looking at the gait and assessing the secondary curves.

The range of motion of the spine is measured in flexion, extension, lateral flexion and rotation. The latter should be either sitting or by holding the pelvis when standing. Assess true spinal movement in forward flexion, for the hips could compensate. Straight leg raising test, passive and active, should be performed, and this could be restricted because of nerve root irritation as in acute disc protrusion. Tight hamstrings with increased popliteal angles could be a feature of spondylolysis with low back pain, especially in a sporty teenager.

One should be able to assess whether pelvic obliquity influences the spine or vice versa. This is discussed in the spinal chapter, as suprapelvic, intrapelvic and infrapelvic types, with intrapelvic causes being assessed by revealing hip deformities or by sitting to identify any true hypoplasia of the hemipelvis (Figure 12.11).

Lower Limbs

Standing examination includes the Trendelenburg test and the block test for limb length inequality.

Trendelenburg Test

Failure of the abductor mechanism, producing a positive Trendelenburg test can be classified as due to instability at the *fulcrum* in DDH; failure of the *lever arm*, as seen in a short or varus femoral neck or pseudoarthrosis and failure of the *power arm* from a neurological cause for weakness of the abductors. A positive test is also seen in severe genu varum. A delayed Trendelenburg test assesses abductor fatigue on loading with time and is positive in residual acetabular dysplasia and coxa vara.

The Trendelenburg test is performed by asking the child to stand on each leg with both hips in extension and the non-weightbearing knee flexed. Normally,

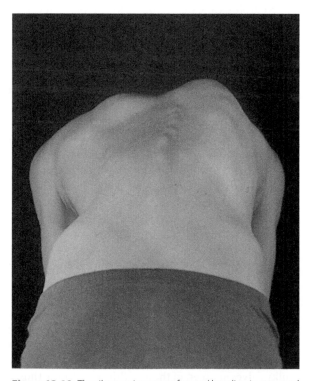

Figure 12.10 The rib prominence on forward bending in structural scoliosis.

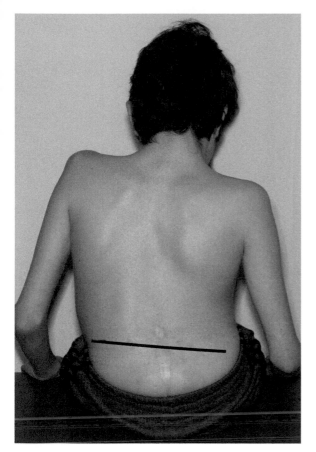

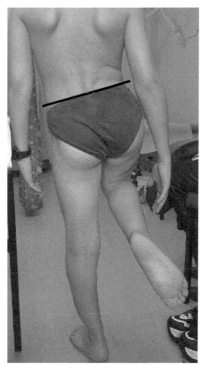

Figure 12.12a The pelvis being elevated when standing on the unaffected or normal left side.

Figure 12.11 Examining the patient sitting to identify any intrapelvic cause of obliquity producing scoliosis.

standing on the unaffected side elevates the pelvis on the opposite side (Figure 12.12a). In a positive test, the opposite side of the pelvis drops, indicating failure of the abductor mechanism (Figure 12.12b). The delayed Trendelenburg test is to make the child stand for 30 seconds to assess the abductor fatigue. When any associated leg length discrepancy is present, levelling the pelvis with blocks prior to performing the Trendelenburg is advisable lest it produces a false positive result.

Limb Length Discrepancy

Limb length discrepancy is assessed by the block test (Figure 12.13). Blocks are of different sizes and the child is made to stand with hips and knees extended and feet together with the shorter side on the blocks. The level of the posterior superior iliac spine (PSIS), the highest point of the iliac crests and the ASIS can

all be used as landmarks. Examination from the back is more accurate. True shortening can be measured this way only if there is no fixed flexion deformity (FFD) at the hip or the knee. If present, the child should be measured in the standing and/or supine position, placing the normal leg in the same attitude as the affected side. The same rule holds good if associated adduction or abduction hip contractures are present. Adduction contracture produces apparent shortening of the limb with the ipsilateral ASIS at a higher level and abduction contracture makes the leg appear longer with the ASIS at a lower level.

To determine whether shortening is above or below the knee, the Galeazzi test is performed with the child lying supine and flexing both the knees at a right angle and the heels together. The mismatch in the knee heights when seen from the side and from the end of the bed will suggest whether the discrepancy is in the femur or tibia (Figure 12.14a,b). Bryant's test can then be used to reveal whether a femoral shortening, if present is supratrochanteric or infratrochanteric by palpating the relative positions of the tips of

223

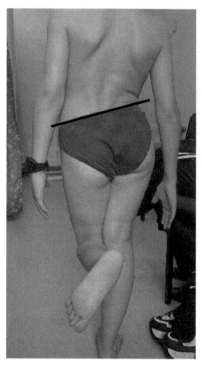

Figure 12.12b When standing on the right leg, there is a positive Trendelenburg test resulting, in this case, from septic arthritis in infancy.

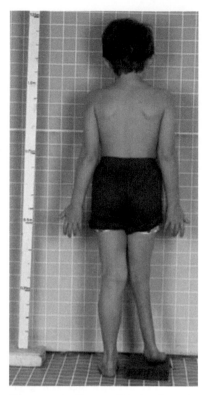

Figure 12.13 The use of blocks of varied heights to measure leg length discrepancy.

the trochanters and ASIS on either side using the thumbs on the ASIS, the middle finger on the tip of the greater trochanter and the index finger perpendicular to the couch. The difference in height between the fingers reveals supratrochanteric shortening.

Rotational Profile

The child may be seen sitting on the floor in the 'W' position, which indicates excessive femoral anteversion (Figure 12.15a).

On walking, the foot and patellar progression angles seen on visual gait analysis will suggest in-toeing or out-toeing, but not necessarily identify the segment for the cause. Remember that muscular forces can also influence this, especially in spastic gait.

Prone examination is the best way to determine the site for the torsional anomalies. With the child prone and flexed at the knees, the feet can be assessed for metatarsus varus (adductus) or other deformities using the heel bisector, or **Bleck's line**, which normally bisects the second toe. The thigh–foot angle reflects tibial torsion and is measured by drawing an imaginary

line along the long axis of the femur and a line bisecting the foot in its resting position. The normal value is 10°–15° of external rotation (Figure 12.15b). Alternatively, the transmalleolar axis can be used in the sitting position by comparing the transcondylar axis of the tibia with the bimalleolar axis, which is usually about 20° of external rotation.

Next, examine the hip for the range of internal and external rotation and perform the **'Gage test'** (Craig test), which determines the femoral anteversion.[9] The leg is used as the lever and the axis of the tibia as a reference. The examiner's thumb is placed on the trochanter and the palm of the hand on the buttock. The angle created by the leg to the imaginary vertical line when the greater trochanter becomes most prominent on rotating the limb from maximum internal rotation to maximum external rotation is the angle of anteversion of the femur. Femoral torsion is described when this is above two standard deviations to the normal. Therefore, there will be excessive internal rotation in femoral torsion and restricted or absent internal rotation in retro-torsion of the hip, as in congenital short femora.

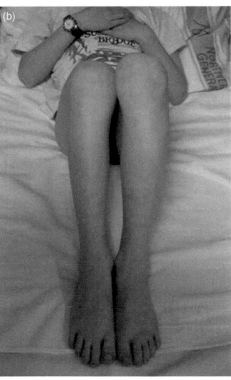

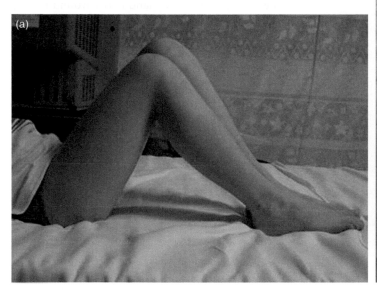

Figure 12.14a,b The Galeazzi sign as seen from the side and from the front in a patient with femoral shortening.

Figure 12.15a Child with femoral anteversion sitting in the characteristic 'W' position.

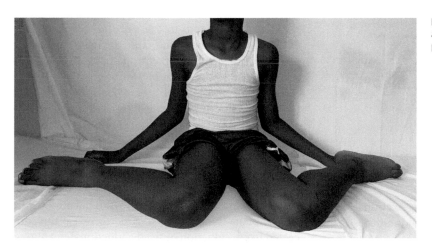

Femoral anteversion at birth is about 40°. It is 20° by the age of 9 and reaches the adult value of 12°–16° by the age of 16 years (Figure 12.15c). It is generally agreed that external rotation if less than 20°, internal rotation more than 70° after the age of 9 years is a relative indication for de-

rotational surgery of the femur provided there are clinical indications in addition. Precise assessments of all the above clinical signs help in the decision making in treatment of gait abnormalities and when in doubt the use of gait analysis is advisable. See Figure 12.15d for summary of steps.

225

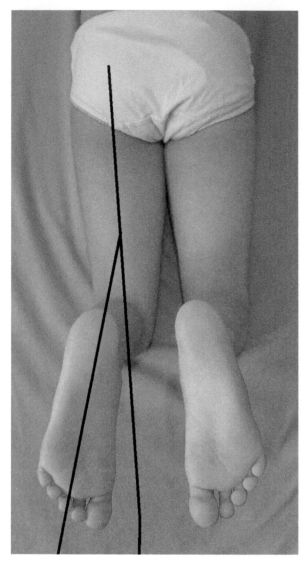

Figure 12.15b The prone examination to assess the thigh–foot angle.

Hip

Look: General inspection on supine examination is for any scars from previous surgery or sinuses from infection. Any asymmetrical creases, especially at the groin extending to the buttock, may be associated with developmental dysplasia of the hip. The attitude of the limb should be assessed, along with any apparent limb length discrepancy. Any effusion in the joint produces a flexion, abduction and external rotation attitude of the limb as in an irritable hip. The limb appears longer with a fixed abduction deformity and the ipsilateral ASIS is at a lower level, a classic presentation of idiopathic chondrolysis of the hip. In adduction deformities the limb appears shorter and the ipsilateral ASIS is at a higher level, a much more common presentation in many problem hip disorders.

Feel: Palpate the bony landmarks around the hip for tenderness, including the greater trochanter. Eliciting palpatory findings of the hip joint per-se is difficult as it is deeply placed. The femoral head may be palpable in the groin in partially treated DDH or in dysplastic hips; this is the 'lump sign'. The femoral head is made more palpable with the limb held in external rotation. The greater trochanter may be broadened in Perthes' disease.

Move: Before assessing range of motion of the hip joint, concealed deformities need to be revealed. The Thomas test is performed to reveal a fixed flexion deformity at the hip (Figure 12.16). This is concealed by an exaggerated lumbar lordosis. The contralateral hip is flexed to its maximum and held there by the child holding the knee, whilst the examiner confirms flattening of the lumbar lordosis using the palm of his or her hand. The child is then asked to gently extend the other leg. The angle created by the thigh segment with the couch is the angle of the FFD. The range of flexion in this hip is determined and the manoeuvre repeated on the opposite side.

The alternative to this test is **Staheli's prone hip extension test** where the child is stabilised at the bottom of the couch in the prone position with both limbs free and supported. The lordosis is then visually flattened by flexing both hips. Then each individual hip is extended and when the buttock starts to rise the angle created by the thigh to the lumbosacral spine is the amount of FFD at the hip (Figure 12.17).

Coronal plane movement is assessed after stabilising the pelvis and confirming that the pelvis is square. Maximum abduction of the unaffected side is a good method of locking the pelvis. When deformities exist in this plane the pelvis is squared to reveal the concealed fixed adduction or fixed abduction deformities. These are quantified and further range of motion in that plane is assessed.

Rotation of the hip in children is best assessed with the hips in extension and the child prone. Rotation with the hip in 90° of flexion can be assessed and documented, but is of less significance. Fixed rotational deformities are always obviously revealed.

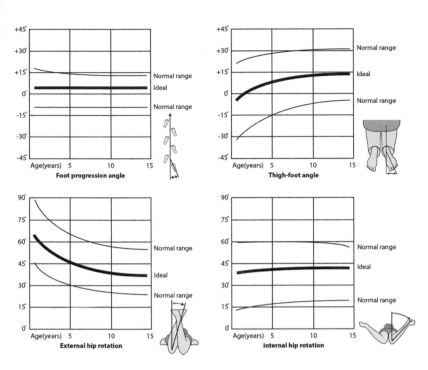

Figure 12.15c The Staheli rotational profile.

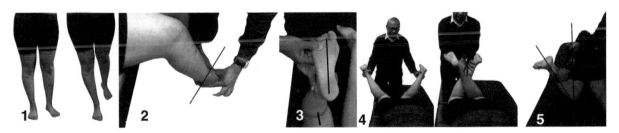

Figure 12.15d The five steps in a rotational profile examination as described above and in the 'Summary' section at the beginning of the chapter.

When examining neonates for *DDH*, the **Ortolani test** (Figure 12.18a,b) is to elicit the 'sign of entry' of the hip from the dislocated position followed by exit to its dislocated position when released. The test is done with the child relaxed on the couch with one hand stabilising the pelvis and the other flexing the knee fully and flexing the hip to 90°. The thumb is on the inside with the outer three fingers on the trochanter. As the hip is abducted, a palpable and audible 'clunk' is a positive test for reduction and when the opposite manoeuvre is performed the 'clunk' of exit is recorded as displacement of the hip.

The **Barlow test** is a provocation test for instability, performed the same way but demonstrating the

'clunk' of exit or give from the acetabular rim by gently pushing backwards with the thumb on the knee and the hip adducted (Figure 12.18c) and returns to the reduced position when released. Please also see (Figure 12.18d).

Dynamic and static ultrasound examination is the gold standard in assessing instability or dysplasia and monitoring progress of treatment up to the age of 6 months. The later classic signs in DDH are those of asymmetrical thigh folds usually the iliogroin crease seen from the front and the back (Figure 12.18e), limitation of abduction and relative shortening of the femur with the knees in flexion (positive Galeazzi sign). The Ortolani and Barlow's tests are not useful after the age of

227

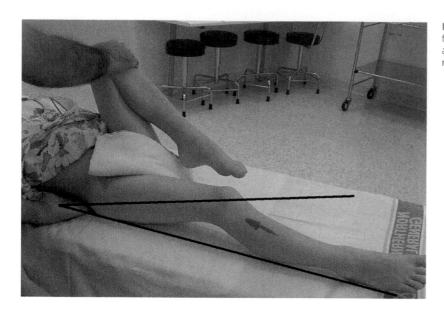

Figure 12.16 Thomas test to reveal fixed flexion deformity of the hip. This child has about 10° of fixed flexion deformity in the right hip.

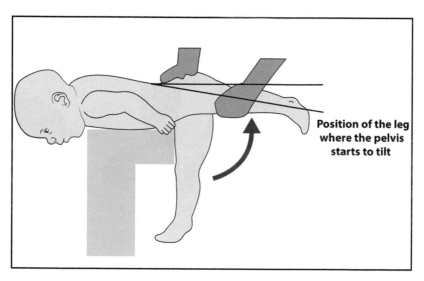

Position of the leg where the pelvis starts to tilt

Figure 12.17 Staheli's prone hip extension test. This test is an alternative to the Thomas test to reveal the fixed flexion deformity of the hip and is more sensitive. Note that the contralateral leg can be flexed and supported during the test to keep the child at comfort.

6 months. A plain AP radiograph of the hips after the age of 6 months can be used to diagnose DDH.

The **telescoping test** is positive in late presentation of dislocated hips. This is elicited with the hip and knee flexed and with the pelvis stabilised. The thigh is loaded downwards and released, feeling the femoral head or trochanter moving vertically.

Children with *Perthes' disease* lose abduction in flexion quite early. They also show features of irritability at the hip and gradually also lack internal rotation. When the hip is flexed the knee deviates towards the ipsilateral shoulder. This clinical sign suggests early femoral head deformity. Spasm can produce deformities at the hip and if complicated with chondrolysis can become fixed. Serial AP radiographs and frog leg lateral views will show the different evolutionary stages in the process of healing, from avascular necrosis with the crescent sign, stage of fragmentation or revascularisation and healing

Children with a *slipped capital femoral epiphysis* have decreased abduction, internal rotation and flexion, whereas they gain adduction, external rotation and extension. Flexing the hip causes the knee to

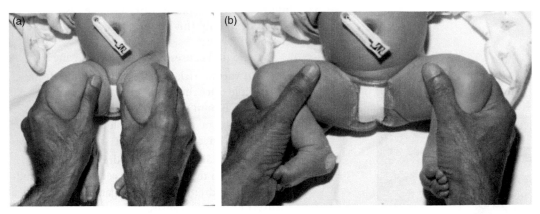

Figure 12.18a,b The Ortolani relocation test for developmental dysplasia of the hip. In this test, the dislocated hip is relocated with a 'clunk'. The manoeuvre is to move the hips from a slightly adducted position into abduction and, at the same time, pushing forwards with the fingers behind the trochanter.

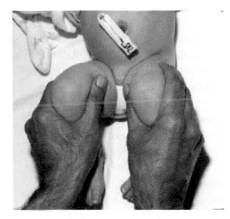

Figure 12.18c The Barlow test for an unstable hip. In this test, an unstable hip is dislocated with a 'clunk'. The manoeuvre is to adduct the hips from a neutral position and then push backwards.

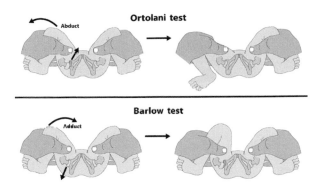

Figure 12.18d Illustration of both Ortolani (left) and Barlow (right) tests.

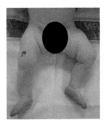

Figure 12.18e The asymmetrical groin crease in late developmental dysplasia of the hip.

deviate towards the ipsilateral shoulder, as in Perthes' disease. The presence of a FFD as well suggests that the hip is developing chondrolysis, a less frequent complication after surgical intervention. An out-toeing gait is one of the presentations, especially in chronic slips.

A frog leg lateral view of the hips will demonstrate the extent of the slip and also show the early slip, which could be missed in the AP film. The percentage of slip can also be measured on this view. The frog leg view is not advisable in those adolescents who cannot weightbear (and therefore the suspicion of having an acute unstable slip as classified by Loder) with the fear of worsening the slip.[10]

229

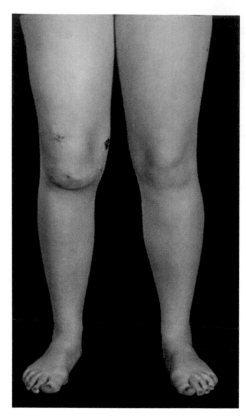

Figure 12.19 Increased girth of the thigh and swelling of the right knee with haemangiomatosis in Klippel–Trenaunay–Weber syndrome.

Knee

Look: Inspect the knee for any swelling. Fullness of the parapatellar fossae suggests a small effusion and a horseshoe swelling of the suprapatellar fossa with larger effusions. Generalised swelling is seen in inflammatory synovitis or haemangiomatosis (Figure 12.19). Localised swellings could result from bursae or bony lumps such as the tibial tuberosity in Osgood–Schlatter's disease. Any colour change with redness and signs of inflammation should be noted. The semi-membranous bursa is commonly seen on the posteromedial aspect of the knee. Coronal plane deformities of genu valgum or genu varum should be assessed standing with the patellae facing forwards. Up to the age of 18–24 months, a moderate degree of genu varum is normal. This then develops into excessive valgus by the age of 3 and normalises to about 7° of valgus by the age of 5–7 years (Salenius and Vankka curve, see Chapter 14). For genu valgum the intermalleolar distance can also be assessed. As a 'rule of thumb' this should be less than 8cm after the age of 7 years.

Pathological causes include the following:

- **Genu varum:** rickets, osteogenesis imperfecta, multiple osteochondromas, achondroplasia, trauma, Blount's disease
- **Genu valgum:** rickets, multiple osteochondromas, renal osteodystrophy, trauma

Popliteal Knee Swellings in Children:

All swellings in the popliteal fossa are termed popliteal cysts in children, with bursae, ganglia and popliteal aneurysm being the causes.

- Semimembranosus bursa is the commonest and is medial to the midline, usually starts above the joint line and lies between the semimembranosus muscle and the medial head of the gastrocnemius. It does not usually communicate with the joint and therefore the swelling does not vary in size. It is best palpated with the knee extended. It is self-limiting and surgical treatment is not necessary.
- A popliteal aneurysm is the least common of the three. It is pulsatile and sometimes bilateral, and examination is only complete by feeling for thrill and auscultating for the bruit.
- A popliteal cyst (called a Baker's cyst in the adult, where it is generally associated with osteoarthritis) is a result of bulging of the posterior capsule and synovial herniation. It is in the midline and at the level of the joint or just below. It communicates with the joint and therefore its size can be variable. No direct treatment is necessary for the swelling. Treatment is usually directed to the underlying pathology in the knee that is producing the fluid.

Feel: The knee is palpated to elicit tenderness at the joint lines for the menisci and bony landmarks (e.g. tibial tuberosity) as well as the patellar undersurface for chondromalacia. For smaller effusions, the bulge test can elicit fluid in the joint and for moderate effusions the patellar tap can be done after squeezing the suprapatellar pouch. A tense haemarthrosis does not have a positive patellar tap.

Move: Active range of motion is best elicited before passive movements. Determine whether there is any FFD of the knee as is seen in discoid menisci. Compare the movements of the good knee with the affected one, both in flexion and extension. Hyperextension at the knee is recorded, as well as symmetry and any associated features of benign hypermobility.

Patellar position, whether high (alta) or low (baja), is noted. Patellar tracking in the sitting position with the legs free can demonstrate lateral squinting and tilting, habitual dislocation or subluxation and persistent dislocation. The patellar apprehension test is elicited by attempting to push the patella laterally in an extended position and then flexing the knee. The child will resist this movement because of discomfort and apprehension if instability exists. Patellofemoral crepitus can be elicited on moving the knee and applying patellofemoral compression against the femoral trochlea.

Ligamentous stability should be tested next. It must be appreciated that ligamentous examination is less accurate in a child. Children's ligaments are more lax compared to adults and thereby laxity can be confused with ligament rupture. It is therefore important to compare with the contralateral side. The sensitivity of picking up ACL ruptures and meniscal tears on clinical examination has been shown in studies to be less in children compared to adults.[11]

The Lachman test with the knee in 20° of flexion determines abnormal movement in the anteroposterior plane and assesses anterior cruciate deficiency as seen in congenital short femur, or longitudinal deficiencies of the lower limbs as well as in the older child who sustains a tear of the anterior cruciate ligament. Posterior sag of the knee can be assessed with the knee held at a right angle to the couch, demonstrating posterior cruciate deficiency as in some longitudinal congenital deficiencies such as proximal femoral focal deficiency (PFFD) or fibular hemimelia. The latter sign is best investigated first, prior to any other signs for cruciate deficiencies. The collateral ligaments are tested with the knee in extension and in 30° of flexion with varus and valgus stress. Ligamentous laxity is associated with many skeletal dysplasias and therefore needs to be recorded.

Foot and Ankle

Look: Examine the feet standing, walking and at rest. On standing the heel is in slight valgus to the long axis of the calf because of subtalar mobility. The arch may be flat (pes planus), normal or high as in pes cavus (Figure 12.20a). Callosities on the sole of the feet inform about the weightbearing pattern and also the soles of the shoes and their uppers. Neuropathic ulcers may be seen in spina bifida and in sensory neuropathic conditions.

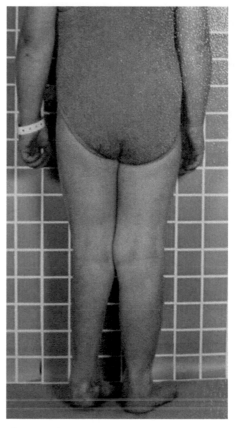

Figure 12.20a Pes cavus secondary to a multiply operated relapsed clubfoot with hindfoot varus and forefoot cavovarus.

Deformities of the toes need to be noted. Curly lesser toes, overriding second toes, overriding fifth toes and hammer and mallet toes are some of the common deformities. Clawing of the toes warrants an examination of the spine to exclude spinal dysraphism (Figure 12.20b), as well as investigations for other conditions such as HSMN and Friedreich's ataxia.[10] Metatarsus adductus or varus may be noted and could be part of a serpentine or skew foot or a residual clubfoot deformity.

Feel: The foot should be palpated over all bony landmarks. Tenderness over the tuberosity of the calcaneum could reflect calcaneal apophysitis (Sever's disease). Tenderness around the second metatarsophalangeal (MTP) joint might reflect Freiberg's disease.

Move: When assessing mobility of the foot, deformities need to be noted. Ankle range of motion in plantarflexion and dorsiflexion, subtalar movement in eversion and inversion and midfoot movement in all planes need to be recorded. Any deformity should

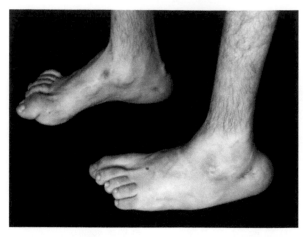

Figure 12.20b Asymmetrical foot deformities with right-sided toe deformities in spinal dysraphism (examine the spine in this situation for external spinal markers).

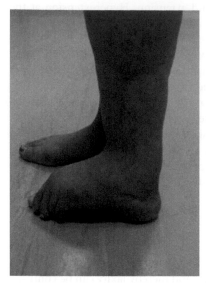

Figure 12.20c Calcaneocavus deformity with the calcaneum loading in a peg-shaped foot.

be assessed as being fixed or correctable, partially or completely. Reduced subtalar movement as in spasmodic peroneal flatfoot is seen in tarsal coalitions in adolescents, and subtalar irritability is seen in seronegative inflammatory conditions as an early presentation.

Flat feet are associated with dropped medial longitudinal arches on standing and valgus heels. When the child is made to stand on tiptoes, they recreate the arch and the heel goes into neutral or varus when there is no underlying abnormality. Similar reconstitution of flexible flat feet can be seen on dorsiflexing the big toe and on standing with external rotation of the tibia; this is otherwise described as the 'Jack test'. Flexible flat feet with tight heel cords need to be identified, as they require treatment by stretching the calf muscles.

Rigid flat feet can be either of the type seen in spasmodic peroneal flat feet of any cause or the rocker bottom seen in congenital vertical talus or in association with other conditions or syndromes such as spina bifida and arthrogryposis multiplex congenita.

Pes cavus can result from plantaris deformities of the first ray of the forefoot, equinocavus or in association with calcaneocavus deformities (Figure 12.20c). Remember to look for a neurological cause in patients presenting with pes cavus and examine the spine for external markers. A general tip: 'If the arch points to the floor, the pathological cause is in the foot generally and if the arch points upwards the pathological cause is higher up.'

Fixed pronation deformities of the forefoot seen in peroneal muscular atrophy can produce a varus posture of the heel on standing. This may be fully correctable. The Coleman block test can be used to elicit this.

The child is asked to stand on a block, which supports the heel and lateral border of the foot, allowing the first metatarsal to drop. The heel should correct to a neutral or valgus position if the hindfoot deformity is mobile and if not, it suggests that the heel varus is driven by the fixed pronation deformity of the forefoot.

Examination of the muscles around the foot and ankle is important and muscle strength should be graded as per Muscle Research Council (MRC) grading. Foot deformities can have varying aetiologies, and may be structural as in congenital talipes equinovarus (CTEV), muscular as in Duchenne muscular dystrophy, peripheral nerve disorders as in peroneal muscular atrophy, lower nerve roots as in spinal dysraphism or caused by upper motor neuron disorders, as in cerebral palsy.

Upper Limbs

Shoulder

Look: Observe the contour of the shoulder from the front, back and side. A high scapula, as in Sprengel's shoulder, can be seen even from the front. The scapula may be hypoplastic and wider sideways. This could be in association with Klippel–Feil syndrome, with shortening and webbing of the neck and a low posterior hairline (Figure 12.21). Webbing of the neck may also be seen in Turner's syndrome.

Abnormalities of the axillary pectoral folds could be because of absence of the sternal part of the pectoralis major, as in Poland's syndrome. Children with hereditary multiple exostoses often have lumps around the shoulder. Unilateral winging of the scapula can be seen in Parsonage–Turner syndrome and, if bilateral in teenagers, could be an early presentation of facioscapulohumeral or scapuloperoneal dystrophies.

Feel: Palpation of the shoulder joint and upper humerus should be performed to elicit tenderness and lumps. Absent clavicles may be seen in cleidocranial dysostosis (Figure 12.22) and defects of the clavicle may be palpable in pseudoarthroses of the clavicle, especially on the right unless with dextrocardia.

Move: Assess the range of motion of the shoulder joint, active first and then passive. The glenohumeral movement is examined by stabilising the scapula and then the scapulothoracic movements without any restriction of the scapula. Children can be asked to clap their hands in forward flexion or over their heads if not cooperative.

Stability of the shoulder is assessed next by stressing the humeral head forwards and backwards and by the sulcus test by pulling on the arm downwards. Multidirectional instability can be demonstrated in the atraumatic groups with bilateral signs and in association with ligamentous laxity. The apprehension test for anterior shoulder instability is performed by attempting to abduct and externally rotate the shoulder. The child resists in a positive test. Quite often, the child can demonstrate the 'clunk' or instability of the shoulder themselves. It is worth getting the child to demonstrate

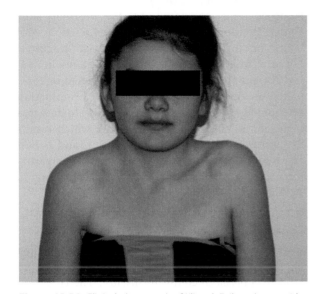

Figure 12.21 Clinical photograph of Klippel–Feil syndrome with a short neck seen from the front with high shoulders and mild webbing. From the back one will also appreciate the low neckline and bilateral Sprengel's shoulders.

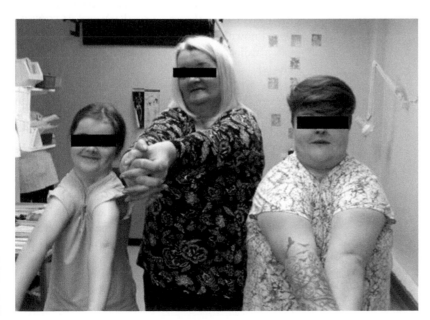

Figure 12.22 Familial condition of cleidocranial dysostosis with absent clavicles and ability to touch the shoulders against each other.

this to see the shoulder action and the direction of instability.

Elbow

Look: The elbow is a relatively easy joint to examine in a child. Swelling and deformities are well seen. In full extension the carrying angle can be assessed and is normally 10°–15° (more in females). Comparison of the unaffected side gives quantification of any deformity. A reduced carrying angle or cubitus varus is seen in malunited supracondylar fractures (Figure 12.23) and, when severe, produces the gun-stock deformity, which looks quite unusual when seen from the back or when the child walks. An increased carrying angle is noted in Turner's syndrome and bilateral symmetrical cubitus varus in Klinefelter's syndrome.

Feel: Palpation of bony landmarks around the elbow is undertaken in a fixed manner. The normal triangular relationship of the epicondyles and tip of the olecranon with the elbow in flexion and the linear relationship with the elbow in extension give clues to assess malunion of the distal humerus or a chronic dislocated elbow. Palpation of the radial head and the assessment of rotation of the forearm may reveal abnormalities of the relationship of the radial head with the capitellum, as in missed Monteggia fractures or congenital dislocation.

Move: Movements of the elbow joint should be recorded and compared to the normal side. Hyperextension can be noted in association with laxity or in malunited supracondylar fractures. Forearm rotation is assessed with the elbow in flexion at right angles. This might be restricted or completely absent in radioulnar synostoses. Examination of shoulder rotation can be used to evaluate varus malunion in supracondylar fractures, which results in increased shoulder internal rotation and is best assessed with the child bent forwards and comparing internal rotation from the back (see also Chapter 3, Yamamoto's test).

Wrist and Hand

Radial club hand may be mild or severe depending on the state of the radius, which can range from mild hypoplasia to complete absence. The condition usually arises sporadically but may be associated with a number of syndromes; for example, TAR syndrome (thrombocytopenia with absent radii, which is always bilateral with the presence of the thumbs), Fanconi anaemia (aplastic anaemia), Holt–Oram syndrome (heart anomalies) and VACTERL (also known as VATER and includes vertebral, anal, cardiac, tracheo-oesophageal, renal and limb defects).

The wrist can be assessed for swellings such as ganglia, classically on the dorsum or the radiovolar aspect. Prominence of the lower end of the ulna with radial and volar deviation of the wrist is seen in Madelung's deformity (Figure 12.24), and may be bilateral in the familial condition of Léri–Weill dys-chondrosteosis, which is associated with short stature or unilateral if acquired, as in post-traumatic physeal arrest of the distal radius. Reverse Madelung's deformity is classically associated in HME due to a short ulna. The wrist can be easily assessed for tenderness, swellings, synovial thickening and any increase in warmth. Movements are assessed and also ligamentous laxity, as seen with hypermobility when the thumb is able to approximate the volar aspect of the wrist.

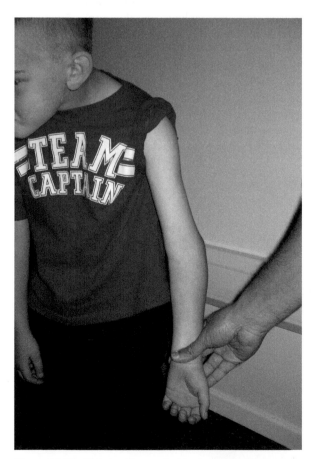

Figure 12.23 Clinical evidence of cubitus varus secondary to a malunited supracondylar fracture of the humerus.

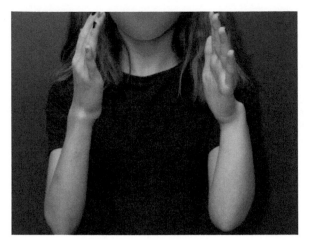

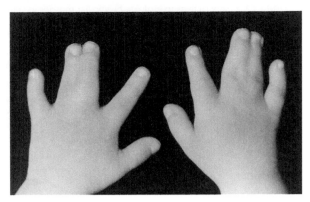

Figure 12.25 Bilateral complete simple syndactyly of both third web spaces.

Figure 12.24 Congenital Madelung's deformity associated with Léri–Weill dyschondrosteosis; prominent ulnar head with volar shift of the carpus, classic on the left.

Generalised systemic disorders can be detected by clubbing or cyanosis of the fingers. Common finger deformities include:

- Kirner deformity – apex dorsal and ulnar curvature of distal phalanx, usually of the little finger
- Clinodactyly – curvature of the digit in the radioulnar plane laterally
- Camptodactyly – flexion deformity of proximal interphalangeal (PIP) joint of the little finger
- Syndactyly – soft tissue or bony connections between the fingers (Figure 12.25)
- Polydactyly – duplication of the digits, pre-axial or post axial, the latter more commonly seen in the Afro-Caribbean population
- Arachnodactyly – 'spider fingers', a condition where the fingers are abnormally long and slender in relation to the palm (Marfan's syndrome).

Finger movements are also a good indication of ligamentous laxity, with hyperextension at the MCP joints. Joint ranges need to be assessed. Neurological examination is important in post-traumatic sequelae when associated with neurovascular injuries. Abnormalities of sensation may be difficult to assess in the younger child. The sweat pattern of the hand can be examined; if lacking, this is an indication of sensory loss. Examining for individual peripheral nerves and documentation of recovery pattern helps in the follow-up.

Any ischaemic sequelae of compartment syndrome need to be identified and differentiated from neurological injury. Asking the child to spread the fingers and demonstrate a 'five', adduct the fingers with the thumb in hand to show a 'four', making a fist and showing the letter 'O' with the thumb and index finger reliably assesses the motor supply of the hand. Strength can be assessed by asking the child to grasp your hand. Test also the pinch and the hook functions.

Neuromuscular Examination

Cerebral Palsy

The sequence of examination should be in one's own style and has to be modified depending on the age of the child, and whether they can stand and walk or not. To start, children younger than 5 years of age can be examined on their parent's lap. The child who can stand and walk can be assessed standing followed by observational gait analysis, sitting and then supine. The child who cannot walk should be first assessed in the wheelchair followed by sitting and finally supine.

Brief upper limb examination: Head and neck control and associated defects need to be assessed. Look for athetoid movements or any abnormal dystonic posturing or other abnormal involuntary movements.

Lower limb assessment: Range of movements should be recorded methodically and muscle testing carried out as per MRC grading, if possible. Leg lengths should be measured with the patient supine, with appropriate positioning depending on pelvic

235

Table 12.2 Special tests to evaluate bi-articular muscles in cerebral palsy

Test	Muscle	Description
Silfverskiöld	Triceps surae	To differentiate the tightness of the gastrocnemius and soleus, with knee in flexion and in extension by dorsiflexing the ankle.
Duncan–Ely	Rectus femoris	Flexion of the hip when knee flexed in prone position.
Hamstring shift	Hamstrings	The difference of angle between the unilateral popliteal angle done with the contralateral hip extended and bilateral popliteal angle. The latter being done flexing the contralateral hip to make the pelvis neutral.
Thomas hip flexion; Staheli's prone hip extension	Iliopsoas tightness	Done in supine and prone position. In neuromuscular cases, the prone test is more sensitive.
Phelps	Gracilis	Prone (or supine) with knees extended, abduct hips and then knees flexed and abduct further. Gain in abduction is a positive test.

obliquity and contractures. Measurement of the true leg length is important in these children. Special tests are required to assess the biarticular muscles (muscles that cross two joints), as these create contractures and need treatment based on their findings (Table 12.2).

Hip: The *Thomas test* is used to elicit the FFD at each hip and further range of motion is measured. *Staheli's prone hip extension test* is a worthwhile alternative test as it is more accurate in children. In the same position, hip rotations can also be assessed. The *Gage test* will determine the angle of femoral anteversion, and femoral torsion is commonly associated with this neuromuscular condition. The *Ely prone rectus femoris test* demonstrates a tight rectus when the buttock elevates as the knee is rapidly flexed. Hip abduction and adduction should be examined with the hips in extension and in flexion (see Chapter 8).

Knee: Spasticity and contracture of the hamstrings can be reliably measured by straight leg raising and assessing the *popliteal angle*. The hip is flexed to 90° and then the knee is extended from the flexed position. The angle created by the front of the leg to the front of the thigh is the popliteal angle (Figure 12.26). Normal values are less than 20°. The *hamstring shift angle* is the average of the unilateral popliteal angle and the bilateral popliteal angle done with the contralateral hip in flexion and placing the pelvis in neutral. This angle gives a better assessment of the tightness of the hamstrings. Any fixed flexion contracture at the knee should be assessed by extending the limb maximally and, if present, will be due to posterior capsular contracture. Quadriceps strength and spasticity can be assessed next. *Phelps' gracilis test* is done with the patient prone, knees flexed and hips abducted. If the hip adducts on extending the knee, gracilis spasm or contracture are confirmed.

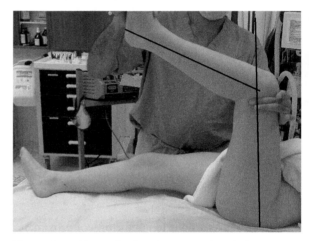

Figure 12.26 The popliteal angle to assess the tight hamstrings.

Foot and ankle: The range of motion at the ankle is recorded. The *Silfverskiöld test* differentiates gastrocnemius contracture from that of the soleus (see Chapter 10). If dorsiflexion of the foot is greater when the knee is flexed than when it is extended, then the gastrocnemius is implicated as the main site of contracture. If there is no change, then contracture of both muscles is present.

Varus of the foot could be due to a spastic tibialis posterior muscle at the hindfoot or the tibialis anterior at the midfoot or both. It could be a dynamic deformity that is more appreciable when the child walks or a fixed deformity. Tibial torsion needs to be assessed in the sitting position using imaginary lines between the proximal condyles and the distal transmalleolar axis. Alternatively, on prone examination the thigh–foot angle gives an accurate clinical measurement of tibial torsion.[4]

(a)

(b)

(c)

(d)

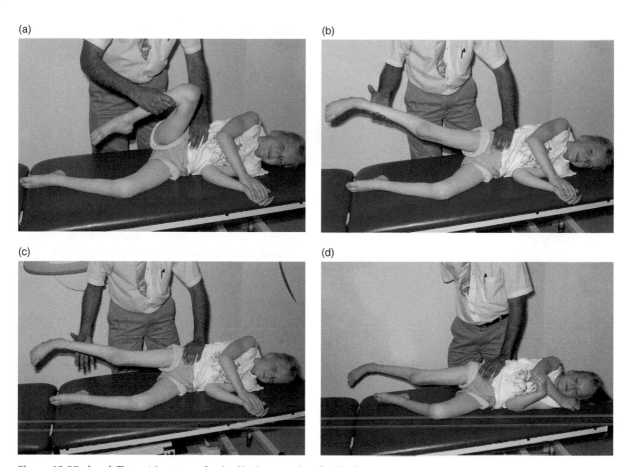

Figure 12.27a,b,c,d The serial sequence for the Ober's test as described in the text.

Other Paralytic Conditions

Knowledge of examining individual muscle groups and for nerve roots is essential in assessing children with paralytic conditions such as poliomyelitis or spina bifida disorders. Sensory dermatomal distribution and knowledge of autonomic systems supplying the bowel and bladder is essential.

Ober's test is used to assess the tightness of the iliotibial band and any abduction contracture at the hip. The test is performed by asking the child to lie on the side opposite to that being tested. The uninvolved hip and knee are maximally flexed to flatten the lumbar spine. The hip to be tested is flexed to 90° with the knee flexed and then fully abducted. The hip is then brought into full hyperextension and allowed to adduct maximally with a controlled drop. In a positive Ober's test, the limb tends to remain in abduction or has a delayed drop, suggesting tightness of the iliotibial band when it is in maximum stretch (Figure 12.27a,b,c,d). The angle

that the thigh makes with a horizontal line parallel to the table is the degree of contracture at the hip. When tight, the iliotibial band produces deformities at the knee of flexion, external rotation and valgus, otherwise called the **'triple deformity'** (Figure 12.28a,b). Gradual posterior subluxation of the knee and secondary deformities of equinus at the ankle, pelvic obliquity, and scoliosis and limb length discrepancy may develop. These are classically seen in residual paralysis after poliomyelitis and transverse myelitis.

Advanced Corner

'Cover Up Test' for Bow Legs

The 'cover up test' is performed on children with bow legs between the ages of 1 and 3 years (Figure 12.29). It involves covering the mid and distal part of the lower leg with the examiner's hand and observing the relationship between the

(a)

(b)

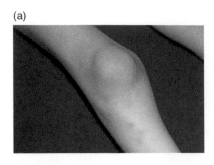

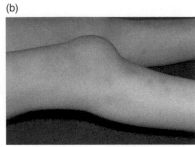

Figure 12.28a,b The triple deformity of the knee seen in the presence of a tight iliotibial band (flexion, valgus and external rotation).

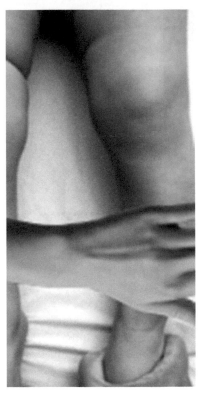

Figure 12.29 'Cover up test'. In a patient presenting with bow legs, the examiner covers the mid and distal parts of the lower leg with their hands. If the proximal part, as in this case, looks to be in valgus alignment compared to the upper leg, then it is likely to be physiological bow legs.

proximal part of the lower leg compared with the upper leg (thigh). This is performed with the patella facing directly forwards. If the proximal part of the lower leg compared with the upper leg is in varus or neutral, then a radiograph should be performed as the child is likely to have infantile tibia vara. If the relationship is valgus, then the child most likely has physiological bow legs.[12]

Irritable and Infected Hip

In irritable hip conditions (transient synovitis), the earliest movement lost is adduction in flexion; normally, there should be at least 20° in this position. Compared to a septic arthritis, in an irritable hip there is some passive movement possible on log rolling

In an acute septic arthritis, the child holds the lower limb in a position of flexion, abduction and external rotation. This is because in this position the hip capsule is at its largest volume and least tension. With septic hip arthritis, there is no active movement, and any passive movement is extremely painful.

The position that the child holds the lower limb and the loss of all movement because of pain is one way to differentiate between a septic arthritis and a transient synovitis. The best way, however, is the use of Kocher's criteria:

> One point is given for each of the following four criteria: non-weightbearing on affected side; ESR > 40; Fever > 38.5°C; white blood cell (WBC) count > 12,000/μl.

The likelihood of septic arthritis increases with scores from 1–4 by the following percentage: 1 (3%); 2 (40%); 3 (93%); 4 (99%).[13]

Recent studies have shown that inability to bear weight and a C-reactive protein (CRP) > 20 mg/l is just as effective at diagnosing septic arthritis.[14]

Assessment of a Child with a Skeletal Dysplasia

A general examination of the child and observation of the parents are both important. Look at the face, hair, presence of hearing aids, hands and feet.

Observe the gait and examine the joints for contractures. Enquire about the respiratory and cardiac systems. Then do a focused examination of various height and length parameters, as these patients frequently have short stature.

Investigation into the child's height starts from birth. Some babies have short length from birth (e.g. achondroplasia) and some have normal birth length and short stature develops with time (e.g. pseudoachondroplasia).[15]

The following are useful measurements (Figure 12.30):

- Total height
- Lower segment length (symphysis pubis to floor)
- Upper segment length (total height minus lower segment length)
- Upper segment to lower segment ratio (birth 1.7:1; puberty 1:1; post-puberty 0.9:1)
- Arm span
- Total height to arm span ratio (1:1 at puberty)
- Sitting height (seat of chair to top of head). Equivalent to upper segment length

Sitting height when compared with standing height (or upper segment to lower segment ratio) classifies skeletal dysplasia in a simplistic way: proportionate or disproportionate (Table 12.3).

Disproportionate short stature can be 'short trunk' or 'short limbed'. Segmental pattern of limb shortening with examples are shown in Table 12.4.

Table 12.3 Skeletal dysplasia in terms of proportions

Pattern	Trunk vs limbs	Clinical examples
Proportionate	Short trunk and limbs	Spondylo-epiphyseal dysplasia congenita (SED-c)
Disproportionate	Normal trunk, short limbs	Achondroplasia Hypochondroplasia
Disproportionate	Short trunk, relatively normal limbs	Morquio syndrome SED tarda (SED-t)

Table 12.4 Skeletal dysplasia in terms of segmental pattern

Pattern	Segments	Clinical examples
Rhizomelic	Proximal (femur and humerus)	Achondroplasia Hypochondroplasia Diastrophic dysplasia
Mesomelic	Middle (radius, ulna, tibia, fibula)	Léri–Weill dyschondrosteosis Chondroectodermal dysplasia
Acromelic	Distal (hands and feet)	Acrodysostosis
Micromelic	When all segments are short (entire limbs)	Kniest dysplasia Roberts syndrome

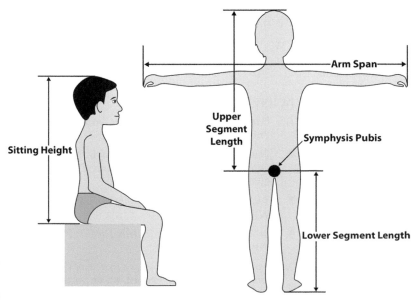

Figure 12.30 Some measurements to assess patients with skeletal dysplasia. Sitting height, arm span and upper and lower segment lengths are demonstrated.

Table 12.5 Spina bifida level and orthosis

Level	Ambulation	Orthosis	Notes
L1/L2	Non-ambulator	HKAFO	High functional level. Hip, knee, foot all not working.
L3	Marginal household ambulator	KAFO	Hip flexion and adduction possible. High risk of hip dislocation. Hip working. Knee not working.
L4	Household ambulator	AFO	Hip and knee working. Ankle and foot not working. Importantly, quadriceps is functioning.
L5	Community ambulator	AFO	Hip, knee and ankle working. Foot dorsiflexion deformity due to unopposed tibialis anterior action.
S1	Normal ambulator	Shoes	Hip, knee and ankle working.

A, ankle; F, foot; H, hip; K, knee; O, orthosis

Examination of Child with Spina Bifida

Spina bifida represents a group of abnormalities in which there is incomplete closure of the spine and membranes around the spinal cord.

They present to the orthopaedic surgeon mainly with lower limb manifestations, although in the spine they can present with scoliosis or kyphosis.

In the lower limb, there can be hip dysplasia or problems of torsion but the majority of these patients develop contractures of the hip, knee or foot and ankle, which affect their mobility.

Knowledge of the spinal level relating to the spina bifida is important for understanding the patient's ability to ambulate.[16] This knowledge can be applied to making decisions on the type of orthosis that will be needed for the child (Table 12.5). In general, for L3 level or above the child is essentially confined to a wheelchair, whereas an L5 can ambulate.

The following is a system for the orthopaedic surgeon to use to assess a spina bifida patient who presents with lower limb problems related to ambulation. The main task of the clinical examination is to establish the level of the disability.

The *look, feel, move, walk* sequence is useful. *Look* is probably the most important.

Look

- Look at the legs generally, describing any wasting or areas of ulceration.
- Look at the spine, describing any obvious dimple, hairy patch, naevus, lipoma or indeed an obvious myelomeningocele.
- Look for the presence of any catheter, which indicates that the patient may have lost control of bladder function.
- Look around for the presence of an orthosis. The type of orthosis is an indicator of the functional level (see Table 12.5).

Feel

- Sensation is difficult to assess in a young patient with spina bifida.

Move

- Movement and assessment of tone, power and reflexes may be difficult but should be carried out if necessary. Most of the required information would have been obtained from inspection.

Walk

- Finally, get the patient to walk +/− orthosis.

References

1. Herring JA. *Tachdjian's Pediatric Orthopaedics*, 4th ed. Philadelphia: WB Saunders, 2008.
2. Benson MKD, Fixsen JA, Macnicol MF. *Children's Orthopaedics and Fractures*. London: Churchill Livingstone, 1994.
3. Tachdjian MO. *Pediatric Orthopedics*. Philadelphia: WB Saunders, 1990.
4. Broughton NS. *Paediatric Orthopaedics*. Philadelphia: WB Saunders, 1996.
5. Apley AG, Solomon L. *Apley's System of Orthopaedics and Fractures*, 7th ed. Oxford: Butterworth–Heinemann, 1993.

6. Alshryda S, Jones S, Banaszkiewicz PA (eds). *Postgraduate Paediatric Orthopaedics*. Cambridge University Press, 2014.

7. Paley D. *Principles of Deformity Correction*. Berlin: Springer, 2002.

8. Bleck EE. *Orthopaedic Management in Cerebral Palsy*. Clinics in Developmental Medicine no. 99/100. Philadelphia: MacKeith Press, 1987.

9. Gage JR, Schwartz, Koop SE, Novacheck TF (eds). *The Identification and Treatment of Gait Problems in Cerebral Palsy*, 2nd ed. Clinics in Developmental Medicine no. 180–181. Oxford: MacKeith Press, 2009.

10. Sivananthan S, Sherry E, Warnke P, Miller M (eds). *Mercer's Textbook of Orthopaedics and Trauma*, 10th ed. London: Hodder Arnold, 2012.

11. Ardern CL, Ekås GR, Grindem H, et al. 2018 International Olympic Committee consensus statement on prevention, diagnosis and management of paediatric anterior cruciate ligament (ACL) injuries. *Br J Sports Med* 2018;**52**(7):422–438.

12. Davids JR, Blackhurst DW, Allen BL Jr. Clinical evaluation of bowed legs in children. *J Pediatr Orthop B* 2000;**9**(4):278–284.

13. Kocher MS, Zurakowski D, Kasser JR. Differentiating between septic arthritis and transient synovitis of the hip in children: an evidence-based clinical prediction algorithm. *J Bone Joint Surg Am* 1999; **81** (12):1662–1670.

14. Singhai R, Perry DC, Bruce CE. The diagnostic utility of Kocher's criteria in the diagnosis of septic arthritis in children: an external validation study. *J Bone Joint Surg* 2018;**94B**(Suppl XXXV).

15. Sung Yoon Cho, Dong-Kyu Jin. Guidelines for genetic skeletal dysplasias for pediatricians. *Ann Pediatr Endiocrinol Metab* 2015 Dec;**20**(4):187–191.

16. Dicianno BE, Karmarkar A, Houtrow A, et al. Factors associated with mobility outcomes in a national spina bifida patient registry. *Am J Phys Rehabil* 2015 Dec;**94**(12):1015–1025.

Examination of the Spine in Childhood

Chapter 13

A. L. Rex Michael and Ashley Cole

Summary of Examination of the Child with Scoliosis

The assessment of the scoliosis patient is very similar to the lumbar spine examination (see Chapter 7).

A. History

B. Clinical Examination

Step 1

Stand and look – most valuable

Step 2

Feel – spinous processes to confirm curves

Step 3

Move – forward bending (lateral flexion)

Step 4

Walk

Step 5

Lie the patient down – neurological exam

In the examination of a patient with scoliosis the following points should be considered, in addition to the above, at each step:

1. On looking, **look** for any stigmata for the cause (e.g. neurofibromata, high arch palate, pes cavus, cutaneous signs of spinal dysraphism, previous thoracotomy or spinal scar, pectus excavatum).
2. When **feeling**, you can assess the frontal plane balance of the spine by using a plumb line.
3. When asking the patient to **move** in forward flexion, look for a rib prominence (structural scoliosis).
4. When performing the **neurological examination**, include the abdominal reflexes as absence or asymmetry may indicate thoracic pathology.

The preceding four points allow for some key questions in the assessment of a scoliosis patient to be answered: Is it associated with any other conditions? Is it balanced? Is it structural? Is there any associated neurological abnormality?

Introduction

The spectrum of conditions of the spine in children includes spinal infection, trauma, tumours, spondylolysis and spondylolisthesis, the adolescent disc syndrome, as well as spinal deformities such as scoliosis.

The clinician should be alerted to the quality and site of any painful spinal symptoms, in terms of whether it is activity related and if there is any neuropathic pain. Worrying symptoms include night pain causing disturbed sleep, continuous and worsening pain requiring regular analgesia and pain interfering with enjoyable activities. *The younger the patient, the more likely it is that a spinal tumour is neoplastic*, with 75% of spinal tumours in the under-6s being malignant, contrasting with less than 33% in over-6s who have spinal tumours.[1]

The benign but painful osteoblastoma and osteoid osteoma occur principally around the thoracolumbar junction and the pain is typically relieved by non-steroidal anti-inflammatory drugs. Although pain is a cardinal feature of spinal malignancy, present in 46–83% of cases, only about one in three cases will present purely with pain and two-thirds will present with neurological problems, such as radicular pain, muscle wasting and weakness and/or a limp. Most children with an underlying neurological or neuromuscular condition will already have a diagnosis, and a previously fit and healthy child who develops new weakness and/or a limp should be suspected of having a spinal tumour or infection until proven otherwise.

The classical triad of fever, spinal pain and spinal tenderness is said to be pathognomonic of spinal infection, but these symptoms are not always present together at the outset and may be insidious in development, resulting often in a late diagnosis of spinal infection. Constitutional symptoms, such as malaise, fever and weight loss, should suggest spinal infection or tumour.

Caution should be exercised when dealing with the teenage male with a painful, stiff, progressive, left thoracic scoliosis, particularly when associated with features such as headache or asymmetrical abdominal reflexes. A syrinx may be present that can be malignant in origin.

There are several paediatric spinal conditions that require different approaches to both the history taking and examination. This chapter covers the following four conditions:

1. Scoliosis
2. Kyphosis/lordosis
3. Back pain (spondylosis/spondylolisthesis/ radicular pain)
4. Torticollis

Scoliosis

History

Patients with no cause for their scoliosis (idiopathic) are divided into two main groups dependent on age: (1) early-onset scoliosis, with development of deformity before the age of 5 years, and (2) late-onset scoliosis, in which the deformity develops after age 5 years, often coming to clinical attention in adolescence, with adolescent idiopathic scoliosis (AIS) diagnosed age 10–18 years.

Respiratory symptoms are more likely to be associated with early-onset scoliosis, reflecting hypoplasia of the pulmonary vascular and alveolar tree secondary to associated chest wall deformity during maximal growth and development of the heart and lungs.

The history should help to determine the problem and the cause:

The problem: Document when and by whom the deformity was first noticed, whether this was some time ago and whether there is a perception of deformity progression. What was noticed and whether this is of concern to the patient is obviously of key importance in AIS, where one of the indications for surgery is to improve trunk cosmesis. Any impact of the spinal deformity at school should be evaluated, as bullying can occur resulting in psychosocial problems.

In wheelchair-bound patients, the first thing noticed by the patient/parents/carers is usually difficulty with sitting balance, especially in those with good upper limb function and cognitive skills. Pressure area problems and particularly hygiene in the skin crease on the concavity of the curve is usually a late feature.

The cause: In apparently fit and healthy children, pain may indicate a cause such as tumour, especially osteoid osteoma, where patients classically have night pain. However, some pain is common in this group and is usually around the area of the curve or in the low back. Worrying features of the pain that may indicate a more sinister cause are:

- Night pain causing difficulty sleeping
- Pain requiring regular analgesia
- Pain causing the patient to be unable to do activities they enjoy
- Any upper or lower limb neurological symptoms

Fit and healthy children presenting with scoliosis may be a first presentation of:

- *Neurofibromatosis*, so any family history of neurofibromatosis, skin lesions or birth marks are relevant and can be evaluated on examination, including looking for axillary freckling.
- *Marfan's syndrome*, so any history of eye or cardiac problems and a very tall, slim patient may suggest this diagnosis and prompt looking for a high-arch palate, heart murmur and abnormally long fingers (arachnodactyly) on examination.
- *Spinal dysraphism*, so any upper or lower limb neurological symptoms, bladder or bowel dysfunction or feet abnormalities (pes cavus/toe clawing) should be noted and evaluated on examination.

It is important to elicit any family history of scoliosis and particularly any family history of other diseases, as this may suggest the diagnosis of a syndrome or neuromuscular diagnosis. A patient with idiopathic scoliosis has a 20% chance of having a first-degree relative with the same condition. Some conditions associated with spinal deformity are autosomal dominant and therefore carry a 50% risk of transmission from parent to offspring. Many syndromes are associated with scoliosis, and this can be a first presentation so referral for genetic evaluation may be appropriate if there is any suspicion.

Growth, and particularly rapid growth velocity, increases the risk of curve progression. The other main risk factor for progression being the size of the curve.

Infants grow most rapidly between birth and 5 years old, although most patients with infantile idiopathic scoliosis will resolve (80%). There is then a small juvenile growth spurt at about 7–8 years of age. In girls, the adolescent growth spurt normally starts between 11 and 12 years of age, reaching peak growth velocity approximately 6 months before menarche (average age 13.1 years in the UK). Girls will then continue to grow at a reducing growth velocity for 2–2.5 years after menarche. The growth velocity chart for boys is similar but takes place 2 years later than for girls and the peak growth velocity is higher.

At first presentation, menarcheal status and estimation from the parents regarding growth is useful. Height should be measured for comparison at subsequent visits. In wheelchair-bound patients, growth estimations are much less reliable and menarcheal status can be misleading. Growth is often delayed, but care must be taken as some syndromes are associated with early growth, e.g. Sotos syndrome.

Examination

The patient must be undressed to expose the lower limbs and trunk, but modesty should be respected, particularly in teenage girls, and the examination can be done in stages. It is often best to examine the trunk first, followed by a neurological examination. The examination should follow the traditional scheme of look, feel, move and special tests.

Look

Stand the patient. The trunk should be inspected from the front, side and rear. Any scars from previous surgery may be relevant (Figure 13.1a).

Sometimes patients with pectus excavatum and carinatum are sent initially to the paediatric spinal surgeon and are associated with conditions know to be associated with scoliosis, e.g. Marfan's syndrome.

Klippel–Feil syndrome, distinguished by a short neck and low hairline, may be associated with congenital scoliosis and/or a small, high-riding scapula (Sprengel's shoulder).

Winging of the scapula can be mistaken for scoliosis.

Any café-au-lait spots or other signs of neurofibromatosis should be noted. Apart from the scoliosis these include neurofibromas, axillary freckling, Lisch nodules and optic gliomas in the eyes.

Stigmata of spinal dysraphism are usually seen in the lumbar spine, especially at the lumbosacral junction but can be hidden in the natal cleft:

- Central lipoma
- Hairy patch
- Dimple (Figure 13.1b)
- Scarring from previous myelomeningocele closure

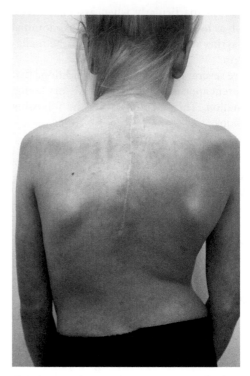

Figure 13.1a Post-operative patient. Note the thoracic midline scar and the café-au-lait patches suggestive of neurofibromatosis.

- Acrochordon (pedunculated skin lesion)
- Haemangioma

The asymmetry of the posterior trunk should be assessed in terms of:

- The convex side(s) and anatomical regions of the curves (thoracic, thoracolumbar and lumbar) (Figure 13.1c,d).
- Shoulder height asymmetry – generally high on the right in a right thoracic curve. When the shoulders are level or high on the side opposite the convexity of the main thoracic curve, suspect a compensatory upper thoracic curve.
- Waist and hip asymmetry (Figure 13.1e). In thoracolumbar scoliosis, the waist is flattened on the convex side of the curve and the hip is prominent on its concave side.
- Frontal plane imbalance. In idiopathic scoliosis, thoracolumbar curves have the greatest tendency to produce frontal plane imbalance with the trunk deviated towards the convex side of the curve (truncal shift).
- Sagittal shape and balance – kyphosis and lordosis. Idiopathic scoliosis is usually

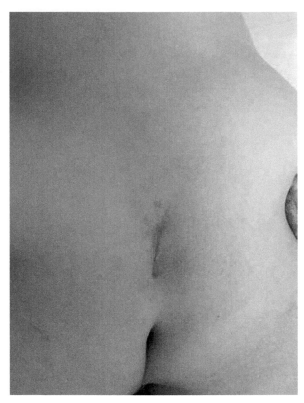

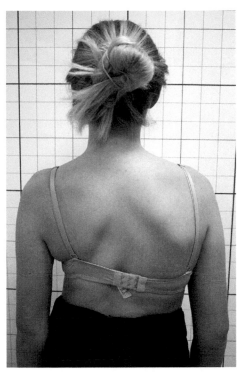

Figure 13.1c Right thoracic adolescent idiopathic scoliosis. Note prominent right scapula and high right shoulder.

Figure 13.1b Dimple at the base of the spine indicating spinal dysraphism.

associated with a reduced thoracic kyphosis, and this is the hardest plane to achieve surgical correction.

- Sagittal plane is assessed by looking at the spine side-on. Comment on:
  - ◦ Neck protraction (chin protruding forwards).
  - ◦ Shoulder protraction – usually on the convex side of a thoracic curve as the scapula slides forwards over the rib prominence.
- Leg length inequality. This can be a cause of postural scoliosis, but scoliosis secondary to leg length inequality can become structural. Ideally reassess with blocks under the short leg to level the pelvis and complete the examination with a level pelvis.

In wheelchair-bound patients, the wheelchair should be inspected to see whether there is a moulded seat, bolster support or whether it is patient controlled, suggesting good cognitive and upper limb function. These patients should be assessed initially sat on the edge of a couch, supported if necessary. The most common curve type is a long C-shaped curve, usually producing marked pelvic obliquity and frontal plane imbalance.

Feel

Feel along the spinous processes to confirm the curve directions and locations. A step in the spinous processes in the lower lumbar spine may suggest a spondylolisthesis that is associated with AIS. Any abnormal masses should be palpated.

At this point, frontal plane balance can be assessed by dropping a **plumb line** from the vertebra prominens (C7), which should bisect the natal cleft (Figure 13.2a). If the scoliosis is not balanced in the coronal plane, the plumb line will fall to one side of the natal cleft (Figure 13.2b).

Move

Rib prominence is evaluated in a forward bending position by **Adam's forward bend test**. This occurs due to rotation of the posterior ribs in the convexity of the curve that becomes more prominent when the spine is

245

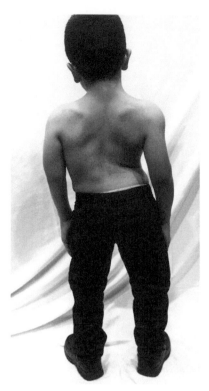

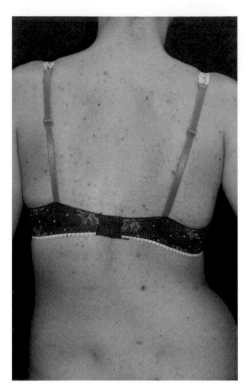

Figure 13.1d Left thoracic scoliosis. Note that the presence of a left thoracic scoliosis is a strong indicator of an underlying neurological problem.

Figure 13.1e Hip and waist asymmetry in thoracolumbar scoliosis.

flexed and can be quantified using a scoliometer (Figure 13.3). This measures the 'angle of trunk inclination' (ATI), which is usually recorded as the maximal angle in the thoracic and lumbar spine.

Lateral flexion can give an idea on correctability or flexibility of the curve. However, this is not an accurate method of making this assessment and is regarded a guess at best by spinal surgeons.

Assessment of curve flexibility is important. In young and light patients, this can be assessed by **suspension**. Another method, though infrequently done, is to place the child in the lateral position on the convex side of the curve on the knee of the examiner.

In larger patients, **prone stretching** is easier. With the patient prone on the couch, ask them to hold the top of the couch tightly and pull on the pelvis, noting the difference in the curve from a standing position.

Walk

Those patients able to walk should be observed walking with lower limbs exposed. In idiopathic scoliosis, this rarely reveals anything unless there is significant pain resulting in a limp or significant leg length inequality. In ambulant patients with syndromes and neuromuscular disease, it is important to assess the effects of the scoliosis on gait and, more importantly, the effects of a potential spinal fusion on gait, especially if the fusion needs to go low into the lumbar spine or even to the pelvis. Patients who rely on increased pelvic rotation during gait may be rendered wheelchair-bound by fusing the spine to the pelvis.

Neurological Examination

Lie the patient down on the couch. A full neurological examination is essential in suspected idiopathic scoliosis, and this should include assessment of upper and lower limb reflexes; Hoffman's sign (flicking the distal interphalangeal (DIP) joint of the index or middle finger looking for flexion of the thumb interphalangeal (IP) joint – this occurs due to dysfunction of the corticospinal tract); ankle clonus; and Babinski reflexes.

Reduction in pain and temperature but a normal appreciation of touch indicates the presence of 'suspended' disassociated sensory loss of a syrinx or intramedullary tumour.

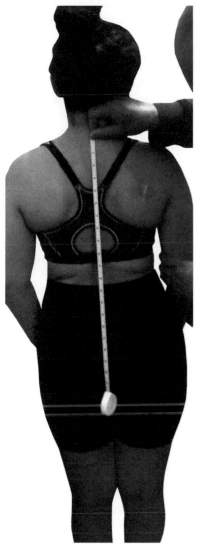

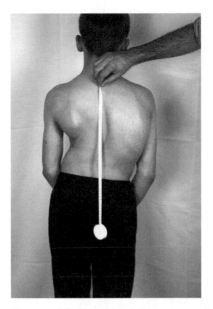

Figure 13.2b If there is imbalance as a result of the magnitude of the curve, the plumb line will fall to one side.

Figure 13.2a Frontal plane balance can be assessed with a plumb line that is dropped from the vertebra prominens (C7) and should bisect the natal cleft.

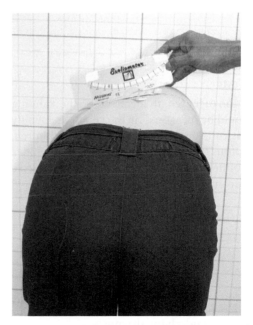

Figure 13.3 Adam's forward bend test showing a right-sided rib prominence quantified using a scoliometer.

Examine the feet for pes cavus and claw toes suggestive of an upper motor neuron problem or spinal dysraphism. Any neurological abnormality should prompt a whole-spine magnetic resonance imaging (MRI) scan.

Assessing the **abdominal reflexes** is an important part of the examination in a patient with scoliosis, as it is one of the few examinations that can give information on thoracic spine neurology (Figure 13.4). This is described in detail in Chapter 7. However, it involves stroking the abdomen radially outwards from the umbilicus in the 2, 4, 8 and 10 o'clock positions. Loss of contraction in the underlying musculature indicates pathology at the level. When abnormal the absent reflex is usually on the convex side of the curve.

247

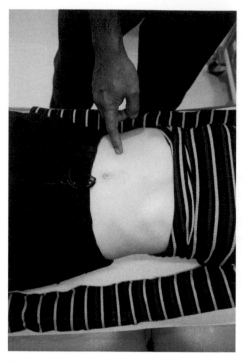

Figure 13.4 Abdominal reflexes. The abdomen is stroked radially outwards from the umbilicus in each quadrant. Absence of underlying muscle contraction may signify thoracic spine pathology.

Additional Tests

Any suggestion of leg length inequality in the standing position should be measured on the couch. Inequality up to 1 cm is considered normal in growing children.

Ligamentous laxity should also be assessed, thinking about connective tissue disorders such as Ehlers–Danlos syndrome.

Kyphosis/Lordosis

History

The history of kyphosis is very similar to that taken for scoliosis:

- Identify the problem.
- Assess for an underlying diagnosis.
- Assess growth potential.
- Evaluate any additional diagnoses that may cause problems with surgery.

These patients will often have back pain in addition to deformity, and, as described above, this needs a careful history to try and determine whether there are any sinister features ('red flags'). If the kyphosis

has developed quickly and is associated with pain, then a pathological fracture secondary to tumour or infection should be considered. In childhood, a kyphosis secondary to previous trauma should give a history of significant injury.

The two types of idiopathic kyphotic deformity are given the eponymous titles of type 1 and type 2 Scheuermann's disease, depending on the region of the spine affected.

Type 1 Scheuermann's disease (lower thoracic) typically presents in the early to mid-teens, whereas type 2 Scheuermann's disease (thoracolumbar) presents in the late teens and early 20s. The presenting features are round back and/or pain over the apex of the deformity. The pain is usually associated with activity and relieved by rest, massage and local heat. Only occasionally and in the more severe degrees of kyphosis do neurological symptoms ensue as thoracic myelopathy.

Just like its scoliotic counterpart, management decisions in Scheuermann's disease are determined to a large extent by the patient's perception of their condition, and this should be explored in the consultation.[2]

Other causes of kyphosis include:

- Myelomeningocele, producing a significant lumbar kyphosis but often not affecting sitting balance
- Neurofibromatosis: this is often a short angular kyphoscoliosis
- Congenital kyphosis
- Achondroplasia: thoracolumbar kyphosis that usually resolves
- Spondyloepiphyseal dysplasia
- Cervical kyphosis
  - ○ Larsen's syndrome
  - ○ Diastrophic dysplasia
  - ○ Osteogenesis imperfecta

In patients presenting with kyphosis, it is important to ask about neurological symptoms in upper and lower limbs, and particularly about early symptoms of thoracic myelopathy such as an unsteady gait, lower limb sensory changes, bladder and bowel dysfunction and subjective lower limb weakness.

Thoracic lordosis is rare and is usually associated with a syndrome such as Marfan's or Beals syndrome. It is an important condition, as the narrowed anteroposterior chest diameter can have a significant detrimental effect on respiratory function, which is usually progressive.

Examination

Look: Inspection should evaluate the kyphosis/lordosis. These deformities are almost always rigid except when combined with neuromuscular disease in wheelchair-bound patients. Juvenile idiopathic kyphosis is more common in teenage boys and acne is often present. This should be noted, as it may increase the risk of infection following a surgical procedure and can be improved with a short course of treatment.[3] Posture is very important, as shoulder protraction and a stooped posture can accentuate a thoracic kyphosis significantly and correcting this may eliminate the requirement for surgery. This posture is often adopted in the teenage population affected by juvenile idiopathic scoliosis. Tight localised kyphosis is typical in neurofibromatosis and congenital kyphosis and has a higher risk of spinal cord compression.

Feel and Move: Palpation and movement are not helpful.

Walk: Gait should be assessed, with a broad-based unsteady gait suggesting myelopathy and spinal cord compression.

Neurological examination: A full neurological examination is essential (see above).

Back Pain

History

Low back pain in childhood is very common, with an increasing prevalence of 27–51%.[4] Whilst it is less common to find a cause for back pain in patients over the age of 10 years and very rare to find a sinister cause, each case should be evaluated in the same way.

In childhood and particularly in teenagers, lumbar disc protrusions do occur and, although they may produce radicular leg pain, they often just give back pain. Radicular pain in childhood is rare and always justifies an MRI scan. If the lumbar spine MRI is normal, then a pelvic MRI should be performed as tumour must be excluded.

A fatigue fracture of the pars interarticularis (spondylolysis) and a forward slip of one vertebra on the vertebra below (spondylolisthesis) are among the most common causes of childhood and adolescent low back pain. However, spondylolysis is seen in 3% of 3-year-olds, 10% of Caucasian adults and up to 50% of Inuits (Eskimo). In most adults with the condition, they are an incidental finding with only a weak or no linkage to back pain.

Painful symptoms associated with these conditions are often reported by individuals who subject their spines to repetitive extension and twisting: ballet dancers, gymnasts and fast bowlers (cricketers). In most, the symptoms will settle with cessation of the provocative activity. Occasionally, the hypertrophic callus at the site of the spondylolysis, can irritate the exiting nerve root and cause radicular pain or sensory disturbance, but rarely motor dysfunction. As most spondylolyses occur at L5, and most spondylolistheses are of L5 on S1, it is the exiting L5 nerve root that is affected.

Thoracic back pain is also common in childhood and may be associated with an increased kyphosis or radiological changes of Scheuermann's disease. Thoracic pain should have a high level of suspicion for sinister pathology and should be investigated with an MRI scan or bone scan for younger patients where the level of suspicion is low.

Rheumatological conditions can present in childhood especially ankylosing spondylitis and juvenile chronic arthritis. The presence of other affected joints or significant early morning spinal stiffness may suggest these diagnoses. There may be a family history of ankylosing spondylitis.

Synovitis, acne, pustulosis (palms and plantar), hyperostosis (sternoclavicular) and osteitis (SAPHO) can present with back pain. The combination of clinical features and anterior vertebral body and endplate erosion suggest this diagnosis.

Neck pain is less common in childhood and should raise suspicion of sinister pathology. Neck clicking is common and can be audible but is not clinically significant. Imaging investigations do not reveal a cause. It is believed to be due to increased mobility of the child's facet joints.

Examination

Look: Inspect for any abnormal masses, overall spinal shape and frontal and sagittal plane balance. A scoliosis may be present owing to muscle spasm secondary to a painful intraspinal problem (such as infection, tumour or even a prolapsed disc) or a paraspinal focus (such as renal tract pathology). The examination should be used to confirm where the patient experiences the pain to define an anatomical level.

Feel: Focal pain should be considered more sinister than generalised pain. Tenderness may be elicited on palpation or percussion.

A spinous process step in the low lumbar spine may suggest a spondylolisthesis. In L5/S1 lytic spondylolisthesis, the step is between the spinous processes of L4 and L5 as the posterior elements of L5 remain in normal position

Move: Spinal movements in the area of concern should be assessed: flexion/ extension and lateral flexion in the lumbar spine; rotation in the thoracic spine and flexion/extension, rotations and lateral flexions in the cervical spine.

Walk: Gait should be observed as a limp may be present and walking may be obviously painful. This suggests sinister pathology such as infection or tumour.

Neurological examination: A full lower limb neurological examination should be performed, especially looking for problems that are unlikely to have been noted by the patient: extensor hallucis longus weakness suggestive of L5 radiculopathy or weakness on tip toe stance suggestive of S1 radiculopathy, reflex abnormalities, including abdominal reflexes, Hoffman's sign if cervical spine pathology is suspected, Romberg's test, ankle clonus and Babinski reflex. The upper motor neuron signs are produced due to the loss of the inhibitory innervation of the reflex arc.

Passive straight leg raise may be restricted because of tight hamstrings, which are common in rapidly growing children, but may also reflect a spondylolysis or spondylolisthesis. A positive stretch test reproducing radicular leg pain or low back pain may suggest a lumbar disc protrusion.

Torticollis

History

It is important to establish the length of time a torticollis has been present. Torticollis since birth suggests sternomastoid tightness, especially if there is a history of a sternomastoid lump, which usually disappears by 4 months. This condition resolves with stretching and positioning and is not painful.

Painful or late-onset torticollis should be considered an urgent condition. Atlantoaxial rotatory subluxation is diagnosed with a CT scan taken with the neck rotated to left and right and is often preceded by an upper respiratory tract infection (Grisel's syndrome).

Examination

Look: In torticollis, the neck tilts to one side (the side of the torticollis) and rotates to the other (Figure 13.5). It

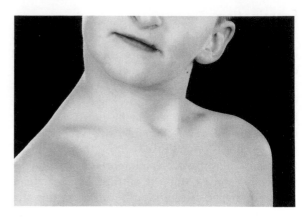

Figure 13.5 Patient with torticollis.

is often difficult to see a tight sternomastoid, but it is always worth checking for scars in the neck and particularly evidence of a previous sternomastoid release (proximally just below the mastoid and distally just above the clavicle). Also seek scars posteriorly that are suggestive of previous surgery to the cervical spine.

Feel: Palpating the sternomastoid may reveal a tight muscle or sternomastoid swelling in congenital muscular torticollis. The absence of a tight sternomastoid may suggest an alternative cause, such as a structural problem in the upper cervical spine (atlantoaxial rotatory subluxation being the most common) or a posterior fossa tumour.

Move: When evaluating movements, it is important to note whether the neck can be tilted to a neutral position or beyond actively and passively, and whether the rotation is correctable.

Advanced Corner

Curve Flexibility in Scoliosis

Curve flexibility is crucial in determining timing of spinal surgery where flexible curves can be observed for longer. This is especially important in juvenile idiopathic scoliosis, where delayed surgery may enable a patient to have a fusion rather than complex growing system. Flexibility of curves may also help predict response to bracing.

Pelvic Obliquity

There are two causes of pelvic obliquity seen with scoliosis:

1. Suprapelvic obliquity is caused by a collapsing neuromuscular scoliosis.

2. Infrapelvic obliquity is caused by unequal spasm in the iliopsoas muscles, the only muscles that cross the pelvis from spine to lower extremity. For practical purposes this will only be encountered in cerebral palsy. This may be correctable or fixed; in the latter, when examining leg length inequality in a supine patient the pelvis cannot be put square to the trunk.

To distinguish between these two causes the patient is laid prone at the end of the couch so that the hips can be flexed over the edge of the couch, negating the hip flexion contractures. Abducting and adducting the hips will correct the pelvic obliquity if the cause is infrapelvic whilst there will be no change if the cause is suprapelvic.

In cerebral palsy, the rarer double curve tends to be well balanced in the frontal plane, reducing the indication for surgery. It is also important to assess neck control, as patients without neck control are more likely to develop proximal junctional kyphosis above a long instrumentation from the upper thoracic spine to the pelvis. Increased thoracic kyphosis is often associated with neuromuscular disease and often causes seating difficulties resulting from anterior imbalance. An increased lumbar lordosis is often seen in long C-shaped scoliosis in cerebral palsy associated with significant lumbar rotation, and this makes surgery much harder as the lumbar spine is very deep.

References

1. Epstein F, Epstein N. Intramedullary tumours of the spinal cord. In McLone D (ed), *Paediatric Neurosurgery: Surgery of the Developing Nervous System*. New York: Grune & Stratton, 1982; pp. 529–540.

2. Murray PM, Weinstein SL, Spratt KF. The natural history and long term follow-up of Scheuermann kyphosis. *J Bone Joint Surg Am* 1993;**75**(2):236–248.

3. Haider R, Najjar M, Der Boghossian A, Tabbarah Z. Propionibacterium acnes causing delayed post operative spine infection: review. *Scand J Infect Dis* 2010;**42**(6–7):405–411.

4. Hwang J, Louie PK, Phillips FM, An HS, Samartzis D. Low back pain in children: a rising concern. *Eur Spine J* 2019;**28**:211–213.

Further Reading

Akbarnia BA, Yazici M, Thompson GH (eds). *The Growing Spine*. New York: Springer, 2011.

Dickson RA, Millner PA. The child with a painful back. *Curr Orthop* 2000;14:369–379.

Paediatric Clinical Cases

Caroline M. Blakey, Shomari Webster-Prince and
James A. Fernandes

Introduction

The spectrum of clinical presentations in paediatric orthopaedics is varied and at times complex. Pathology may be focal or may form part of a generalised disorder or syndrome, the clues to which can often be found on observation alone.

The aim of this chapter is to allow the reader to identify signs from the clinical appearance and by utilising the skills gained in the preceding chapters, to understand how these can be applied. Examination is directed according to these clues alongside an understanding of normal development in children.

A selection of paediatric orthopaedic pathology is presented here where the power of observation is stressed.

Disorders of Torsion and Alignment

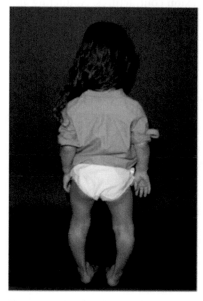

Figure 14.1b After the age of 2 years, symmetrical genu varum of this degree is likely to be associated with generalised pathology. There is short stature and disproportionate short limbs, seen with a skeletal dysplasia.

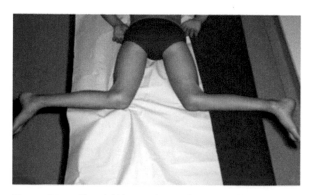

Figure 14.1a This child has evidence of increased femoral anteversion with 90° of internal rotation. External rotation will be reduced. Derotation osteotomy must be justified with significant clinical symptoms; it should not be a prophylactic procedure, and never before the age of 9 years.

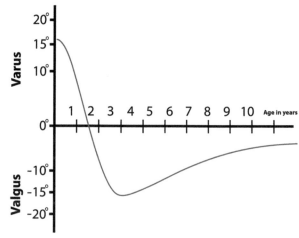

Figure 14.1c Salenius and Vankka depicted the natural tibiofemoral alignment in children. The graph can be helpful in describing to parents the natural history of alignment.

Alignment of the lower limbs change with growth. This normal variation is depicted in the Salenius and Vankka curve (Figure 14.1c), with physiological varus seen in infancy, progressing to maximal valgus alignment around the age of three. Internal tibial torsion will accentuate physiological genu varum.[1] Torsional alignment also changes with age. Femoral neck anteversion is as high as 40° in infancy but reduces to 10°–15° on reaching maturity. The tibia rotates laterally from 5° at birth to around 15°. After the age of 9, changes in alignment and torsion are not expected.

Significant asymmetry suggests pathological development, and alignment greater than two standard deviations from normal warrants further review.

Pathological disorders affecting coronal alignment include metabolic disease (e.g. rickets) and skeletal dysplasias, and this suspicion is highlighted if the height of the child is below the 25th centile. Blount's disease is idiopathic progressive proximal tibia vara, resulting in internal tibial torsion, procurvatum of the tibia and, in severe cases, development of lateral thrust in gait. Post-physeal injury growth arrests are also asymmetrical in their presentations.

Key Points

- In the assessment of coronal plane deformities, a cursory general examination of height for short stature, asymmetry or generalised deformity is wise. Ask about onset of the deformity and progression, family history and nutritional concerns. Consider bone profile, endocrine referral or genetic review where there is evidence of a generalised disorder.

- A full-length standing radiograph, with patella forwards mimicking the clinical examination allows assessment of overall alignment, tibial metaphyseal angle for assessment of tibia vara and an assessment of the physeal region for evidence of rickets or dysplasia. Further radiographs may then be required.

- Brace treatment may be used in early tibia vara (Blount's disease). Hemiepiphysiodesis or osteotomy is indicated if tibia vara progresses or presents late. Overcorrection of the deformity will accommodate recurrence. The use of external fixation in older children is likely to be required to correct the multiplanar deformities.

- Cozen's phenomenon is post-traumatic genu valgum resulting after incomplete proximal tibial fractures in children. Management of proximal tibial fractures includes varus moulding with knee in extension and counselling the family of possible deformity. Guided growth may be appropriate where there is incomplete resolution.

- Persistent femoral anteversion in isolation rarely requires treatment. Computed tomography (CT) imaging is helpful in diagnosis and planning, but treatment decisions should be based on clinical assessment including the effect on range of movement and gait. There may be associated hip dysplasia. Reduced anteversion or retroversion may result in impingement and joint degeneration and more commonly requires surgical intervention

Short Stature and Skeletal Dysplasia

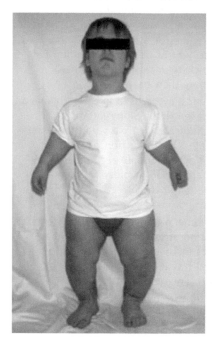
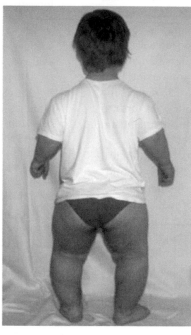

Figure 14.2a An adolescent with achondroplasia. Trunk height is normal but there is shortening of the proximal limb segments with overall reduction in height. This is rhizomelic shortening. Other features of achondroplasia include frontal bossing, spinal gibbus and short and broad (trident) hands.

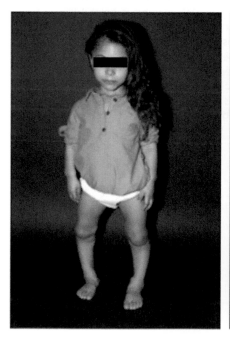
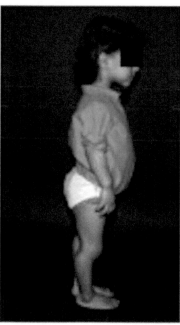

Figure 14.2b(i,ii) This 6-year-old has pseudoachondroplasia. There is disproportionate short limb dwarfism with 'knobbly' appearance of the knees, but no craniofacial dysmorphism. With this condition, growth rate is initially normal but falls after the first to third year. There may be varus or valgus malalignment of the lower limbs.

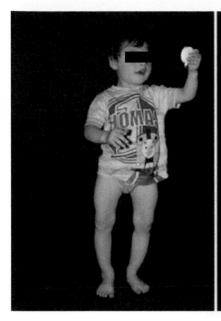 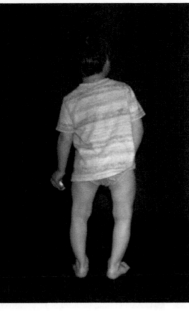

Figure 14.2c A 3-year-old with X-linked hypophosphataemic rickets. Remember to look at family members for signs of hereditary disorder.

Short stature may be familial, the result of hormone deficiency, primary systemic disease, dysmorphic syndromes such as Turner or Prader–Willi syndrome, or skeletal dysplasia. Skeletal dysplasias include a heterogeneous group of disorders, the commonest of which is achondroplasia. More than 400 dysplasias have been genetically identified.

In addition to short stature, features of skeletal dysplasia include deformity of the limbs or axial skeleton, ligamentous laxity, localised dysmorphism and joint contractures.[2]

Retardation of growth may be proportionate, where the upper segment is equal to the lower segment, or disproportionate. Remember the ratio of the upper to lower segment changes with age.

Key Points

- Short stature is defined as height for age that is less than two standard deviations below average for that gender.

- Establishing the diagnosis includes examination of absolute height and growth velocity. Determine the age at which growth became affected. Slowed growth may not be evident from birth. Examine the height of both parents.
- Examine the trunk to extremity ratio by comparing sitting to standing height. Carefully assess body proportions and define the affected segment: rhizo- (proximal), meso- (middle), acro- (distal), see Chapter 12, Advanced Corner.
- Look for other features of dysplasia including facial dysmorphism, abnormalities of the eyes or dentition that may suggest collagenopathy.
- Laboratory screening tests may be required to exclude systemic endocrine or renal disease.
- A skeletal survey is performed if dysplasia is suspected.
- Establish the stability of the cervical spine before any intervention.

Lower Limb Deficiencies

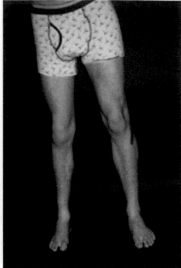

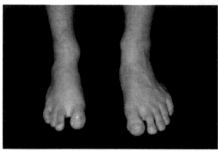

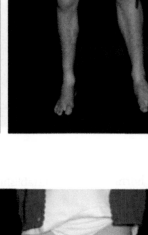

Figure 14.3a(i,ii) A 15-year-old with right-sided fibular hemimelia, a post-axial longitudinal deficiency. There is absence of the right lateral ray and a leg length discrepancy with hypoplasia.

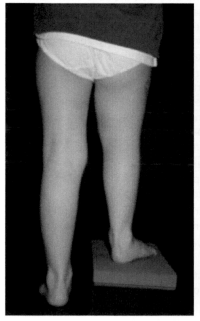

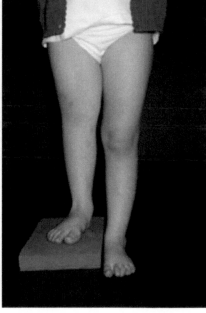

Figure 14.3b(i,ii) This 7-year-old has proximal femoral focal deficiency (PFFD) another longitudinal post-axial deficiency.

Limb deficiencies can be described as longitudinal or transverse. Longitudinal deficiencies can be further divided into pre- or post-axial. Congenital femoral deficiencies cover the spectrum of developmental failure to include congenital short femur and proximal focal femoral deficiencies (PFFD).

Fibular deficiency is the most common congenital longitudinal deficiency of the lower limb. The fibula may be hypoplastic or completely absent. Classification is based on the portion of fibula remaining. There is associated tibial shortening and often femoral deficiency. Associated findings include genu

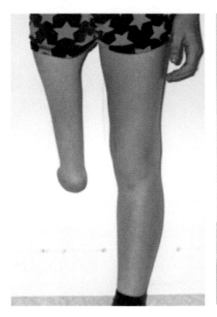
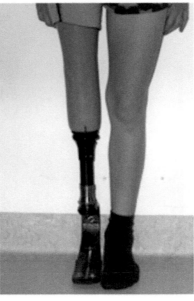

Figure14.3c(i,ii) Severe PFFD with previous hip reconstruction and Syme's amputation. The right knee has been fused.

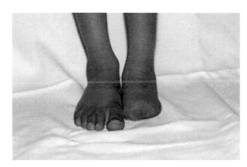

Figure 14.3d A 7-year-old who was born prematurely, with necrotic amputation of the left forefoot. This would be considered an acquired transverse deficiency.

valgum secondary to hypoplasia of the lateral femoral condyle, cruciate ligament deficiency, patellar instability, a ball and socket ankle, tarsal coalition and equinovalgus foot deformity.

Transverse deficiencies may be congenital or acquired (the latter as in meningococcal sepsis), traumatic or post-surgical. Amniotic band syndrome may cause congenital terminal deficiencies, annular constrictions, or acrosyndactyly.

Key Points

- A multidisciplinary approach is required to provide reassurance and education for the family.
- A 'block test' is a useful way of measuring leg length in these patients where bony landmarks may not be standard.
- The aim of treatment is optimal function for the child. Projected limb length discrepancy, the severity of the anomaly at the hip, and the presence of a functional foot help to guide management.
- In more severe deformities with a non-functional foot, or when significant lengthening is required, ablative reconstruction may be more appropriate. A Syme's amputation is preferred. The ankle may function as a knee joint in rotationplasty. In unsalvageable limbs aim to allow prosthetic fitting by walking age.
- Mild length discrepancy may be managed by orthosis alone. Larger discrepancies may warrant epiphysiodesis of the contralateral limb, multiple lengthening procedures or a combination of both surgeries.
- Surgery aiming to address length discrepancy must consider stability of the adjacent joints.
- Coronal plane deformity must also be addressed whether or not the lower limb is salvaged.
- Calculate projected leg length discrepancy (LLD) plotting sequential imaging and skeletal age. Acquired deficiencies will be progressive rather than proportionate. Shapiro classified the progression of leg length discrepancy.

Tibial Bowing

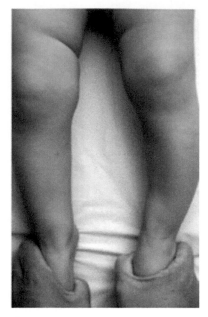

Figure 14.4a A 10-month-old with neurofibromatosis type 1 (NF1). There is anterolateral bowing of the left tibia.

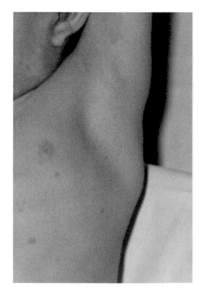

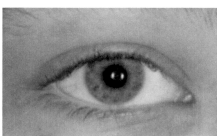

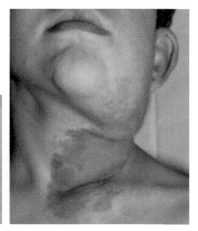

Figure 14.4b(i,ii,iii) Some of the associated manifestations of NF1 when one sees a child with a congenital anterolateral bow or pseudoarthrosis of the tibia. These are axillary freckling, Lisch nodules, café-au-lait spots and a large plexiform neurofibroma as shown above.

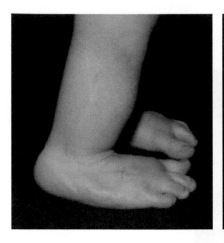 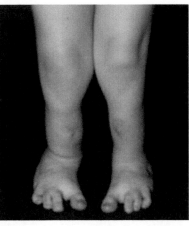

Figure 14.4c(i,ii) A 6-year-old with bilateral fibular hemimelia. The fibula is absent and there is a four-ray foot. There is persistent tibial kyphus consistent with anteromedial bowing. Note the dimple associated with the tibial kyphus.

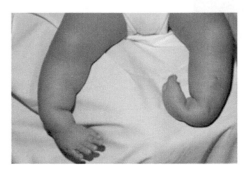

Figure 14.4d An 11-month-old with bilateral tibial hemimelia, a pre-axial longitudinal deficiency. The left foot has only two rays and is considered non-functional.

Tibial bowing can be classified according to the direction of the tibial apex. Identify the plane of the deformity and any associated anomalies.

Anteromedial bowing of the tibia may be seen with partial or complete agenesis of the fibula (fibular hemimelia). There may be associated equinovalgus foot posture.

Anterolateral bowing is associated with neurofibromatosis, in isolation and with fibrous dysplasia. The bowed tibia may fracture and fail to unite.

Posteromedial bowing is associated with a calcaneovalgus foot deformity. It is not completely benign, but the outcomes are generally favourable. The foot posture will improve as the bowing resolves, but residual leg length discrepancy may require intervention later in childhood.[3]

Key Points

- Projected limb length discrepancy and severity of foot deformity help to guide management. With limb deficiencies, consider ablative reconstruction in the presence of a non-functional foot with fewer than three rays.
- In general terms, if shortening is expected to be greater than 2 cm, equalisation is appropriate. The technique will depend on whether deformity correction is also required. Posteromedial bowing can be expected to spontaneously correct, but there may be residual length discrepancy.
- Anterolateral bowing can be considered the precursor to pseudarthrosis of the tibia. A large proportion (50–55%) are associated with neurofibromatosis.
- Bracing may prevent further bowing or fracture but fracture non-union (the pseudarthrosis) is extremely difficult to manage. Specialist management includes excision of the hamartoma, intramedullary and/or external fixation with bone and periosteal grafting.
- Additional causes of tibial bowing may include fibrous dysplasia, tibial hemimelia, osteogenesis or metabolic conditions, e.g. rickets. In conditions such as rickets, correction of the deformity can be expected with optimised medical treatment and early surgery is not indicated.

Disorders of the Upper Limb

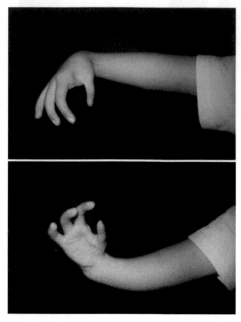

Figure 14.5a A 5-year-old with radial club hand, a preaxial upper limb deficiency with centralisation and pollicisation.

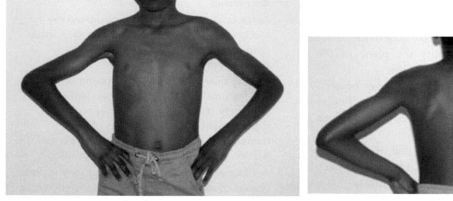

Figure 14.5b(i,ii) An 11-year-old with obstetric brachial plexus palsy post-anterior release and latissimus dorsi transfer. Look for asymmetry of muscle bulk, operative scars and assess neurological function.

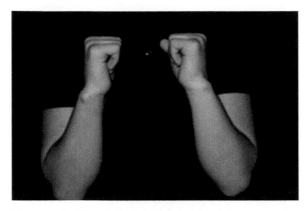

Figure 14.5c Bilateral distal radial growth arrest due to secondary post meningococcal septicaemic sequelae (acquired Madelung's) treated previously with distal ulnar physeal ablation. The ulnar heads remain prominent secondary to the radial deformity.

Paediatric upper limb conditions can be categorised based on their aetiology. Congenital conditions can be classified under Swanson's classification (Table 14.1).

As with the lower limb, certain deformities are associated with generalised conditions. Radial aplasia characteristically is bowing of the shortened forearm with the hand deviated radially, often orthogonal to the forearm. The thumb may be absent and bilateral in over half of the cases. It is associated with conditions such as VACTERL (vertebral, anal, cardiac, tracheo-oesophageal, renal, limb), Fanconi's anaemia, Holt–Oram syndrome or thrombocytopenia absent radius (TAR). Upper limb deficiencies should prompt evaluation of the whole child as in the lower limb.

Table 14.1 Swanson's classification

Type	Common examples
Failure of formation	Transverse deficiency: congenital amputation Longitudinal deficiency: radial club hand
Failure of differentiation	Radioulnar synostosis, camptodactyly, syndactyly
Duplication	Polydactyly: pre/post-axial
Overgrowth	Macrodactyly
Undergrowth	Thumb hypoplasia
Constriction ring syndrome	Amniotic bands
Generalised skeletal abnormalities	

Malunited fractures frequently result in angular deformities and restriction in range of movement if not carefully managed. The majority of growth comes from the physis at the wrist and shoulder. Commonly seen is the gunstock deformity of a malunited supracondylar fracture. Lateral condyle fractures are at risk of non-union and can result in progressive cubitus valgus with secondary ulnar nerve problems.

The upper limb is often given less focus in neuromuscular disorders. Weakness and contractures can result in significant disability. Consideration should be given to optimising function and proprioception, and prevention of secondary deformity.

Key Points

- Treatment of radial aplasia is initially conservative with passive stretching and splinting but later operative intervention is required, including carpal centralisation, corrective ulnar osteotomy and pollicisation.
- Congenital Madelung's deformities are associated with Léri–Weill dyschondrosteosis. This a rare condition in which there is a partial growth arrest of the distal radius. It usually presents in adolescence with progressive deformity including increased ulnar inclination and volar tilt. Bilaterality occurs in about half of the cases. Treatment includes distal ulnar physeal ablation and excision of the Vickers ligament with physeal bar excision and interposition grafting. In the presence of ulnar abutment, ulnar shortening or radial lengthening may be appropriate.
- Physical and occupational therapy plays a vital role in the upper limb. Strengthening functioning muscles, preventing joint contractures and occupational therapy usually is the mainstay. Surgical options may include tendon transfers, release of soft tissue contractures and corrective osteotomies to optimise function. Nerve transfers may be indicated in brachial plexus palsies.
- Early prosthetic use in upper limb deficiencies may preclude bimanual function. Children are very adaptable and can be surprisingly functional despite significant anomaly. Allow for natural adaptations.

Generalised Deformity and Disorders

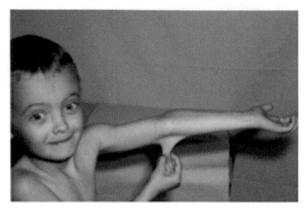

Figure 14.6a There are multiple forms of Ehlers–Danlos syndrome, most are autosomal dominant (AD) inheritance. The skin is lax and fragile. There may be problems with wound healing. Joint laxity results in dislocation and deformity. Soft tissue fragility can cause vascular aneurysms.

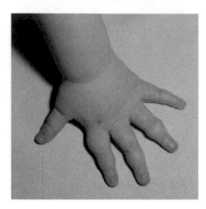

Figure 14.6b Ollier's syndrome describes multiple enchondromas in the metaphysis of long bones. Limb length equalisation, hemiepiphysiodesis and corrective osteotomies may be required to address the angular deformities and growth retardation that results. In Maffucci syndrome, haemangiomas are also present. The risk of malignant transformation is higher in this group.

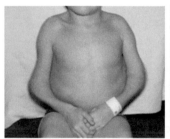
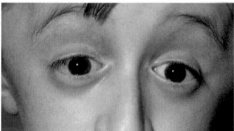

Figure 14.6c(i,ii) Osteogenesis imperfecta results from defective type I collagen, which may be quantitative or qualitative. Silence classified four genetic phenotypes, but the numbers now recognised are much greater. The spectrum of disorder is from mild increased fracture risk to incompatibility with life. Abnormalities of type I collagen results in defective dentition, sclera, and soft tissues, weakness of bone with multiple fractures and deformity.

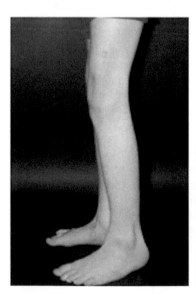
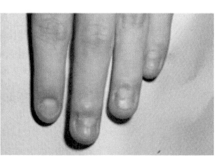

Figure 14.6d(i,ii) Nail-patella syndrome (NPS), or onycho-osteo-arthrodysplasia, characteristically affects the nails, elbows and knees with pathognomonic posterior iliac horns seen on viewing a pelvic X-ray. The patellae are hypoplastic or absent. Nails are dystrophic and discoloured. There may be antecubital webbing, but other elbow deformities include congenital dislocation of the radial head.

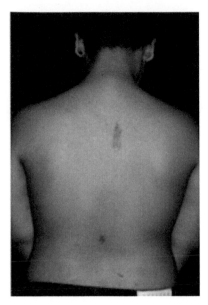

Figure 14.6e Features of McCune–Albright syndrome include the jagged-edged 'coast of Maine' café-au-lait spots, precocious puberty and polyostotic fibrous dysplasia, which may present with deformity or multiple fractures requiring orthopaedic intervention.

Paediatric orthopaedics presents with multiple clinical conditions and syndromes that may result in deformity or dysfunction. Others are innocuous or normal variants and will remain asymptomatic. Determining the difference is critical for reassurance of the child and parents, appropriate follow up and intervention.

Generalised disorders of the musculoskeletal system include thousands of disorders that may present with focal or global deformity. Children may present with delayed motor development, deformity or pain. The deformity may be the major presenting problem but establishing the underlying diagnosis, such as clubfoot in arthrogryposis, is imperative.

Key Points

- Assessment of the child with deformity requires a systematic examination.
- The history should include pre- or perinatal complications, developmental milestones, family history including background of consanguinity.
- Investigation of a possible skeletal dysplasia includes a recommended series of radiographs including the lateral skull and lateral thoracic spine.
- Global examination should look for dysmorphia, height for age, proportion and symmetry, skin changes, laxity or contracture.
- There may be multiple fractures, deformity or atypical response to treatment. Look for contractures or laxity and instability.
- Weakness should prompt a full neurological assessment, consider creatinine kinase levels in the presence of toe walking especially in boys (Duchenne muscular dystrophy).

Deformities of the Paediatric Foot

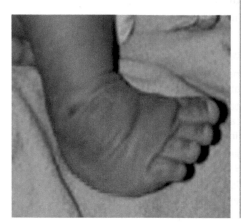

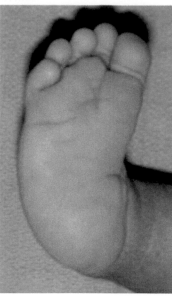

Figure 14.7a(i,ii) An infant with congenital talipes equinovarus (CTEV), which includes cavus, forefoot adduction, hindfoot varus and equinus.

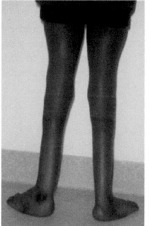

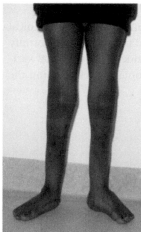

Figure 14.7b A 6-year-old with VACTERL syndrome, a genetic disorder associated with multisystem anomalies. Limb malformations such as CTEV are seen. The child has had surgical correction but shows signs of recurrence on the left with increased cavus, hind foot varus and a curved lateral border.

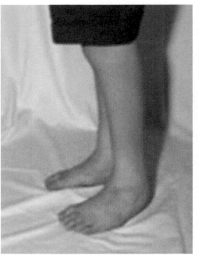
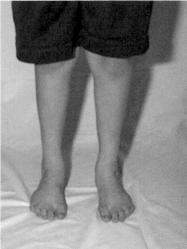
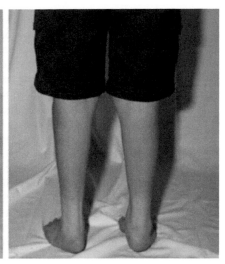

Figure 14.7c(i,ii) Signs of recurrence can also be seen in this 10-year-old by with idiopathic CTEV treated in infancy. Recurrence can be associated with poor orthotic compliance post-correction.

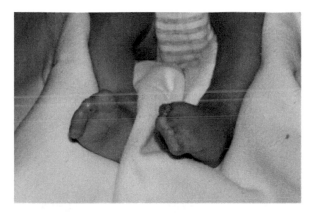

Figure 14.7d Acrosyndactyly associated with Apert syndrome.

Congenital foot deformity includes the equinovarus deformity of clubfoot, metatarsus adductus, calcaneovalgus and congenital vertical talus. Congenital talipes equinovarus (CTEV) responds well to serial manipulation and casting, but requires compliance with orthotics until the age of 4 years. Calcaneovalgus is the commonest foot deformity at birth, usually supple and is likely to resolve with a gentle stretching program.

Flexible flat foot is physiological in children. The medial longitudinal arch develops only by the age of 5 or 6 years. A painful rigid flat foot is pathological as with tarsal coalitions, or the rocker bottom rigid flat foot seen with congenital vertical talus. Cavus feet are commonly associated with neurological abnormalities or spinal dysraphism and rarely idiopathic.[4] Charcot–Marie–Tooth presents with bilateral cavovarus foot deformity later in childhood, as the weak tibialis anterior and peroneus brevis are overpowered by the tibialis posterior and peroneus longus muscles. A progressive unilateral cavovarus foot raises concerns for spinal cord lesions.[5]

Foot deformities are common amongst children with neuromuscular disorders and may be progressive. Equinus, planovalgus, equinovarus or equinocavovarus deformities are seen. Principles of management depend on the severity of deformity, level of symptoms and disability of the child. The primary goal in ambulant children is to improve gait efficiency.

Key Points

- Whilst many are idiopathic, foot deformities in a newborn may be associated with limb deficiency, spinal dysraphism, dysplasia (e.g. diastrophic dwarfism), neurogenic conditions or a more global syndrome (Larsen's, arthrogryposis, constriction band syndrome). It is critical to establish a diagnosis, as treatment may be directed to more urgent anomalies, or there may be modification to the method of deformity correction.

- The exact site of the deformity needs to be determined. Mistakes in early clubfoot management could be considered a lack of understanding of the fulcrum of deformity and mechanics of the foot.

265

Ponseti philosophy of serial manipulation and casting involves correction of cavus or plantaris of the first ray followed by adduction, varus and hindfoot deformity correction. In contrast manipulation of persistent metatarsus adductus moulding is directed over the cuboid.

- Surgery for paediatric foot deformity should be considered only when conservative measures fail. The flexible flat foot can be considered physiological and can generally be observed. Orthotics may provide symptomatic relief but will not alter foot shape and are not indicated in asymptomatic patients. The principles of surgery, when indicated, involve correcting the deformity whilst maintaining motion where possible, minimising the risk of recurrence and reducing pain.
- Cavus feet should prompt neurological assessment. When surgery is indicated, soft tissue rebalancing procedures are generally performed before osteotomies or fusions of more rigid deformities. The Coleman block test determines whether the deformity is hindfoot or forefoot driven.

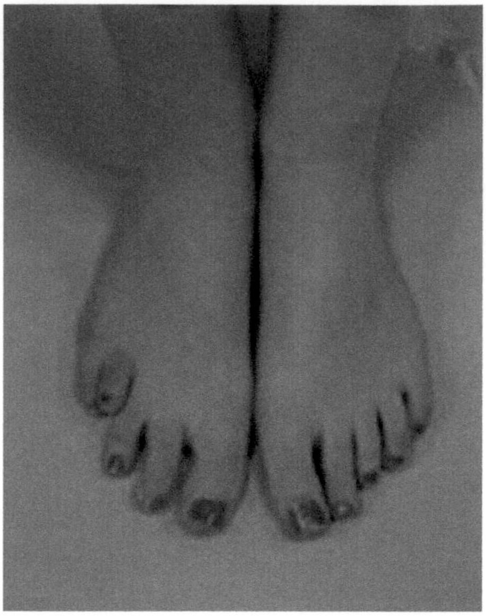

Toe Deformities

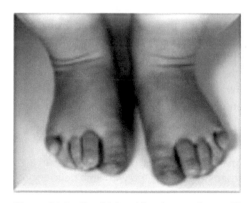

Figure 14.8a The third and fourth are curly toes. The fifth toe is overriding. The second toe is usually normal and is lifted to accommodate the space taken up by the curly toes.

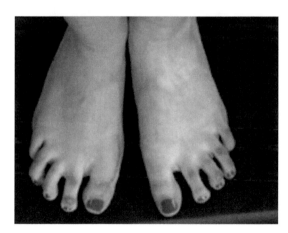

Figure 14.8b Short fourth metatarsal with symptoms of metatarsalgia.

Figure 14.8c Adolescent hallux valgus post-surgical correction with evidence of a scar.

Toe deformities may be congenital or developmental. The commonest sagittal toe deformity are curly toes. They tend to affect the third to fifth toes and are bilateral, symmetrical and familial. They are usually asymptomatic, but can be a problem with shoewear, putting on socks or when the nail is weightbearing.

An overriding fifth toe may present at birth or develop during childhood with symptoms similar to curly toes. It is hyperextended at the metatarsopha-langeal (MTP) joint and flexed at the IP joint. Often the toe is hypoplastic and there may be a rotational component so that the nail faces laterally.

Short fourth or third and fourth metatarsals can produce metatarsalgia and may need surgical lengthening to realign the parabola of the forefoot.

Hallux valgus is thought to affect around a quarter of adolescents, it is predominantly idiopathic. There may be a family history. The great toe is laterally deviated with pronation of the hallux, often associated with pes planus and metatarsus primus varus. The distal metatarsal articular angle (DMMA) is increased.

Key Points
- Conservative measures usually suffice for curly toes. Overriding fifth toes are more likely to end up requiring surgery.
- Generally, surgery for curly toes and overriding fifth toes are done after age 3 years when the toes are bigger and when some may have resolved.
- Tendon balancing procedures are useful in the flexible deformities. After the age of 12 years the deformity is more rigid and bony procedures may be necessary.
- Open flexor tenotomy via volar approach is the commonest procedure for curly toes. The most important part of the operation is to close the incision so that it does not cause contractures across the skin crease.
- Girdlestone's flexor to extensor transfer is performed less often as it produces a toe stiff in extension.
- There are many different approaches for the overriding fifth toe, but any surgical procedure must include a complete division of the extensor tendon with a wide capsular release including the collateral ligaments. Correction of the skin contracture is commonly performed by a double racquet handle incision (Butler procedure).

- The management of hallux valgus in adolescents is initially conservative, including accommodative shoe wear, with a cautious approach to surgical intervention. Conservative measures will not halt progression of the deformity.
- The risk of recurrence is significantly higher in adolescent hallux valgus before physeal closure.
- With a grossly abnormal DMMA, the scarf osteotomy is a powerful diaphyseal osteotomy that can be combined with an Akin closing wedge osteotomy to achieve correction.
- The risk of recurrence in the presence of open physes is high, and correction should be delayed until skeletal maturity where possible.[6]

References

1. Staheli, LT. *Practice of Paediatric Orthopaedics*, 2nd ed. Philadelphia: Lippincott, Williams and Wilkins, 2006.

2. Shapiro F. *Paediatric Orthopaedic Deformities*. Vol. 1, *Pathobiology and Treatment of Dysplasias, Physeal Fractures, Length Discrepancies, and Epiphyseal and Joint Disorders*. Cham: Springer International, 2016.

3. Shapiro F. *Paediatric Orthopaedic Deformities*. Vol. 2, *Developmental Disorders of the Lower Extremity: Hip to Knee to Ankle and Foot*. Cham: Springer International, 2019.

4. Ford SE, Scannell BP. Pediatric flatfoot. *Foot Ankle Clin* 2017;**22**(3):643–656.

5. Kedem P, Scher DM. Foot deformities in children with cerebral palsy. *Curr Opin Pediatr* 2015:**27** (1):67–74.

6. Agrawal Y, Baja SK, Flowers MJ. Scarf-Akin osteotomy for hallux valgus in juvenile and adolescent patients. *J Pediatr Orthop B* 2015;**24**(6):535–540.

Further Reading

Alshryda S, Jones S, Banaszkiewicz P (eds). *Postgraduate Paediatric Orthopaedics. The Candidate's Guide to the FRCS (Tr & Orth) Examination*. Cambridge University Press, 2014.

Joseph B, Nayagam S, Loder RT, Torode I. *Paediatric Orthopaedics: A System of Decision-Making*. London: Hodder Arnold, 2009.

McClure, PK, Herzenberg, JE. The natural history of lower extremity malalignment. *J Pediatr Orthop* 2019;**39**(S6, Suppl1):S14–S19.

Chapter
15

Spine Clinical Cases

Daine Clarke, James A. Fernandes and Jonathan A. Clamp

Introduction

Spinal pathology can present with a wide variety of clinical features.

Manifestations of spinal pathology extend beyond the axial skeleton and so a comprehensive multisystem examination may be required. In particular, a neurological examination should be performed. Frequently, spine pathology is part of a congenital disorder.

Significant pathology may be present with very little abnormality clinically apparent with the spine. For example, cervical myelopathy will be identified with a careful neurological assessment and the pathology cannot be identified by local examination of the cervical spine.

Thoracic Kyphosis

The head is no longer centred over the pelvis – a positive sagittal imbalance. There is no compensatory lumbar hyperlordosis. There is also an area of hyperpigmentation over the apex of the deformity, likely secondary to chronic skin irritation whilst seated.

Global sagittal balance is radiographically represented by a vertical plumb line from the posterior aspect of the anterior arch of C1 to the posterior superior aspect of the S1 vertebral body and is affected by changes in the cervical lordosis, thoracic kyphosis or lumbar lordosis. The normal thoracic kyphosis is 20°–45°. An exaggerated thoracic kyphosis displaces the centre of gravity anteriorly, i.e. positive sagittal imbalance. To regain balance, there is often a compensatory hyperlordosis of the cervical and lumbar spine. Pelvic tilt (retroversion) can further compensate.

Examination of a patient with an apparent thoracic deformity, as with all other spinal deformity, includes an assessment of gait, coronal and sagittal alignment, flexibility of the deformity (can it be reduced by the patient standing upright?) and a neurological assessment. Flexibility of the deformity

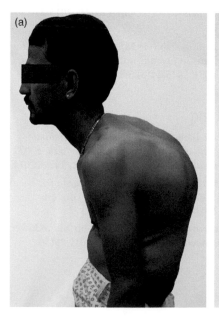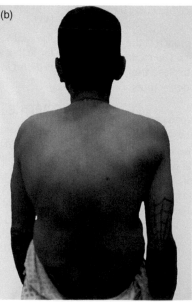

Figure 15.1a,b Clinical photographs of an adult male showing significant thoracic kyphotic deformity. Patients present with chronic back and neck pain, stiffness and, rarely, breathing problems.

will give an indication of whether it is structural or non-structural (a 'postural roundback'). Forward flexion will often reveal a sharp thoracic deformity in a structural kyphosis as opposed to the rounded deformity of a postural kyphosis.

Key Points

- Common causes of structural exaggerated kyphosis include:
  - Scheuermann's disease (most common cause)
  - Post-traumatic
  - Post-infective (discitis, vertebral body osteomyelitis including tuberculosis (TB))
  - Inflammatory disorders (ankylosing spondylitis)
  - Tumours
  - Congenital deformities (mucopolysaccharidoses)
  - Iatrogenic (post-laminectomy, particularly in the cervical spine)
- Scheuermann's disease is a rigid hyperkyphosis >45° caused by anterior wedging >5° across three consecutive vertebrae. It affects the thoracic spine and is seen especially in males. Onset is usually in the pre-teen age group. It tends to be painful. The cause is not known but is thought to be because of abnormal collagen aggregation causing abnormal anterior end plates.
- Postural kyphosis is usually flexible and can be differentiated from Scheuermann's disease radiologically.

- With kyphosis, patients may develop tightness in their hamstrings, iliopsoas and anterior shoulder muscles, which may become apparent on clinical examination.
- Treatment is usually conservative with physiotherapy and analgesia. Surgical correction of deformity using posterior pedicle screw constructs (± anterior release) is indicated for failure of conservative treatment of symptoms and unacceptable cosmetic deformity in curves >70°.[1]

Ankylosing Spondylitis

In ankylosing spondylitis, apart from that mentioned in Figure 15.2a,b, clincal findings will include tenderness over the sacroiliac joints, positive sacroiliac joint provocation tests (e.g. flexion, abduction, external rotation (FABER)) and decreased range of movement of the lumbar spine.

Loss of lumbar lordosis and increased thoracic kyphosis are typically the earliest signs. Early in the disease, the patient stands with a slightly flexed hip and knee in order to be upright. Later, the hips may develop a fixed flexion deformity and, together with the loss of compensation from the lumbar spine, the patient may assume a stooped posture. This loss of compensatory lumbar spine movement must also be kept in mind when interpreting the findings of Thomas test, as the patient may be unable to fully

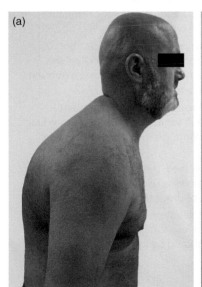
(a)

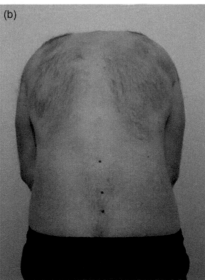
(b)

Figure 15.2a,b In this clinical photograph (a) the patient stands with his heels and buttocks against the wall. Note the kyphotic deformity of the upper thoracic spine and the relative forward position of the head, indicating positive sagittal imbalance. The second photograph (b) shows reduced forward flexion on performing Schober's test. These are features of ankylosing spondylitis affecting the spine.

flatten the lumbar spine on the couch when assessing for fixed flexion deformity of the hip.

Schober's test (and more accurately the modified Schober's test) will indicate reduced spinal forward flexion with an increase of less than 5 cm on measurement. Lateral flexion is also reduced.

Assessment of the functional deformity of the cervical spine is performed by the measurements outlined below. To take these measurements the patient stands with buttocks and heels against a wall, the hips and knees fully extended and the neck in a neutral or fixed position (Figure 15.2c).

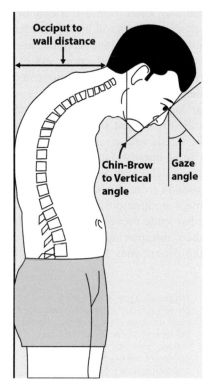

Figure 15.2c ○ **Chin-brow to vertical angle** (CBVA) – the angle between the vertical and a line drawn between the brow and the chin.[2]
○ **Gaze angle** – a CBVA of between −10° and +10° has the best horizontal gaze.[1]
○ **Occiput-to-wall distance.** Should be 0–2cm.

Reduced **chest expansion** is another clinical sign seen with ankylosing spondylitis. This is assessed in the following way: Ask the patient to put their hands on their head. The tape measure is placed around the chest at the level of the fourth intercostal space. The patient is asked to exhale fully, and the measurement is noted. Then the patient is asked to maximally inhale and the measurement taken again. Normal chest expansion is an increase by 3–7.5 cm.

Key Points

- Ankylosing spondylitis is one of the seronegative spondyloarthropathies. It is more common in Caucasians with a male predilection and commonly presents within the first three to four decades of life. The majority of patients are HLA-B27 positive (>90%). It is characterised by generalised inflammation with an affinity for the axial skeleton, hips and sacroiliac joints. The sacroiliac joint is usually involved early in the course of the disease.
- Other seronegative spondyloarthropathies such as psoriatic arthropathy can present in a similar manner and looking for a psoriatic patch may be helpful in making the diagnosis.
- A rigid spine and relative osteopaenia increases the risk of fracture from low-energy trauma, e.g. fall from standing height. Fractures are most common in the cervical region and at the C7/T1 junction.
- High risk of neurological deficit with fractures either secondary to haematoma or translation due to long lever arm.
- Suspect missed fractures in rapidly worsening kyphosis.
- Fractures are often difficult to detect on X-rays. Never exclude a fracture unless computed tomography (CT) and/or magnetic resonance imaging (MRI) have been performed.
- Immobilise the cervical spine in a position of comfort to accommodate the usual kyphosis – a flat position may cause a significant extension deformity at the fracture site.
- Surgery is indicated to improve patient's quality of life if sagittal balance affects visual fields, swallowing, pulmonary mechanics or ambulation.
- If the hip is involved, then a hip replacement may be indicated. However, warn the patient about the increased risk of dislocation (mainly anterior).
- There is some debate with regards to sagittal realignment before total hip replacement (THR). The decision should be individualised.[3]

Lumbar Spondylolisthesis

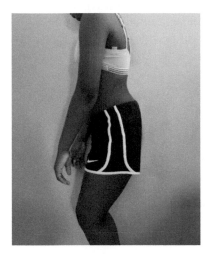

Figure 15.3a This clinical photograph of an adolescent reveals an exaggerated lumbar lordosis. On closer inspection, there is flattening of the buttocks with hip and knee flexion to compensate for the deformity. The patient has a high-grade spondylolisthesis at L5/S1.

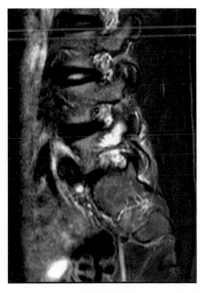

Figure 15.3b MRI scan (STIR sequence) of a different patient showing intense oedema within the pedicle consistent with a stress response/fracture in the adjacent pars.

In a high-grade slip, causing a kyphotic lumbosacral junction, the lordosis in the cranial segments will increase to restore balance of the spine in the sagittal plane. The pelvis will help to compensate by retroversion, requiring additional hamstring effort, hence the spasm. Pelvic retroversion is limited by tight iliofemoral ligaments and so hip flexion is recruited to allow more retroversion. This requires knee flexion to put the feet back on the floor under the pelvis.

Key Points

The causes of spondylolisthesis are classified by Wiltse:

- o Congenital dysplastic pars defect
- o Lytic defect in the pars – spondylolysis (most common at L5, hence L5/S1 spondylolisthesis)
- o Degenerative (most common at L4/5)
- o Traumatic
- o Iatrogenic (following decompression)
- o Pathological

- Lytic and degenerative account for majority of cases.
- A lytic pars defect (stress fracture in the pars interarticularis) often follows repeated hyperextension stresses, e.g. in gymnasts and cricket fast bowlers. It presents with focal pain worse with activity.
- A spondylolysis may result in a spondylolisthesis and the severity of this is quantified by Meyerding's classification: Grade I slip 0–25%; Grade II slip 25–50%; Grade III slip 50–75%; Grade IV slip 75–100%; Grade V slip >100% (spondyloptosis). High-grade slips (III or above) are rare.
- Spondylolysis is treated with activity modification, analgesia and rehabilitation.
- Failure of conservative treatment can be addressed surgically by a direct pars repair with screw fixation (if no listhesis and normal L5/S1 disc) or fusion of the motion segment if these criteria are not satisfied.
- A high-grade slip is stabilised to prevent progressive deformity (kyphotic lumbosacral junction) and neurological deficit (L5 nerve root, from traction injury).
- Reduction of high-grade slips is controversial due to the risk of neurological damage. In situ fusion is preferred if the spine is balanced. Surgical approach is posterior or combined anterior and posterior.[4]

Spinal Metastases

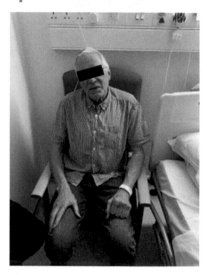

Figure 15.4a Clinical photograph showing a 70-year-old with head tilted to the right. He has noticed a progressive tilt of his head to the right as depicted (he states, 'The world is no longer level'). Clinical history reveals recent onset progressive upper axial neck pain, much worse on movement and he now is unable to drive. He describes recent weight loss. This patient has metastatic disease. The primary lesion is usually breast, lung, prostate, renal or haematological (myeloma). The patient must be examined for these.

Neurological dysfunction occurs in 5–10% of patients with metastatic spinal disease.[3] Symptoms and signs of cervical radiculopathy are less common but those of central canal narrowing and cord compression (weakness, lack of dexterity, balance disturbance) more so. Spinal cord compression is more common in the subaxial area rather than the atlantoaxial region. Long tract signs may be seen, but sphincter disturbance is a late finding and signifies poor prognosis.[3]

The reason why neurological deficit is less common in the atlantoaxial region is that the spinal canal at the C1 and C2 levels is the largest in the spine (Steel's rule of thirds). As a result, signs and symptoms are often those of mechanical instability rather than neurological due to spinal cord compression.

Key Points

- Deformity in the lower cervical spine is usually gradual angulation (kyphosis) due to vertebral body collapse.
- Investigations includes MRI of the whole spine and staging CT scan (chest, abdomen, pelvis).
- An unstable spine is declared when, under physiological load, the structural compromise is sufficient to cause significant pain, deformity or neurological deficit (Punjabi and White definition of instability).[5]
- A biopsy may be required – consider CT-guided biopsy if appropriate.
- Multidisciplinary team (MDT) input is crucial, and surgery should be performed before radiotherapy or the risk of delayed wound healing and infection is high.
- Surgery is indicated for:
  - Neurological deficit
  - Instability pain
- Surgical approach is usually posterior decompression and stabilisation with pedicle screw construct (if the patient has a prognosis of at least 3 months) and consideration of anterior column augmentation (cement) or reconstruction (cage) if the prognosis justifies this.

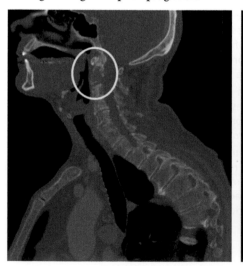

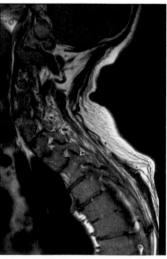

Figure 15.4b(i,ii) A CT scan reveals a large lytic lesion in the odontoid peg and a T1 sagittal MRI scan confirms diffuse low signal infiltration in the region of the right C2 lateral mass.

Cervical Myelopathy

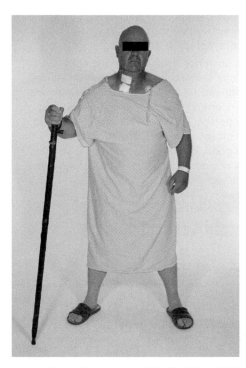

Figure 15.5a Clinical photograph showing a middle-aged man with a wide-based gait and using an independently sourced walking aid. Note the anterior cervical dressings indicating recent surgery.

With cervical myelopathy clinical findings include the following (see also Chapter 7):

- Sensory changes: proprioception loss and global numbness
- Finger escape sign
- Grip and release test
- Signs of upper motor neuron lesion:
    - Hyperreflexia
    - Clonus (>3 beats)
    - Babinski reflex
    - Hoffmann's sign
- Gait abnormalities: Romberg's test positive, broad-based gait
- L'hermitte's sign: posterior column dysfunction

Be aware of the differential diagnoses and the fact that they can coexist:

- Multiple sclerosis in younger patient age 20–40 years.
- Amyotrophic lateral sclerosis (ALS) similar age group (age 40-60 years).
    - Tongue fasciculation is a classic finding.
    - Other findings include fasciculation and atrophy of upper limb with diminished reflexes.
    - Absence of pain and sensory changes.

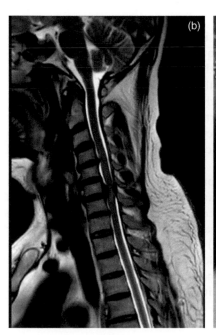
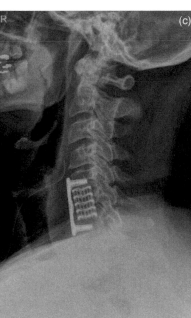

Figure 15.5b,c An MRI scan(b) confirms the diagnosis. T2 mid-sagittal image showing large C6/7 disc protrusion causing spinal cord compression and myelomalacia changes. (c) Post-operative image demonstrating C6 corpectomy and discectomy used to decompress the cord and reconstruct the anterior column.

Cervical spondylotic myelopathy refers to an upper motor neuron disorder due to compression of the spinal cord in the cervical region as a result of degenerative changes. Patients generally complain of difficulty with fine motor activities, weakness, clumsiness and disturbances in gait. There may be paraesthesia to the upper limbs and neck pain.

Pathoanatomy is related to both static and dynamic factors causing narrowing of the spinal canal and the resultant compressive effect on the cord.

Static

- Congenital narrow canal
- Age-related disc degeneration and annular bulging
- Hypertrophy or folding of ligamentum flavum due to loss of disc height
- Loss of cervical lordosis or development of kyphosis (spinal cord gets stretched over disk bulges or bone)
- Ossified posterior longitudinal ligament (OPLL) can occur in conjunction with cervical spondylosis

Dynamic

- Segmental instability caused by facet joint and ligamentous degeneration
- Development of stiff segments and compensatory hypermobile segments

---

Key Points

- Patients rarely volunteer a clear history – often specific questions which are easy to understand are required to identify the symptoms, e.g. can you button up a shirt?
- Don't miss subtle signs – slip-on shoes, no buttons, no belt – patient can't manage so they adapt!
- Surgery is principally designed to prevent progression and can't guarantee recovery, so intervention is often early.
- When examining a patient immediately following anterior cervical decompression (anterior cervical discectomy and fusion (ACDF) surgery), look for hoarseness (recurrent laryngeal nerve damage) and Horner's syndrome (sympathetic chain damage) because of possible damage to structures at risk.

- Compression with a kyphotic deformity is best addressed through an anterior approach to address deformity and adequately decompress. A posterior decompression requires cervical lordosis to facilitate the cord falling away from an anterior compressive lesion.
- After a posterior laminectomy the cord can fall posteriorly causing a traction neuropraxia on the (shortest) C5 root and resulting weakness. This is referred to as post-operative C5 palsy. It usually presents soon after surgery with deltoid and/or biceps weakness. The prognosis is usually good, but the recovery time is variable.[6] It does not occur with anterior decompressive procedures.

Rheumatoid Cervical Spine

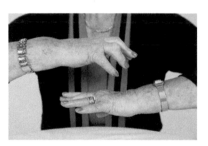

Figure 15.6a This 70-year-old presents with neck pain. She has signs of rheumatoid arthritis in her hand.

Cervical spine involvement in rheumatoid arthritis (RA) is less frequent than involvement of the peripheral joints of the hands and feet. The patient can present with the complications of cervical spine involvement, which carries a significant risk of morbidity and mortality. The clinical examination must therefore be focused on detecting signs of instability and neurological deficit associated with cervical myelopathy.

The most common clinical findings are neck pain and reduced range of movement. The neck pain is usually in the craniocervical junction. There may be an occipital headache (in atlantoaxial instability or cranial settling) which is due to compression of the greater (posterior ramus of C2) and lesser (anterior ramus of C2) occipital nerves as they pass between C1 and C2. In addition, ear or mastoid pain may be due to compression of the greater auricular nerve.[7]

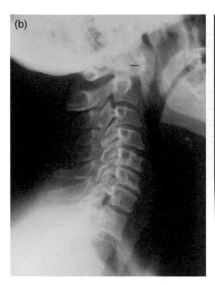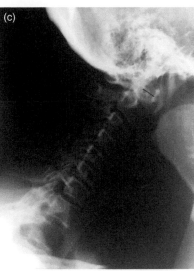

Figure 15.6b,c Lateral cervical spine radiographs in neutral and flexion showing an increased anterior atlantodens interval in flexion.

Look for symptoms and signs of cervical myelopathy such as lack of dexterity and balance disturbance. The pre-existing hand deformities can make it difficult to decide if signs are neurological or mechanical and the examination can be inconclusive. For example, when eliciting Hoffman's reflex, concurrent deformities and stiffness of the hand may hide a positive response.

With regards to cervical instability the patient may describe a sensation of the 'head falling forward' with flexion. Clinical examination may reveal a palpable 'clunk'.

The patterns of cervical instability in RA (from most frequent to least) are atlantoaxial instability (AAI), subaxial subluxation (i.e. below C2) and basilar invagination. The correlation between instabilities and clinical signs and symptoms is poor. Patients with subaxial subluxation tend to be younger.[8]

Key Points

- There is a high incidence of asymptomatic instability in rheumatoid arthritis; therefore, radiographic assessment should be considered.
- Radiographic assessment should include flexion-extension lateral radiographs, as dynamic instability may not be apparent on neutral radiographs (Figure 15.6b,c).[9,10]
- Disease-modifying agents and biological agents are unable to prevent the progress of cervical disease once it has started. In contrast, these agents are effective in treating peripheral joint manifestations.[11]
- Surgery is usually indicated for symptoms and signs of cervical myelopathy.
- In the upper cervical spine:
  - Occipitocervical fusion is indicated in patients with basilar invagination.
  - C1/C2 fusion is used mainly for AAI, and does not treat basilar invagination; 50% of cervical rotation is lost.
  - Anterior (trans-oral) procedures may be required.
- In the lower cervical spine, anterior or posterior approaches may be used. The objective is decompression of the neural elements and stabilisation of the affected motion segments – fusion is required.[12]

Adolescent Idiopathic Scoliosis

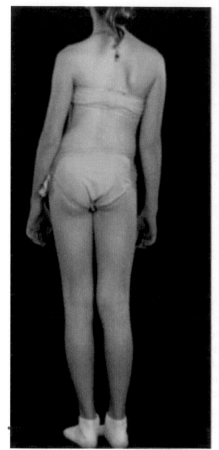

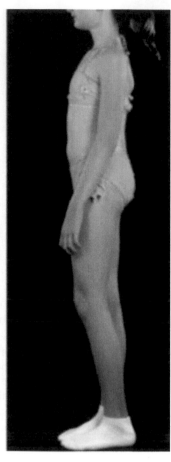

Figure 15.7a Clinical photograph of a patient with adolescent idiopathic scoliosis (AIS). Note on clinical inspection:

- Coronal plane deformity
- Asymmetry of the shoulders
- Prominence of the ribs on the right
- Waistline asymmetry
- Truncal shift to the right
- Hypokyphosis

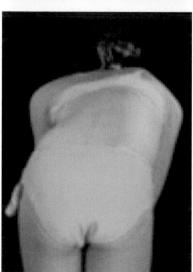

Figure 15.7b Clinical photograph showing Adam's forward bend test. This exaggerates the right rib prominence (hump). The deformity from a structural curve will become exaggerated with the forward bend test – rib prominence with thoracic curves, loin prominence with lumbar curves.

When examining a patient with structural scoliosis, there are other clinical findings to look for:

- Limb length discrepancies
- Pelvic tilt if neuromuscular scoliosis, e.g. cerebral palsy
- Signs of spinal dysraphism – dimple, naevus, hairy patch, lipoma, obvious myelomeningocele or surgical scars.
- Skin changes (café-au-lait patches or neuromas in neurofibromatosis)
- Neurological examination including abdominal reflexes. Asymmetrical reflexes indicate possible neuraxial anomalies, e.g. syrinx.
- Gait abnormalities

Key Points

- Scoliosis is a complex three-dimensional deformity of the spine typified by a curve in the coronal plane measuring over 10° using the Cobb angle.
- Scoliosis is either congenital, neuromuscular or idiopathic (idiopathic accounts for 80% of cases). Idiopathic scoliosis is now divided into early onset (<10 years) and late onset (>10 years). Early onset scoliosis (EOS) has the potential to affect pulmonary development and should be monitored and treated if required.

Adolescent Idiopathic Scoliosis

- Onset is 10 years and over (previous subdivisions of idiopathic scoliosis were infantile, juvenile, adolescent – now changed to early and late onset to reflect importance of relevance to pulmonary development). It is more common in females (4:1), and right thoracic curves are the most common.
- Curve growth is more rapid the earlier the age of onset, before and around the time of menarche, in early Risser stage and with larger curves.
- Assessment requires standard PA and lateral radiographs. Bending films are used to define non-structural curves (bend to <25°), plan surgery and indicate likely degree of correction.
- Management:
  - Scoliosis requires follow-up until skeletal maturity.
  - Bracing is for curves of 25°–40° and skeletal immaturity (Risser 0–2, Figure 15.7c).

- Bracing is not widely used because of poor compliance, i.e. wearing it less than 23 hours/day renders it significantly less effective.
- Effectiveness of bracing is dependent on number of hours worn with a minimum of 23 hours required. Bracing is cumbersome for patients in the tropics and equatorial regions.
- Recent resurgence in bracing after Bracing in Adolescent Idiopathic Scoliosis Trial (BrAIST).[13]
- Curves are classified using Lenke classification, which focuses on curve location, sagittal profile and coronal balance
- The indications for surgery are curves >40°–50° with risk of progression.
  - Posterior correction of deformity and instrumented fusion using pedicle screw constructs is the standard procedure.
  - All structural curves should be included in the fusion.
- Patients who are Risser Stages 0 and 1 are highly likely to progress.
- At skeletal maturity, if Cobb angle < 30° the curve is unlikely to progress; if 30°–50°, progression variable; if >50°, curve progression is at a rate of 0.5°–1° per year.

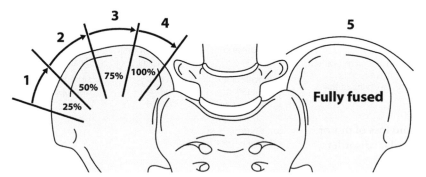

Figure 15.7c The Risser classification is used to grade skeletal maturity radiologically based on the level of ossification and fusion of the iliac crest apophysis. Stage 0 = no ossification; Stage 1 = up to 25% ossification of the iliac crest etc., up to Stage 5 where the iliac crest is fully fused.

Neuromuscular Scoliosis

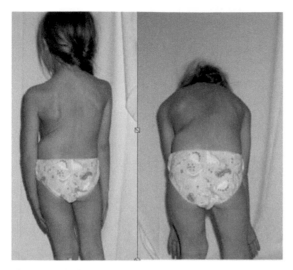

Figure 15.8a,b Long right-sided C-shaped curve usually seen in neuromuscular conditions. This child has a lower motor neuron pathology secondary to transverse myelitis.

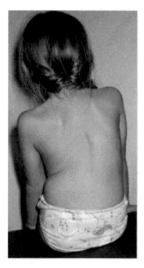

Figure 15.8c Curves tend to be long and are often associated with pelvic obliquity. Due to the underlying condition, there is often a failure to develop compensatory curves and the flexibility of the curve decreases with time.

Due to muscle weakness, imbalance and loss of motor tone or control seen in neuromuscular disorders, scoliosis is a common feature.

The curve pattern often varies from idiopathic cases and the commonest pattern is the C-shaped curve as in Figure 15.8c, especially in non-ambulant patients.

Additional examination should include:

- Nutritional status
- Neurological status, intellectual function, head control and ambulatory status
- Pelvic obliquity and curve flexibility
- Infrapelvic causes of pelvic obliquity inclusive of hip contractures

Key Points

The Scoliosis Research Society classifies the underlying causes into 'Neuropathic' and 'Myopathic' (Table 15.1).

- The goal of treatment is to prevent respiratory deterioration, maintain a balanced spine over a stable pelvis, facilitate seating and maintain mobility as long as possible.
- Conservative management is often unsuccessful due to the progressive nature of the condition and lack of effectiveness of orthoses.
- There is a higher mortality and morbidity rate with surgical intervention than idiopathic scoliosis but surgery is the most effective method of treatment.

Table 15.1 Scoliosis Research Society classification

Neuropathic		Myopathic
Upper motor neuron	**Lower motor neuron**	
Cerebral palsy	Viral myelitis	Muscular dystrophy
Spinal cord trauma	Spinal muscular atrophy	Arthrogryposis
Spinal cord tumour	Traumatic	Congenital hypotonia
Syringomyelia	Dysautonomic disorders	Myotonia dystrophy
Spinocerebral degeneration: a. Friedreich's ataxia b. Charcot–Marie–Tooth disease	Werdnig–Hoffman disease	Fibre-type disproportion

Pelvic Obliquity

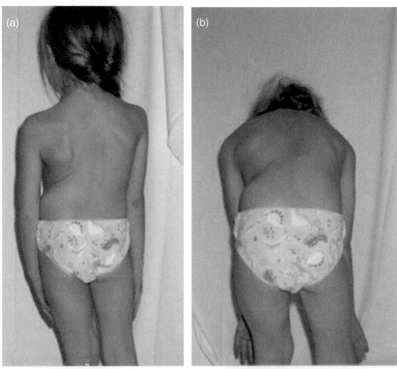

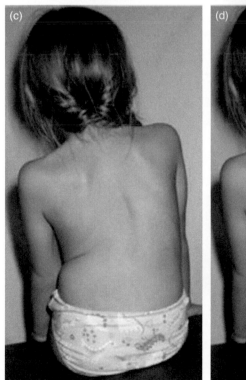
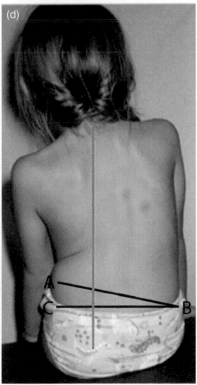

Figure 15.9a–h (a) Suprapelvic cause of obliquity with equal leg lengths.
(b) Decompensated plumb line to the right with a right-sided rib prominence.
(c,d) Note that the pelvic obliquity does not correct with sitting.

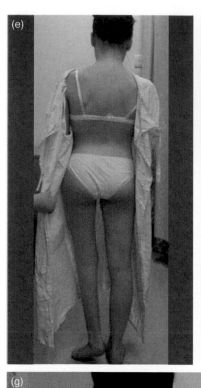

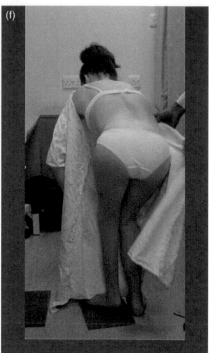

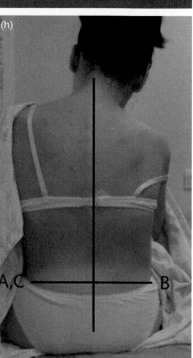

Figure 15.9a–h (cont.)
(e) Infrapelvic cause for obliquity of the pelvis.
(f) Blocks used to negate the leg length discrepancy and forward bending to appreciate the curve.
(g,h) Sitting position shows pelvis level.

Pelvic obliquity is a failure of the pelvis to maintain a horizontal position in the frontal plane and, as a result, the tangential line connecting the highest point of both hemipelvises falls at an angle to the midline.

Superiorly, pelvic obliquity may act as a driving force for a compensatory scoliosis to maintain coronal balance. Alternatively, pelvic obliquity may be due to a long scoliotic deformity of the spine such as in neuromuscular scoliosis.

The pelvis in most cases operates as a single unit due to its strong ligamentous connections. Its position in the coronal and sagittal planes will have an effect on its attachment, i.e. the hips inferiorly and the spine superiorly.

Pelvic obliquity may change the force vectors acting on the hip and may increase the risk of hip dislocation. It also affects sitting position and may asymmetrically increase pressure over the ischial tuberosity. This can be painful in patients with intact sensation or result in pressure ulcers in insensate patients. Additionally, it may affect coronal balance and increase the difficulty of maintaining an upright-seated position without the assistance of the upper limbs especially in non-ambulators.

Assessment of Pelvic Obliquity

Pelvic obliquity can be subdivided depending on whether the cause is infrapelvic as due to limb length discrepancy (LLD) or hip contractures, suprapelvic driven by scoliosis and intrapelvic when there is an intrinsic pelvic mismatch in heights of the two hemipelvises. Sometimes a patient can have more than one of these causes; this is especially seen in congenital paediatric cases with spinal and pelvic abnormalities.

Assess the position of the interspinous (interanterior superior iliac spine (ASIS)) line in relation to the midline of the body with the prerequisite that the legs are parallel to the midline of the body.

Assess pelvic obliquity in both standing, sitting and recumbency position to aid in differentiating functional from structural causes.

If a structural cause is present, try to differentiate between suprapelvic and infrapelvic cause. In infrapelvic, the position of the lower limbs will assist in correcting obliquity. An adduction contracture raises the ipsilateral pelvis with an apparent

shortening, whereas an abduction contracture will lower the hemipelvis and produce an apparent longer limb. Variation in limb position does not have an influence on pelvic obliquity if the cause is suprapelvic and the examiner has to assess the patient standing from the back.

One has to differentiate intrapelvic obliquity that may be due to conditions such as congenital malformations of the hemipelvis or post-pelvic oncological resections. This can be determined whilst sitting, as the heights of the hemipelvis are asymmetrical.

Assess the patient for secondary deformities including scoliosis and contractures of the hip. Measure limb length (as discrepancy can result in pelvic obliquity) and range of movement of the hip (as pelvic obliquity can affect hip stability). Finally, assess the gait looking for a short leg or a Trendelenburg gait.

Key Points

- Pelvic obliquity may be related to non-structural or structural causes. Structural causes may be suprapelvic, intrapelvic or infrapelvic. On some occasions, multiple causes may coexist.[14]

- Non-structural pelvic obliquity is most likely due to a limb length discrepancy. This will correct if the patient is seated and will also correct (together with the compensatory scoliosis) when the patient is asked to stand on blocks.

- A structural pelvic obliquity is a fixed deformity that persists in all positions and cannot be passively corrected.

- Suprapelvic cause of structural pelvic obliquity is most likely due to neuromuscular or congenital scoliosis. This is not the case in AIS, as the curve does not extend to the pelvis.

- The main infrapelvic cause of structural pelvic obliquity is hip contracture and LLD.

- Assessing contractures around the hip, especially in the child, is best accomplished with the patient in the prone position. During this position, the reducibility of the obliquity may also be assessed.

Congenital Conditions of Cervical Spine

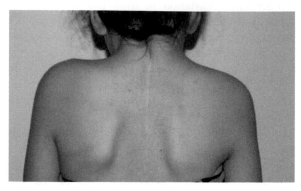

Figure 15.10 Clinical photograph depicting a short neck and low hairline of Klippel–Feil syndrome. Also note mild webbing and bilateral Sprengel shoulders and surgical scar from previous omovertebral bar excision.

In Klippel-Feil syndrome, less than 50% of patients have the classic clinical triad of low posterior hairline, short webbed neck and decreased cervical range of movement.[15]

The common clinical finding is painless decreased range of cervical movement, the extent of which depends on the number of spontaneously fused segments. Rotation is usually affected more than flexion-extension.

Because of the omovertebral connections in a Sprengel shoulder the range of shoulder movement is also decreased.

Look for associated conditions:[16]

○ Torticollis
○ Scoliosis
○ Spina bifida occulta
○ High-riding scapula secondary to Sprengel deformity
○ Auditory impairment, which may be conductive, sensorineural or combined
○ Cleft palate and other craniofacial anomalies
○ Associated VACTERL (vertebral, anal, cardiac, tracheo-oesophageal, renal, limb) anomalies: 30% renal and genitourinary, 15% cardiac

Differential diagnoses include the following:

○ Congenital muscular torticollis
○ Multiple synostosis (GDF6 deficiency)
○ Ankylosing spondylitis
○ Juvenile rheumatoid arthritis

Key Points

- Klippel–Feil syndrome is a congenital fusion of two or more cervical vertebrae. It is due to failure of formation or segmentation of cervical vertebrae during the third to eighth weeks of gestation. It may be due to spontaneous mutation or autosomal dominant or recessive inheritance. As such, it represents a heterogenous group of features that must be looked for when assessing the patient.

- Management involves that of associated conditions, e.g. cervical radiculopathy. Spinal surgical intervention may be required for associated instability (craniocervical junction, C1–C2) or applying the usual principles for degenerative pathology.

- Consider avoiding contact sports in those patients with long fusions or single open interspace between two fused segments.

References

1. Sardar ZM, Ames RJ, Lenke L. Scheuermann's kyphosis: diagnosis, management, and selecting fusion levels. *J Am Acad Orthop Surg* 2019;27(10):e462–e472.

2. Song K, Su X, Zhang Y, et al. Optimal chin-brow vertical angle for sagittal visual fields in ankylosing spondylitis kyphosis. *Eur Spine J* 2016;25 (8):2596–2604.

3. Kubiak EN, Moskovich R, Errico TJ, Di Cesare PE. Orthopaedic management of ankylosing spondylitis. *J Am Acad Orthop Surg* 2005;13 (4):267–278.

4. Crawford CH 3rd, Larson AN, Gates M, et al. Current evidence regarding the treatment of pediatric lumbar spondylolisthesis: a report from the Scoliosis Research Society Evidence Based Medicine Committee. *Spine Deform* 2017;5(5):284–302.

5. White AA 3rd, Johnson RM, Panjabi MM, Southwick WO. Biomechanical analysis of clinical stability in the cervical spine. *Clin Orthop Relat Res* 1975(109):85–96.

6. Thompson SE, Smith ZA, Hsu WK, et al. C5 palsy after cervical spine surgery: a multicenter retrospective review of 59 cases. *Global Spine J* 2017;7(Suppl 1):64s–70s.

7. Passos Cardoso AL, Da Silva NA, Daher S, De Moraes FB, Do Carmo HF. Evaluation of the cervical spine among patients with rheumatoid arthritis. *Rev Bras Ortop* 2010;45(2):160–165.

8. Zhu S, Xu W, Luo Y, Zhao Y, Liu Y. Cervical spine involvement risk factors in rheumatoid arthritis: a meta-analysis. *Int J Rheum Dis* 2017;20(5):541–549.

9. Clarke D, Neil I, Vaughan K, Smith T. Radiographic recognition of cervical instability in rheumatoid arthritis. *West Indian Med J* 2017. doi:10.7727/wimj.2017.103.

10. Roche CJ, Eyes BE, Whitehouse GH. The rheumatoid cervical spine: signs of instability on plain cervical radiographs. *Clin Radiol* 2002;**57**(4):241–249.

11. Mallory GW, Halasz SR, Clarke MJ. Advances in the treatment of cervical rheumatoid: less surgery and less morbidity. *World J Orthop* 2014;**5**(3):292–303.

12. Gillick JL, Wainwright J, Das K. Rheumatoid arthritis and the cervical spine: a review on the role of surgery. *Int J Rheumatol* 2015;**2015**:252456.

13. Weinstein SL, Dolan LA, Wright JG, Dobbs MB. Effects of bracing in adolescents with idiopathic scoliosis. *N Engl J Med* 2013;**369**(16):1512–1521.

14. Mayer L. Fixed paralytic obliquity of the pelvis. *J Bone Joint Surg* 1931;13(1):1–15.

15. Tracy MR, Dormans JP, Kusumi K. Klippel-Feil syndrome: clinical features and current understanding of etiology. *Clin Orthop Relat Res* 2004;**424**:183–190.

16. Copley LA, Dormans JP. Cervical spine disorders in infants and children. *J Am Acad Orthop Surg* 1998;**6**(4):204–214.

Upper Limb Clinical Cases

Simon Robinson, John E. D. Wright and Vijay Bhalaik

Chapter

16

Introduction

Upper limb presentations can involve a single joint or multiple joints. Frequently, pathology of one location will affect the function of the entire upper limb. Therefore, this needs to be taken into consideration on assessment. In addition, cervical spine pathology can present with clinical signs in the upper limb.

Examination of the shoulder follows the *look, feel, move* sequence, whereas in the elbow and wrist, this is *look, move, feel*. The process of hand examination is dependent on what the provisional diagnosis is after performing the screening manoeuvre.

The Hand

Dupuytren's Disease

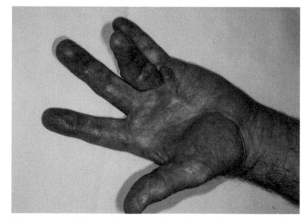

Figure 16.1a The ring finger has a flexed attitude. This will be fixed as there is a pretendinous cord in the palm in keeping with Dupuytren's disease. Both the metacarpal phalangeal joint (MCPJ) and proximal interphalangeal joint (PIPJ) are flexed.

Dupuytren's patients are classically of northern European heritage, male and middle to older age.

Cords usually start on the ulnar aspect of the palm and often progress radially.

Assessment of the degree of deformity of the MCPJ, PIPJ and distal interphalangeal joint (DIPJ) are important in managing the condition and for outcome of surgical management. Assess for cords to the other digits, commissural cords and for Garrods pads.[1] If there is an adduction deformity, a commissural cord may be palpated in the first webspace.

If the patient is young, always assess for the stigmata of Dupuytren's diathesis, as there may be associated Ledderhose disease (sole of foot) or Peyronie's disease (penis).

Key Points

- Differential diagnoses for a flexed attitude of the fingers include Dupuytren's disease, extensor tendon rupture, sagittal band rupture, late trigger finger, dislocated MCPJ and posterior interosseous nerve (PIN) palsy.

  ○ Dupuytren's disease has a classical fixed flexion deformity due to the pathological cord.

  ○ Extensor tendon rupture is usually passively correctable.

  ○ Being able to hold the MCP joints extended when passively corrected may therefore indicate a sagittal band rupture.

  ○ Trigger finger has a classical history with a palpable flexor nodule.

  ○ Dislocated/subluxed MCPJs are usually associated with features of inflammatory arthropathy.

  ○ Patients with PIN palsy are unable to extend the fingers at the MCPJ or retropulse the thumb.

- The treatment options for Dupuytren's disease depend on the deformity and the impairment to activities of daily living. The management ladder escalates from watchful waiting, night splints, needle fasciotomy, collagenase injection, fasciotomy, fasciectomy, dermofasciectomy to amputation.

Rheumatoid Hand

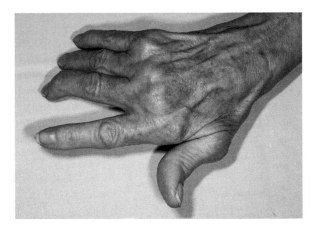

Figure 16.1b(i) This clinical photograph demonstrates a patient with swollen metacarpophalangeal (MCP) joints, finger deformity at the middle finger distal interphalangeal (DIP) joint and previous wrist surgery as seen by the well-healed dorsal longitudinal scar. The ulnar three fingers sit in a flexed and ulnarly deviated posture. This patient has the stigmata of a symmetrical inflammatory polyarthropathy in keeping with rheumatoid disease.

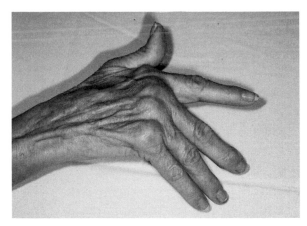

Figure 16.1b(ii) Right hand of this patient with rheumatoid disease with 'dropped fingers' and the inability to extend the ulnar three fingers. The picture also demonstrates subluxation of the extensor tendons. It is important to assess whether this is a fixed or passively correctable deformity.

The reasons for the dropped fingers in the rheumatoid patient are extensor tendon rupture, sagittal band rupture, subluxed or dislocated MCPJs and posterior interosseous nerve palsy.

Key Points

- Remember to perform a functional hand assessment in the rheumatoid hand.
- Reasons for ulnar deviation:
  - Synovitis within the MCP joints leads to attenuation of the capsule and ligaments, causing an unstable joint that may sublux and even dislocate.
  - The hand radially deviates at the wrist and the fingers deviate ulnarly, creating a Z-deformity altering the line of pull of the extrinsic tendons.
  - The extensor tendons slip ulnarwards and into the groove between the MCP joints. This then leads to the pull of the extensors becoming a flexor when the line of pull subluxes past the transverse axis of the MCP joint.
- Non-surgical management includes watchful waiting, splinting and hand therapy.
- Surgical management would depend on the MCP joints. Centralisation of the extensor tendons with sagittal band reconstruction is an option with or without MCP joint replacement. If there is significant wrist deformity, this may need to be corrected first to improve the alignment of the pull of the tendons.[2]

Finger Deformity

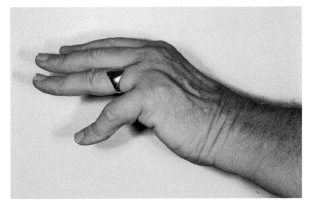

Figure 16.1c The little finger demonstrates a Boutonnière deformity. Assess whether this is a flexible or fixed deformity and then assess the function. Assess for any other manifestations of a symmetrical inflammatory polyarthropathy.

The mechanism by which this deformity occurs is failure of the central slip, allowing subluxation of the lateral bands until they are volar to the centre of rotation of the PIP joint, changing an extension force into a flexion one. This central slip rupture may occur due to capsular expansion in inflammatory arthropathy or trauma, which may be blunt trauma or a laceration.

The acute central slip rupture can be diagnosed using Elson's test (Chapter 5).

Key Points

- Acute management is usually in the form of splinting but may include surgical repair. The flexibility of the joint is key for deciding management of a chronic Boutonnière deformity.
- For a chronic flexible Boutonnière deformity, a Fowler (terminal tendon) tenotomy is an option, although there are reconstructive options with variable results.[3]
- For a fixed Boutonnière deformity, hand therapy to regain movement is preferred. If this fails, then fusion procedures may correct the deformity to a more functional position.

Congenital Hand Deformity

Associated conditions include: VACTERL (vertebral, anal, cardiac, tracheo-oesophageal, renal, limb) / VATER, TAR, Fanconi's anaemia and Holt–Oram syndrome, so look for other features associated with these syndromes.

Examine the hand to assess for either a hypoplastic thumb, a previous pollicisation procedure (which is most likely in this case (Figure 16.1d), given the dorsal curvilinear scar) and/or a centralisation procedure. It is important to assess function of this limb, as improving function is the main surgical aim. Assessing the elbow and the contralateral upper limb is also important.

Key Points

- Swanson's classification was initially used, but the Oberg–Manske–Tonkin (OMT) classification has superseded this.[4,5] The OMT divides these deformities into three groups: Malformations; Deformations; Dysplasias. Malformations are the most common and are further subdivided on whether the whole limb is involved or just the hand alone, and whether the primary insult involves one of the three axes of limb development and patterning or is non-axial.
- Surgery would usually be performed at 6 to 12 months of age if function is compromised. Centralisation and thumb reconstruction/ pollicisation are the common options here.

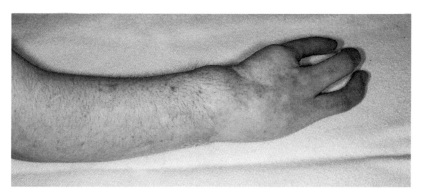

Figure 16.1d Congenital deformity of the upper limb where there is a radial longitudinal deficiency.

Wasting in the Hand: Ulnar Nerve

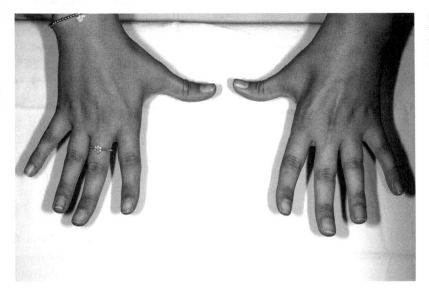

Figure 16.1e There is marked wasting of the first dorsal interosseous muscle along with evidence of wasting of the intrinsic muscles in the left hand compared to the right.

The diagnosis in the case above is ulnar nerve neuropathy, although brachial plexus injury and cervical nerve root entrapment are differential diagnoses. The nerve roots for the hand intrinsic muscles are C8/T1. Therefore, in order to differentiate this from an ulnar nerve lesion, examination should assess the sensation of the medial border of the forearm (T1 dermatome), which will be affected in a nerve root lesion as opposed to an ulnar nerve lesion.

To detect whether the ulnar nerve lesion is high or low, some proximally innervated muscles need to be tested. If they are intact, then the compression is low, most likely in Guyon's canal. Flexor carpi ulnaris (FCU) and flexor digitorum profundus (FDP) to the little finger are the two muscle that can be tested that have proximal innervation. If there is significant clawing, then it is more likely the compression is low (ulnar paradox).

Key Points

- Sites of ulnar nerve entrapment: medial intermuscular septum; medial head of triceps; arcade of Struthers; medial epicondylar osteophytes, aponeurosis of the two heads of FCU; deep flexor/pronator aponeurosis; Guyon's canal (zones 1–3).
- Non-surgical management of cubital tunnel syndrome includes splinting/prevention of elbow flexion, activity modification and NSAIDs. Success depends on the severity of the compression. Surgical management encompasses decompression of the nerve at the site of compression +/− treat the cause +/− transposition.

Wasting in the Hand: Median Nerve

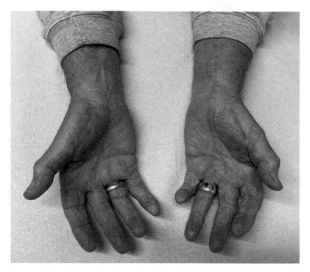

Figure 16.1f This patient has a scar in keeping with carpal tunnel release of the left hand along with thenar muscle wasting.

The diagnosis in the case above is median nerve compression in the carpal tunnel. However, a differential diagnosis of a C6 lesion, brachial plexus lesion or polyneuropathy should be considered. Stigmata of trauma should be looked for, which may indicate previous management of an acute median nerve compression.[6]

With regards to differentiating between C6 root lesion and median nerve compression, testing sensation is of limited benefit. There may be weakness of wrist extension with a C6 lesion, but this is not so with median nerve compression.

This patient had carpal tunnel syndrome so it would be expected that flexor carpi radialis (FCR) and flexor digitorum superficialis (FDS) to the index finger would have normal power. Assess the power of the intrinsic muscles of the hand supplied by the median nerve, which should be weak.

In addition, feel the sensation of the autonomous area of the median nerve (radial aspect of index finger at level of DIPJ) and sensation of the thenar eminence to differentiate between a low or high median nerve lesion. In carpal tunnel syndrome, sensation over the thenar eminence should be preserved.

Special tests: Tinel's test over the carpal tunnel, Durkan's compression test or Phalen's test (see chapter 5). Being aware of the sensitivity and specificity of these tests will aid your diagnosis.

Key Points

- If not a classical picture, then request nerve conduction studies. A Martin–Gruber anastomosis may confuse the clinical findings.
- Management depends on the clinical findings and may range from addressing the cause (hypothydroidism/weight loss/oedema), splinting, corticosteroid injection to carpal tunnel release.

Bony Swellings in the Hand: Multiple Enchondromas

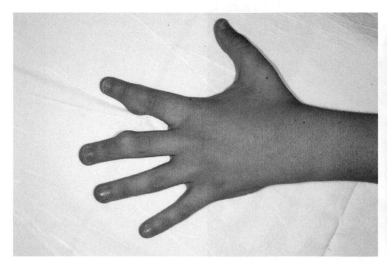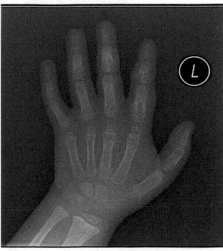

Figure 16.1g(i,ii) This 10-year-old patient has two swellings located over the ulnar border of the index finger middle phalanx and the radial border of the middle finger middle phalanx. The rest of the hand appears normal. This is an example of multiple enchondromas.

With multiple enchondromas (Ollier's disease), the lesions are located asymmetrically in the skeleton, with wide variation with regards to size and number. Involvement may range from a single hand to the entire skeleton. In any one patient, it tends to favour one side of the body. As a result of growth plate damage, other presenting clinical features include deformities and leg length discrepancy.

The main differential diagnosis of a patient presenting with multiple bony lumps to the hand is osteochondromas or hereditary multiple exostosis (HME). This differentiation may be difficult clinically, but with HME other lumps may be seen in relation to the metaphyses of long bones and some flat bones. Radiology will differentiate the two. Osteochondromas will arise from the bone surface, whereas enchondromas are located in the centre of the bone.

Key Points

- The diagnoses of Ollier's disease or Maffucci's syndrome need to be considered with multiple enchondromas. Maffucci's syndrome is associated with haemangiomas and a much higher risk of malignant transformation (Ollier's <30%; Maffucci's up to 100%).

- Management depends on whether these enchondromas were symptomatic. If they were symptomatic or had caused a pathological fracture, then the best option would be curettage and bone graft.

Post-operative Tendon Transfer

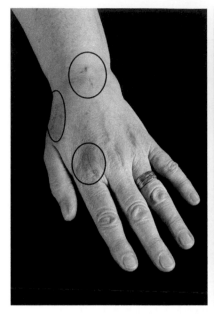 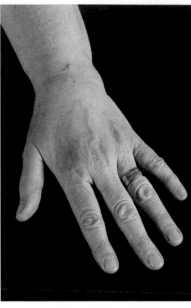

Figure 16.1h(i,ii) (i) This patient has a pattern of scars compatible with having had an extensor indicis (EI) to extensor pollicis longus (EPL) transfer. (ii) The thumb is clearly demonstrating active retropulsion.

In this case, the pattern of scars is classic, and if identified on inspection look for an underlying cause for the tendon rupture. For example, examine the elbows for rheumatoid nodules and other scars. There may also be a scar from a volar locked plate, as EPL rupture can occur if screws penetrate the third dorsal compartment.

Retropulsion is the specific movement of the thumb performed by extensor pollicis longus. This is tested by asking the patient to put the hand flat on a surface and raise the thumb away from the surface.

In a patient who demonstrates lack of retropulsion, it is important to demonstrate independent index and little finger MCPJ extension with the middle and ring fingers flexed. This shows the patient has expendable tendons (EI and extensor digiti minimi (EDM)) for consideration of a tendon transfer.

Key Points

- EPL rupture most commonly occurs with inflammatory arthritis, where there is attritional rupture around Lister's tubercle. It is also associated with patients who have an undisplaced distal radius fracture (ischaemic cause) as well as a complication of volar locked plates.

- Following an EPL rupture, surgery can be delayed as some patients find the lack of retropulsion is not limiting. The patient also needs to be aware of the rehabilitation required following surgery before agreeing to it.

- An advantage of using EIP for tendon transfer is that EIP has a similar amplitude and direction of pull compared to EPL.

- When examining a patient with an EPL rupture, test also for the presence of palmaris longus, as this tendon can be used to augment a direct repair or can be used as a free graft.

The Wrist

Radial-Sided Wrist Pain: Carpometacarpal Joint Arthritis

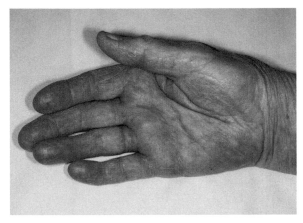

Figure 16.2a This patient has some squaring of the base of the thumb and the thumb is sitting in a partially opposed posture. This points to the first carpometacarpal (CMC) joint as the primary pathology. With symptomatic first CMC joint osteoarthritis the grind test will be positive and palpating the joint will be tender.

Assessing radiocarpal movement, especially radial and ulnar deviation will help ascertain if the scapho-trapeziotrapezoidal (STT) joint is symptomatic as well and should be used to guide management.

The point of tenderness is usually the site of the pathology. Therefore, knowledge of the surface anatomy of this area will help with the differential diagnosis.

Joints: Thumb CMC joint osteoarthritis, STT joint osteoarthritis, radiocarpal osteoarthritis (scaphoid fossa secondary to scapholunate advanced collapse (SLAC) wrist).

Tendons: De Quervain's disease, intersection syndrome, FCR tendonitis.

Nerves: Superficial radial nerve neuroma, Wartenberg's syndrome.

Key Points

- With CMC joint arthritis, radiographs (including Gedda type view) are generally all that is required to confirm the diagnosis.
- Management can be escalated from simple analgesia, splints and hand therapy to corticosteroid injections and then surgical

intervention. Surgery may involve trapeziectomy +/− soft tissue reconstruction, arthroplasty or arthrodesis, depending on the patient's requirement.[7]

Stiff Wrist

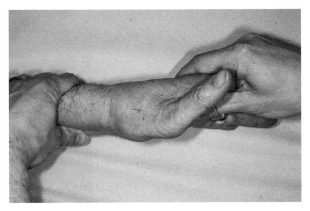

Figure 16.2b This patient demonstrates minimal active and passive flexion-extension at the wrist.

Differential diagnoses include wrist osteoarthritis (SLAC) / scaphoid non-union advanced collapse (SNAC)), ankylosed wrist secondary to inflammatory disease, a stiff total wrist arthroplasty or following a partial wrist fusion. Evidence of previous surgery (dorsal wrist scars heal well and may not be seen unless inspected for closely) and plain films aid differentiation here.

For further assessment of this patient, assess finger movement and pronation and supination of the forearm. Assess grip strength.

Key Points

- If a patient has failed conservative measures such as analgesia, splinting, hand therapy and injections, then surgical management is appropriate.
- Wrist denervation is a possible first-line option (if a wrist block has been successful) before consideration of movement preserving surgery or total wrist fusion (depending on the pathology).[8] The indications for these options need to be understood and discussed with the patient.
- The distal radioulnar joint (DRUJ) needs assessing pre-operatively and, if symptomatic, may require surgical intervention at the same time.

Lack of Forearm Rotation

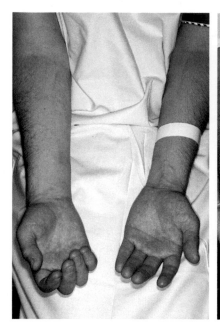
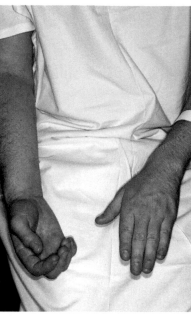

Figure 16.2c(i,ii) This patient demonstrates lack of active right forearm pronation. This requires the wrist and elbow to be assessed.

To assess pronation and supination, the elbows should be tucked into the side in order to minimise any compensation from the shoulder. Examine the other movements at the elbow and the wrist joint to determine whether the pathology is at the proximal or distal radioulnar joint.

Palpate for the presence and location of the radial head and look for any subluxation of the ulnar head at the DRUJ. Assess for the integrity of the triangular fibrocartilage complex (TFCC). This patient had pain and deformity at the wrist rather than the elbow.

Differential diagnosis of a patient that presents with reduced forearm pronation and supination includes:

Acute: Trauma to radial head/DRUJ dislocation.

Chronic: Malunion, DRUJ instability, post-traumatic synostosis, heterotopic ossification.

Congenital: Radial head dislocation, congenital proximal radioulnar synostosis.

Key Points

- A recurrent dislocator of either the DRUJ or the radiocapitellar joint should have the Beighton score for hyperlaxity assessed.
- If the radial head is dislocated, it is important to assess the shape of the radial head (loss of concavity) and the capitellum. Has the radial head ever been in joint? If not, check the knees and the hands for evidence of nail-patella syndrome.

The Elbow

Elbow Osteoarthritis

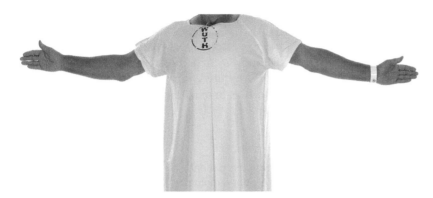

Figure 16.3a There is loss of right elbow extension due to osteoarthritis. The right elbow is held with a flexed attitude of approximately 30°.

Assess for scars, previous trauma, deformity, stigmata of inflammatory polyarthropathy and evidence of neurological deficit.

It is particularly important in the elbow to assess passive movement after active movement, as this will help determine whether there is a mechanical cause to the block.

There are many causes of loss of extension in the elbow. These include intra articular causes such as osteoarthritis, loose bodies and intra articular mal- or non-union. Extra-articular causes include heterotopic ossification and prominent metalwork.

Key Points

- Non-operative management includes analgesia, physiotherapy and injection therapy.
- Operative management may be open or arthroscopic. Open procedures may range from arthrolysis to the OK procedure, radial head excision to elbow arthroplasty.
- The surgical options are very patient dependent. Joint-preserving procedures are the ideal management in a young, higher demand patient such as a manual worker.
- Elbow arthroplasty is usually reserved for the lower demand or older patient.

Olecranon Bursa

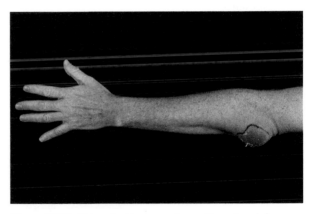

Figure 16.3b This patient has a swollen erythematous left olecranon bursa. The key to managing this patient is establishing whether the bursa is infected.

The cause of an olecranon bursitis may be traumatic (acute/chronic), inflammatory (gout/rheumatoid arthritis) or infective. Rarer differential diagnoses would include olecranon fracture, triceps rupture or septic arthritis.[9] A plain radiograph would usually suffice to look for any prominent spurs, inflammatory arthropathy or chondrocalcinosis.

Risk factors include any profession that involves repetitive elbow use/pressure / leaning on the elbows. Middle-aged males are most commonly affected. Patients with impaired immunity are at a higher risk (e.g. diabetes, HIV, alcoholism, uraemia).

Key Points

- Around one-third of olecranon bursitis cases are infective. Any signs of systemic illness, significant cellulitis or pus would suggest this. Look for an abrasion or puncture wound.
- Management can include rest, compression, NSAIDs, antibiotics and aspiration. Aspiration is not advisable for the vast majority of cases as it can lead to the introduction of infection or a sinus, which is very difficult to treat.
- Aspiration or drainage samples should be sent for microscopy, crystal analysis and white blood cell count along with Gram stain and culture. *Staphylococcus aureus* is this most common infective organism.
- Careful surgical technique along with splinting the elbow in an extended position after decompression helps decrease wound healing problems.

The Shoulder

Post-traumatic Shoulder Stiffness

It is important to determine whether this loss of movement is both active and passive. If so, then the possibilities are: glenohumeral osteoarthritis (primary or secondary), frozen shoulder, stiff shoulder arthroplasty or a locked posterior shoulder dislocation. The patient's age and history will generally determine the cause.

If active external rotation is restricted and further passive movement is possible, then the possibilities are weak/ruptured infraspinatus or a neurological cause such as brachial neuritis or Parsonage–Turner syndrome.

Key Points

- Given this patient's age, osteoarthritis is most likely but radiological confirmation is required before differentiating between osteoarthritis and a frozen shoulder (Figure 16.4a(ii)).
- Surgical management would most likely be arthroplasty in this patient's age group. Clinical assessment of the rotator cuff and deltoid along with radiological assessment of glenoid version and depth would help decide between hemiarthoplasty, anatomical shoulder replacement or reverse shoulder replacement. Given the patient's age, many surgeons may currently choose a stemmed reverse total shoulder replacement as a single or staged procedure.[10]

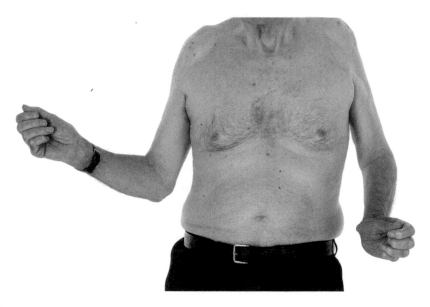

Figure 16.4a(i) This 79-year-old patient has limited external rotation of the left shoulder compared to the right. The deltoid is flattened and there is a well-healed anterior shoulder scar in keeping with a deltopectoral surgical approach.

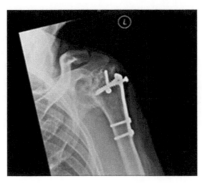

Figure 16.4a(ii) The plain film shows post-traumatic osteoarthritis in this patient's case. Treatment depends on the level of symptoms. Non-surgical management would include optimising analgesia, physiotherapy, glenohumeral joint injections or suprascapular nerve blocks.

Painful Shoulder Arthroplasty

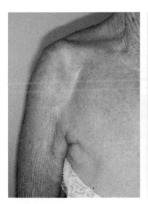

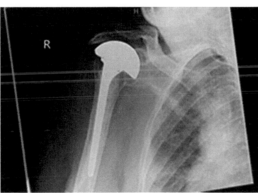

Figure 16.4b(i,ii) (i) This 75-year-old patient has a painful right shoulder after a previous hemiarthroplasty. (ii) Plain radiograph confirms the rotator cuff has failed and the superior glenoid is eroding.

On inspection, this patient has a well-healed scar in keeping with the deltopectoral approach to their right shoulder. Active then passive range of movement should be assessed, as a stiff shoulder may cause pain. Differential diagnoses include infection, loosening, soft tissue failure and implant failure.

Look for any evidence of erythema or swelling to raise the possibility of a significant infection. Low-grade infections such as *Cutibacterium acnes* (previously *Propionibacterium acnes*) are difficult to exclude.

Assessment of the rotator cuff is also important in hemiarthroplasties and anatomical total shoulder replacements, especially supraspinatus and subscapularis. This can be challenging if movement is painful or stiff.

Key Points

- Initial investigations would include plain radiographs, which would confirm the implant, along with blood investigations (full blood count (FBC), urea and electrolytes (U&Es), inflammatory markers).[11]
- Definitive biopsy sampling may be required along with removal of the implant. This is followed by computed tomography (CT) scan assessment of the glenoid and humeral bone stock, which is a consideration before undertaking a revision shoulder arthroplasty.

Massive Rotator Cuff Tear

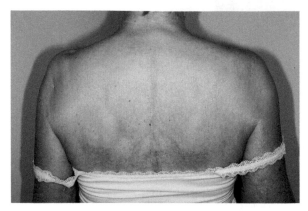

Figure 16.4c This 85-year-old woman has marked infraspinous fossa wasting of the left shoulder along with evidence of a previous shoulder arthroscopy portal. This patient has a massive rotator cuff tear, which has led to cuff tear arthropathy.

Differential diagnoses include rotator cuff tear, rotator cuff tear arthropathy, pain inhibition/disuse or a neuropathic cause (Parsonage–Turner syndrome, suprascapular nerve injury, brachial plexus injury, disc prolapse).

Supraspinous fossa wasting is difficult to assess at this angle. In massive tears, at least the supraspinatus and infraspinatus tendons are torn. Wasting will be evident in both muscles.

In this case, both deltoids also appear a little flattened. Sometimes a subcutaneous effusion may be seen which is due to the joint fluid escaping from the torn capsule.

Active elevation may not be possible (pseudoparalysis). With elevation of the arm, prominence of the humeral head anteriorly may be seen (anterosuperior escape).

Usually there is at least 30° of passive abduction possible beyond the active movement. If there is painful passive movement of the shoulder, it is likely that the patient has developed a rotator cuff arthropathy.

Weakness of external rotation is a common feature. This is demonstrated by a positive 'lag sign' and 'hornblower's sign'.

Key Points

- Plain radiographs often give the examiner enough information to diagnose a chronic rotator cuff tear or cuff tear arthropathy.

Ultrasound and or magnetic resonance imaging (MRI) scans can give further information with regards to cuff tear retraction and fatty atrophy. CT scan is useful for assessing glenoid bone stock.

- Prior to surgery, it is important to confirm that the deltoid and the axillary nerve are intact if a reverse shoulder arthroplasty is to be performed.

- Surgical management for this 85-year-old patient would most likely be a reverse shoulder arthroplasty (after appropriate pre-op planning). More conservative options of arthroscopic debridement +/− biceps tenotomy may help but are less reliable. Rotator cuff repair is an option before any significant arthropathy is present, but as the patient's age increases and the size of the tear increases, the chances of a successful repair diminish. Narrowing of the acromiohumeral distance also diminishes the likelihood of a successful repair.[12]

Scapular Winging

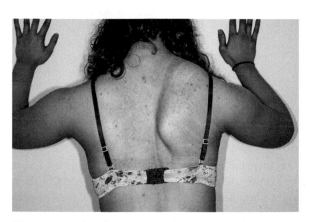

Figure 16.4d This clinical picture shows a young female patient with marked winging of her right scapula whilst performing a wall press. She demonstrates medial scapular winging in keeping with long thoracic nerve or serratus anterior pathology.

When scapular winging is seen, it is important to assess the muscles that stabilise the scapula such as the serratus anterior, trapezius and the rhomboids. Scoliosis should also be looked for and excluded.

Long thoracic nerve palsy may be a clue that there is a brachial plexus injury, and this must be looked for, especially the pre-ganglionic signs.

Classification of winging:[13]

- ○ Medial winging (more common): serratus anterior palsy, long thoracic nerve palsy, repetitive stretching/compression/trauma/ brachial neuritis or Parsonage–Turner syndrome (more pain).
- ○ Lateral winging: trapezius palsy, iatrogenic injury within posterior cervical triangle (spinal accessory nerve).
- ○ Winging + generalised weakness: facioscapulohumeral dystrophy (FSHD).

Key Points

- With FSHD, the patient can present with shoulder prominence due to scapular winging. They have limited arm abduction and flexion but selective sparing of the deltoid. In the face, there is incomplete eye closure, loss of forehead wrinkling and a transverse smile. Characteristically, the patient is unable to whistle.
- If there is a small, superior, winged scapula, the diagnosis is likely to be a Sprengel shoulder associated with Klippel–Feil syndrome.
- Treatment for winging would depend on the symptoms and functional limitation:
  - ○ *Medial*: 6–24 months of conservative management. Physiotherapy to keep movement. Most get better over time. Nerve exploration or pectoralis major transfer are options.
  - ○ *Lateral*: Nerve exploration, Modified Eden– Lange procedure (transfer of levator scapulae and rhomboid minor) or scapulothoracic fusion.
  - ○ *Sprengel shoulder*: Woodward procedure (detachment of the trapezius and rhomboids, excision of omovertebral bone/ fibrous bands, relocation of the scapular inferiorly and reattachment of muscles).

Swelling around the Shoulder

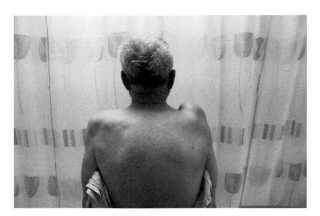

Figure 16.4e This man has a large swelling on the superior aspect of his right shoulder. It is fluid filled, transilluminates and is in keeping with a ganglion or bursa.

This represents a **geyser sign,** which is a subcutaneous swelling superficial to the acromioclavicular joint (ACJ) and is a result of fluid escaping from a chronic full-thickness rotator cuff tear through a degenerate ACJ (Figure 16.4e).

Marked bilateral infraspinous fossa wasting is apparent. The active movement in the shoulder is usually minimal in these cases along with limitation of passive external rotation.

Key Points

- Plain radiographs (true AP and axial) confirm the above diagnosis.
- Non-surgical treatment includes watchful waiting. Avoid aspiration if possible due to the high risk of recurrence.[14]
- Surgical management: Treat the underlying cause if indicated. ACJ excision or excision +/– ACJ capsular repair may help. A rotator cuff tear in this setting is usually irreparable. Reverse total shoulder replacement if indicated would likely treat the cause. Surgical excision of the swelling is associated with a high recurrence rate.

Upper Limb Amputation: Trans-humeral Amputation

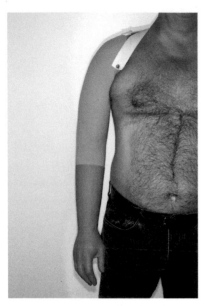

Figure 16.4f Patient with a right upper limb prosthesis. This patient had a transhumeral amputation. When assessing a patient with a prosthesis, both the patient and the prosthesis require examining.

The levels of upper limb amputation in ascending order are transphalangeal, transmetacarpal, transcarpal, wrist disarticulation, transradial, elbow disarticulation, transhumeral, shoulder disarticulation and forequarter amputation. Transphalangeal account for almost 80% of upper limb amputations.

Inspect the residual limb for oedema, which is common after amputations. Contractures and local residual limb problems such as bone prominence and neuromas must also be looked for. Assess for sensation, as numbness is common.

It is important to consider a reason for the amputation, e.g. scars signifying trauma or signs of Horner's syndrome indicating a possible flail limb. Eighty per cent of acquired upper limb amputations are a result, directly or indirectly, of trauma. The other 20% are mainly due to tumour and vascular complications of disease.[15]

Look at the adequacy of length of the amputation residual limb. Transhumeral amputations need to be 4–5 cm proximal to the elbow joint to allow for the prosthetic elbow lock mechanisms to appear equal to normal elbow location of the opposite arm. If more proximal amputation is required, at least 5–7 cm of residual length is needed for glenohumeral biomechanics.

Key Points

- When assessing these patients, if the patient is complaining of pain think of phantom pain or residual pain, which is usually musculoskeletal and due to remodelling of scar tissue, muscle and fascia. Ask whether there are any concerns about cosmesis and body asymmetry that may alter the centre of gravity, leading to pain and discomfort in other parts of the body.
- If this was a shoulder disarticulation, the scapula should be retained to prevent disfigurement of the back.
- Prostheses are made up of the following parts:
  - Interface/socket
  - Suspension mechanism
  - Struts – structures that recreate the limb length
  - Articulations (if needed)
  - Terminal device

References

1. Black EM, Blazar PE. Dupuytren's disease: an evolving understanding of an age-old disease. *J Am Acad Orthop Surg* 2011;**19**:746–757.

2. Papp SR, Athwal GS, Pichora DR. The rheumatoid wrist. *J Am Acad Orthop Surg* 2006;**14**:65–77.

3. Burge P. Mini-symposium: the elective hand (iii): the principles of surgery in the rheumatoid hand. *Curr Orthop* 2003;**17**:17–27.

4. Swanson AB. A classification for congenital limb malformations. *J Hand Surg Am* 1976 Jul:**1**(1)8–22.

5. Tonkin MA, Oberg, KC. The OMT classification of congenital anomalies of the hand and upper limb. *Hand Surg* 2015;**20**(03):336–342.

6. Floyd WE, Earp BE, Blazer PE. Acute median nerve problems in the setting of a distal radius fracture. *J Hand Surg Am* 2015;**8**(40):1669–1671.

7. Berger AJ, Meals RA. Management of osteoarthrosis of the thumb joints. *J Hand Surg Am* 2015;**40**(4):843–e850.

8. Bain GI, McGuire DT. Decision making for partial carpal fusions. *J Wrist Surg* 2012;**1**:103–114.

9. Elliott J. Olecranon bursitis. In Stanley D, Trail IA (eds), *Operative Elbow Surgery*. Edinburgh: Churchill Livingstone, 2012; pp. 547–554.

10. Wiater JM, Fabing MH. Shoulder arthroplasty: prosthetic options and indications. *J Am Acad Orthop Surg* 2009;**17**:415–425.

11. Rangan A, Falworth M, Watts, AC, et al.; BESS PJI Group. Investigation and management of periprosthetic joint infection in the shoulder and elbow: evidence and consensus based guidelines of the British Elbow and Shoulder Society. *Shoulder Elbow* 2018;**10**(1S):S5–S19.

12. Rashid MS, Cooper C, Cook J, et al. Increasing age and tear size reduce rotator cuff repair healing rate at 1 year. *Acta Orthop* 2017 Dec;**88**(6):606–611.

13. Martin RM, Fish DE. Scapular winging: anatomical review, diagnosis, and treatments. *Curr Rev Musculoskelet Med* 2008;**1**:1–11.

14. Singh R, Hay B, Hay S. Management of a massive acromioclavicular joint cyst: the geyser sign revisited. *Shoulder Elbow* 2013;**5**:62–64.

15. Ovadia S, Askari M. Upper extremity amputations and prosthetics. *Semin Plast Surg* 2015;**29**(1):55–61.

Lower Limb Clinical Cases

Faiz Shivji, Thomas Kurien, Karen Robinson and Fazal Ali

Introduction

Patients with orthopaedic lower limb pathology will usually present with pain on walking. Frequently, deformity is also present. It is important to remember to examine these patients first in a standing position. This should be followed by observing the alignment and leg length. Then observe the patient whilst walking, as gait is usually affected.

Always remember to observe the posterior aspect of the lower limb whilst standing, as pathology can be missed once the patient lies on the couch. Undressing the patient to observe the spine to see if there is a compensatory curve or to see if the spine is the source of a neurological pathology is also important.

Hip

Fixed Flexion of the Hip

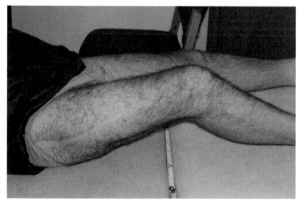

Figure 17.1a Patient with hip and knee flexion whilst supine with a large lateral scar from the proximal to distal thigh. Thomas test confirms a fixed flexion deformity of the hip of 20°.

Most cases of fixed flexion deformity at the hip are due to osteoarthritis. Other causes include inflammatory, post-traumatic or neurological conditions.

Look for hyperlordosis of the spine, as this can mask a fixed flexion deformity of the hip when the patient is standing or lying on a couch. The patient uses this manoeuvre to stand upright or to lie flat in bed. Thomas test is performed to eliminate this compensation from the lumbar spine by flexing the contralateral hip and thereby tilting the pelvis and flattening the lumbar spine.

A false impression of fixed flexion of the hip may be seen in a patient who has a fixed flexion deformity of the knee. In this case, when performing Thomas test it is important to bring the patient to the foot of the couch (or to hang the leg over the side of the couch), as doing so will eliminate the effect of the fixed knee flexion.

Key Points

- In osteoarthritis, flexion contracture is usually associated with adduction contracture, and this will give the impression of apparent shortening.
- When measuring true leg lengths, remember to 'square' the pelvis and place the normal limb in a similar position as the affected limb.
- When performing a hip replacement in a patient with a fixed flexion deformity of the hip due to osteoarthritis, the following points should be considered:
  - In addition to the standard surgical technique for total hip arthroplasty (THA), the surgeon may need to consider additional procedures to restore leg length, offset and range of movement.
  - If the hip is ankylosed and difficult to dislocate, a neck cut in situ may be required.
  - Soft tissue releases include a full release/excision of contracted capsule, release of iliopsoas and release of rectus femoris.
  - The hip may also have a fixed external rotation contracture that may result in difficulty repairing the posterior capsule and piriformis during closure.

Hip Arthrodesis

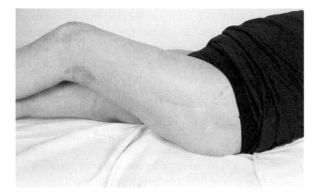

Figure 17.1b This patient is lying on a couch with flexion of the left hip. There is a lateral scar and no movement in that hip. This patient previously had an arthrodesis of the hip. As standard, the hip is fused in 20° of flexion, 0°–5° adduction, 5°–10° external rotation.

The effect of hip fusion is an increased load on adjacent joints with the lower back, ipsilateral knee and contralateral hip (in that order) being most affected. Consequently, the most common presenting complaint of these patients is lower back pain 20–30 years after arthrodesis and this is also the most common indication for conversion of an arthrodesis to a THA.

This patient will stand with an increased lumbar lordosis (to compensate for the hip fused in flexion) and pelvic tilt. They will walk with left sided 'hip-hiking' (raising of the hemipelvis) and circumduction during mid swing.[1] There will be true shortening as a result of the surgical arthrodesis and this is best assessed by the 'block test' whilst standing. There will also be further apparent shortening when lying on the couch because of the flexed and adducted hip.

These patients find walking more difficult, with an estimated 50% reduction of efficiency of gait due to increased energy expenditure and oxygen consumption.

Key Points

- Hip arthrodesis was traditionally indicated for young, active, high-demand patients when the results of arthroplasty were suboptimal in terms of function and survival. However, in modern times, arthrodesis is considered a salvage procedure for chronic infection both in native (e.g. tuberculosis or septic arthritis) and replaced hips.

- A popular technique is Cobra head plating. This uses a lateral approach with trochanteric osteotomy, preparation of joint surfaces, pelvic osteotomy and fixation with the Cobra head part of the plate fixed in the pelvis.[2]
- Avoid fusion in abduction, as it creates a pelvic obliquity and can exacerbate back pain.
- Conversion to THA is possible but only in the presence of abductor function. The abductor complex may have been stripped or superior gluteal nerve damaged during the initial surgical approach. In addition, no hip movement for years would result in wasting of any remaining abductor muscle.
- Inadequate abductor function leads to a Trendelenburg gait and an increased risk of dislocation. Preoperative abductor integrity should be assessed by electromyography (EMG).[3]
- The surgical approach during conversion to THA may require a trochanteric osteotomy and/or adductor tenotomy. A constrained acetabular component should be considered. Ipsilateral knee pain and back pain resolve in roughly 50% of patients after THA. Complications including failure, loosening, dislocation and sciatic nerve palsy occur in around 20% of patients.

Knee

Knee Parameniscal Cyst

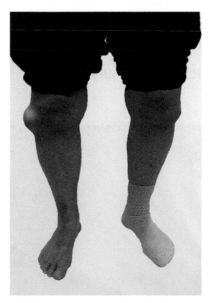

Figure 17.2a There is a large 5 x 8 cm swelling at the level of the knee joint on the lateral side. This is a lateral parameniscal cyst.

Examine the knee to determine whether there is a degenerate meniscal tear. Joint line tenderness and the presence of the swelling along the joint line are important in confirming the diagnosis. In general, medial meniscal cysts are more common that lateral meniscal cysts.

The differential diagnosis of a soft tissue swelling in this location could include neoplasm (e.g. lipoma, sarcoma, liposarcoma, synovial haemangioma), bursitis (e.g. lateral collateral ligament (LCL), iliotibial), nerve sheath ganglion cyst (e.g. common peroneal) and abscess.

In this case, due to the location of the cyst on the lateral side, it will be important to assess the common peroneal nerve.

Key Points

- Parameniscal cysts arise at the joint line or posteromedially in the form of a Baker's cyst (between semimembranosus and the medial head of gastrocnemius).
- They are caused by a meniscal tear (usually horizontal or complex), resulting in synovial fluid extruding out through the meniscus via a one-way valve mechanism. Vertical or radial tears result in perimeniscal cysts (within the meniscus).
- If symptomatic, arthroscopic meniscal debridement with marsupialisation of the tract can be performed. This could be combined with cyst excision (open excision if large). A trial of aspiration and injection of steroid may be considered before surgery.[4]

Posterior Sag Secondary to Posterior Cruciate Ligament (PCL) Injury

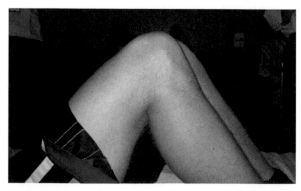

Figure 17.2b A posterior sag can be seen on the right knee. The presence of this sag can be emphasised by placing the pen on the tibial tubercle.

If a posterior sag is identified, the posterior draw test will be positive. A positive quadriceps active test will confirm the sag. In all patients in whom a PCL injury is suspected, a dial test should be performed because of the association with injury to the posterolateral corner.

Remember also to assess the common peroneal nerve and the distal vascular status, as the high-energy injuries that result in a PCL injury can be associated with neurovascular damage.[5]

Key Points

- When looking for a posterior sag, be aware that some patients may have an abnormally prominent tibial tubercle on the contralateral side; therefore, it may give a false positive posterior sag. This could be a result of previous Osgood–Schlatter disease or previous tibial tubercle osteotomy.
- Initial treatment for isolated PCL injury consists of PCL bracing for 6–12 weeks with range of movement exercises and quadriceps strengthening.
- Surgical reconstruction (commonly using allograft) is indicated in multi-ligament injuries or isolated injuries with persistent functional instability.
- Chronic PCL insufficiency is associated with medial and patellofemoral compartment chondropathy as a result of increased contact pressures in those compartments in flexion due to posterior subluxation of the tibia.[6]

Varus Knee Osteoarthritis

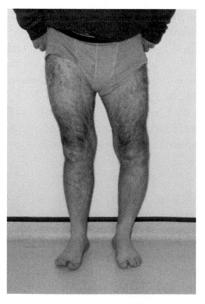

Figure 17.2c This 50-year-old patient has left medial compartment knee arthritis leading to a varus deformity of the knee.

The patient in Figure 17.2c has pelvic obliquity due to apparent shortening of the leg. When walking, the patient is likely to have a varus thrust/lurch. On further examination, it is important to exclude hip pathology and to quantify the range of movement, correctability of the deformity and integrity of the collateral and cruciate ligaments as these examination findings are important in planning further treatment.[7]

Key Points

- Important points in the history necessary for planning treatment include occupation and expectations from treatment.
- In all arthritic knees the range of movement of the knee should be assessed especially looking for a fixed flexion deformity which can be corrected during total knee replacement (TKR) surgery.
- The examination findings should enable the examiner to choose the most appropriate option for a young patient with unicompartmental osteoarthritis: non-operative with possible injections and/or off-loading braces, osteotomy surgery, medial unicompartmental knee arthroplasty (UKA) and total knee arthroplasty (TKA).[8]
- Mechanical axis radiographs are essential in planning surgical treatment.
- Osteotomy surgery (usually medial opening wedge high tibial osteotomy) is suitable for patients with primary tibia vara, a mechanical axis passing through the medial compartment, and isolated medial osteoarthritis (OA).[9]
- Medial UKA is most suitable for isolated anteromedial OA with an intact anterior cruciate ligament.
- TKA is suitable for bi/tri-compartmental OA and/or ligament insufficiency.
- Correctability of the varus deformity is important to identify. Non-correctable deformities may require significant medial release, which may not be suitable for medial UKA and therefore require TKA or osteotomy.
- Significant varus thrust may indicate LCL laxity/insufficiency, which may require a constrained TKA.

Valgus Arthritic Knee

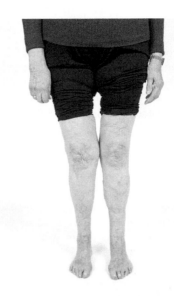

Figure 17.2d This patient has a valgus deformity of both legs, giving a classic 'knock kneed' appearance, due, in this patient, to osteoarthritis of the knees affecting mainly the lateral compartments.

Remember to look for signs of rheumatoid arthritis, as a valgus knee is more common in a patient with rheumatoid disease than with osteoarthritis. This is important because the surgical options for treating knee arthritis are influenced by rheumatoid disease.

During examination of gait, there may be a valgus thrust. It is therefore important to assess the integrity of the medial collateral ligament to see if valgus thrust is due to the lateral compartment wear or laxity of the medial collateral ligament (MCL).

Key Points

- Lateral femoral and tibial deficiencies, contracted lateral soft tissue structures, attenuated medial soft tissue structures and multiplanar deformities may all be present to some degree in the valgus arthritic knee.

- Other causes of a valgus knee must be considered, in addition to the more common causes of primary osteoarthritis and rheumatoid disease. These include rickets and renal osteodystrophy. If a scar is seen, then consider previous open lateral meniscectomy, previous trauma with malunion (e.g. lateral tibial plateau fracture) or an over-corrected high tibial osteotomy.

- Surgical options for lateral compartment arthritis consist of:

  o Osteotomy surgery: Usually a medial closing wedge distal femoral osteotomy is suitable to increase the distal femur varus and shift the mechanical axis to the medial compartment. Osteotomy is only suitable in unicompartmental arthritis. It may be preferred in younger, active patients who wish to continue active work or sports. Ten-year survival rates of 80–90% have been reported.[10]

  o Lateral UKA: Fixed bearing UKAs may be used in patients with isolated lateral compartment arthritis. Due to the potential for bearing spin-out and failure, mobile bearings are not used. Unicompartmental knee replacements are not recommended for those patients with a significant valgus deformity and medial collateral ligament laxity due to instability post-op.[11]

  o Total knee arthroplasty: TKAs potentially allow full correction of the valgus deformity and any fixed flexion using bony and soft tissue procedures. Ligament laxity can be compensated for by the use of constrained implants.
  TKA will be the surgical option of choice in the rheumatoid patient. In these patients a posterior stabilised implant is preferred as the PCL is usually deficient.

- Correction of severe valgus and fixed flexion deformities during TKR can tension the common peroneal nerve (CPN). It is therefore important to examine this nerve in the immediate post-operative period. If CPN palsy occurs, remove bandages and flex the knee as an emergency treatment. Consider CPN decompression if symptoms persist.

Knee Arthrodesis

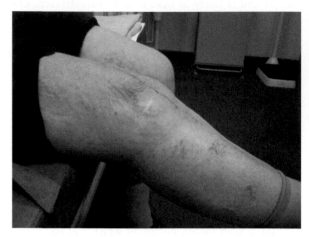

Figure 17.2e This patient, when asked to sit on the edge of the couch, assumes the position shown in the photograph. They have a fused right knee and are therefore unable to bend it.

Assess the patient for the standard position of fusion, which should be 5°–7° of valgus, 15° flexion and slight external rotation matching the contralateral side. A slightly shortened limb allows easier clearance during the swing stage of gait and as such, on walking, the patient will exhibit no knee movement and a short-leg gait.[12]

When examining a patient with an arthrodesed knee, it is important to examine the adjacent joints as there will be a 'knock on' effect on these joints, particularly the lumbar spine, ipsilateral hip and contralateral knee. Pain in these joints is usually the most common presentation of a patient with previous knee arthrodesis.

As there is likely to be a leg length discrepancy in trying to achieve the fusion, leg length should be measured in segments or on blocks with the patient standing.

Key Points
- Indications for knee arthrodesis include failed TKA (infection, bone loss, loss of extensor mechanism), septic arthritis, osteomyelitis, fracture fixation with subsequent infection, neuropathic joint and post-tumour resection. Contraindications include active infection.

- Fusion can be achieved using external fixation, plate or intramedullary fixation.
- Note that if previous treatment resulted in shortening of the leg, it will be better to perform the arthrodesis in full extension rather than in slight flexion.
- Non-union is the most common complication. Therefore, instability at the arthrodesis site must be looked for on assessing these patients.
- Conversion to TKA is possible to improve the patients function. Sufficient soft tissue quality/coverage and an intact extensor mechanism are prerequisites before proceeding. Patients should be made aware of the high complication rate including infection, persisting stiffness, limited flexion, amputation and pain, especially if they currently have a painless arthrodesis. Constrained implants are likely to be necessary due to the significant soft tissue releases required. Tibial tubercle osteotomy may be required to gain access to the knee in addition to a VY quadricepsplasty to improve flexion.[13]

Post-patellectomy

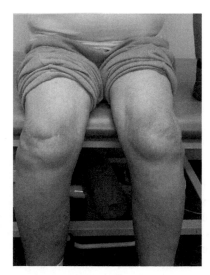

Figure 17.2f This 76-year-old patient presents with right knee pain. Inspection shows a well-healed transverse scar following a patellectomy 30 years ago. He has now developed arthritis of his knee.

Following patellectomy, the altered magnitude and direction of forces on the knee can lead to increased stresses on the knee and consequently degenerative changes. Other causes of degenerative changes include loss of the protection of the trochlea by the patella and the physical abrasion of the trochlea surface by the repaired tendon.

Instability may occur, as in patellectomy patients the extensor mechanism does not restrain the femur from anterior translation in the same manner as it does in patients with an intact patella. Also, the repair results in a change in alignment of the quadriceps and patella tendons and may aggravate anteroposterior instability if the cruciate mechanism is already damaged or absent.

As such, patients can present with pain, swelling, stiffness, instability and, characteristically, difficulty ascending and descending stairs.

On examination, palpation would confirm absence of the patella with thickening of the repaired tendon. There is up to 60% weakness of quadriceps function after patellectomy.[14]

Flexion and extension of the knee may reveal a laterally subluxing tendinous repair. There is a reduced range of movement with decreased flexion, which is especially noticeable in the stance phase of gait.[15] The patient usually has an extensor lag where active straight leg raising will show a deficit which can be passively corrected.

Key Points

- In modern-day knee surgery, it is very rare to perform a transverse incision over the knee. When this is seen, it is usually due to surgery performed a long time ago in which the main indications were patella fracture fixation and patellectomy. Patella tendon repairs were also performed through a transverse incision, but these were located lower than those for patella surgery.
- Previous indications for patellectomy include patella fracture, patellofemoral arthritis, patella instability, infection and anterior knee pain (usually chondromalacia patellae).
- Patellectomy is rarely performed now. Current indications include very comminuted fractures, osteomyelitis and tumour.
- The most common reasons for patients to present post-patellectomy are symptoms related to arthritis, instability and a subluxing repaired extensor mechanism.

- Patellectomy is one of the indications for a posterior stabilised TKA. Due to the mechanical disadvantage of the previous patellectomy, it is suggested that a prosthesis with more constraint be used, such as a posterior stabilised implant.[16]
- TKA following patellectomy demonstrates slightly worse results and a higher complication rate, including knee flexion which is reduced.[17]

Rotational Abnormalities

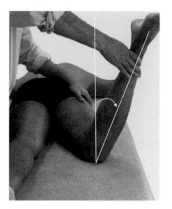

Figure 17.2g(ii) Femoral anteversion, Gage test. On rotating the hip with the knee flexed to 90°, palpate for the point at which the trochanter becomes most prominent. The angle of femoral anteversion is between the axis of the tibia and the vertical axis.

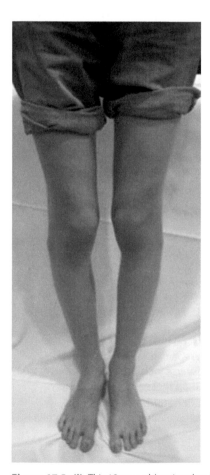

Figure 17.2g(i) This 19-year-old patient has inward-facing ('squinting') patellae with their feet pointing in a neutral position. This is a case of miserable malalignment syndrome.

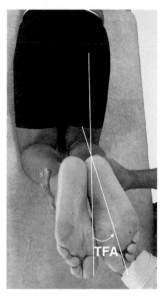

Figure 17.2g(iii) Thigh–foot angle (TFA). This is the angular difference between the axis of the thigh and the axis of the foot.

patella is a result of increased femoral anteversion combined with external tibial torsion, which explains why the feet point in a neutral position. In these patients, the axis of flexion of the knee is not in the line of progression.

Further examination should consist of a gait assessment commenting on patella and foot progression angles and a rotational profile examination. In the prone position, the hips should be assessed for excessive femoral anteversion (Figure 17.2g(ii)) and tibiae assessed to confirm external tibial torsion.

Patients with miserable malalignment syndrome can present as a young adult, and not necessarily in childhood, with anterior knee pain. Malalignment of the

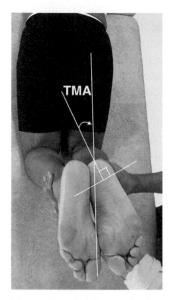

Figure 17.2g(iv) Transmalleolar angle (TMA). This is the angular difference between the transmalleolar axis and the axis of the thigh.

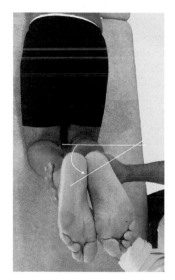

Figure 17.2g(v) Another method of measuring the TMA is the angle between the transmalleolar axis and the bicondylar axis of the tibia.

Figure 17.2g(iii,iv,v) demonstrates various ways of assessing tibial torsion. The TFA assesses the tibial and hindfoot rotational status combined. The TMA assesses the tibial rotation alone. The difference between the two (TFA and TMA) is therefore a measure of hindfoot rotation.

Key Points

- Metatarsus adductus may be present in some patients with miserable malalignment. When assessing for this in the prone position, it is important to allow the foot to fall into its natural position and not to manually position it, as this will lead to inaccuracy in assessment.
- Frequently, this condition is associated with increased joint laxity, further compounding the problem.
- The vast majority of patients do not require surgical intervention. Surgery should be performed to address functional limitations rather than to treat calculated angles.
- Operative management consists of derotational osteotomies of the femur (intertrochanteric, subtrochanteric, supracondylar) or tibia (proximal or supramalleolar) with plate/nail fixation. Usually, if surgery is undertaken for miserable malalignment, it is four-level. Most commonly, in the femur the osteotomy is intertrochanteric and in the tibia it is supramalleolar.[18]

Foot and Ankle

Hallux Valgus

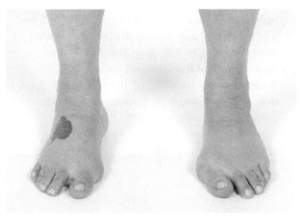

Figure 17.3a This patient has bilateral hallux valgus deformities, with the left side affected more significantly. Each hallux is laterally deviated and pronated.

These patients should always be examined weightbearing, as the hallux valgus deformity, as well as lesser toe deformities, are more evident on weightbearing.

Hallux valgus is a complex deformity that results in transfer of forces to the lateral aspect of the foot, thereby causing callosities, sesamoid tenderness and other lesser toe deformities. A callosity beneath the second metatarsal head is an indirect sign of first ray instability.

When examining the patient there are specific findings that will influence surgical decisions and these mut be particularly inspected for:

- On testing passive movement of the first metatarsophalangeal joint (MTPJ), manually correct the hallux valgus deformity and assess the range of movement, as this can be predictive of the movement that will be obtained following surgical correction.
- Reduced and painful range of movement or a positive grind test may influence arthrodesis. Fusion is further advised with gout, cerebral palsy, rheumatoid arthritis and generalised joint laxity.
- Movement of the hallux interphalangeal joint and progression of arthritis in this joint can be adversely affected by fusing the MTP joint.
- Mobility at the first tarsometatarsal (TMT) joint would suggest a Lapidus procedure (first TMT joint arthrodesis with additional soft tissue corrective procedure such as adductor hallucis release from the proximal phalanx, lateral capsule release and medial capsule imbrication) should be performed. The first TMT joint is key to supporting the medial arch. Instability will give rise to flat foot, transfer metatarsalgia and hallux valgus. Assessing the stability of the first TMT joint is not easy and must be compared with the contralateral side and with the lesser

metatarsals of the ipsilateral side. Stability in the plantar and dorsal directions is assessed, but the important finding is elevation of the first metatarsal above the second.

- The neurovascular status must be evaluated, as surgery is contraindicated in the presence of poor vascular supply. The dorsomedial cutaneous nerve must be tested for. Up to 44% of patients can have decreased sensation in its distribution as a result of the bunion. This is also a nerve that is frequently damaged with surgery; therefore, its pre-operative status should be documented.[19]

> **Key Points**
>
> - When examining a patient with hallux valgus look for any identifiable risk factors such as:
>   - **General:** rheumatoid arthritis; cerebral palsy; generalised joint laxity.
>   - **Intrinsic:** first TMT joint instability; second toe deformity or amputation; pes planus.
>   - **Extrinsic:** shoe-wear: those with narrow shoe box.
> - In general, with mild hallux valgus (hallux valgus angle, HVA, <25°) a distal osteotomy can be performed (e.g. Chevron osteotomy). With moderate disease (HVA 26°–40°), perform a proximal osteotomy +/– distal (e.g. scarf and Akin). For severe hallux valgus (HVA 41°–50°), a double osteotomy is performed.[20]

Rheumatoid Feet

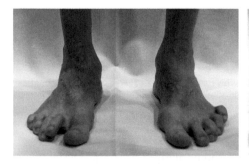
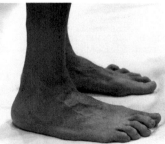

Figure 17.3b(i,ii) This patient has rheumatoid arthritis with visible deformities to the feet. On both sides, multiple toes are extended at the MTP joints and flexed at the proximal interphalangeal (PIP) joints and DIP joints, consistent with claw toe deformities. The right second/third toe deformity is known as a crossover toe. On the soles of the feet, there are likely to be callosities due to dislocations of the MTP joints. The right foot shows collapse of the midfoot.

Description of the rheumatoid foot should follow a sequence based on knowledge of the likely deformities, as described below.

The forefoot is a common source of patient symptoms and signs. Hallux valgus deformity is common. MTP joint synovitis leads to plantar plate and collateral ligament destruction and dorsomedial subluxation of the toe in relation to the metatarsal. Due to this subluxation, the interosseous muscles become ineffective extensors with a subsequent flexor overload. This leads to a flexible claw toe deformity that can progress to a rigid deformity. Hyperextension of the lesser toes pulls the fat pads from under the metatarsal heads into a location distal to it. Hence, the metatarsal heads become exposed, leading to pain ('walking on marbles') and callosity formation.[21]

Although the majority of patients will have radiographic evidence of midfoot involvement, with midfoot collapse, symptomatic arthritis is uncommon.

The hindfoot should be inspected from behind to assess for the presence of rheumatoid nodules. Swellings consistent with tenosynovitis affecting the posterior tibial tendon or peroneal tendons may be seen. The hindfoot may be in valgus and there may be a 'too many toes' sign due to talonavicular uncovering from forefoot abduction (planovalgus foot). Patients may be unable to heel raise.

Key Points

- The vast majority of patients with rheumatoid arthritis have foot and ankle pathology. However, the entire patient should be examined as cervical spine and upper limb severity correlates with the foot and ankle severity. Involvement of the upper limb may affect compliance of weightbearing instructions following foot and ankle surgery.
- Treatment for foot deformities should focus on which symptoms predominate. Options include orthoses and surgery. Orthotics may be functional, where flexible deformities are corrected, or accommodative, where rigid deformities are cushioned and supported.
- Hallux valgus deformities may be treated with fusion of the first MTP joint. Hammer and claw toes can be treated with PIP joint/distal interphalangeal (DIP) joint fusions. Lesser metatarsal issues may be treated with surgical resection of the metatarsal heads. Talonavicular, subtalar and ankle fusion procedures may be used to correct deformity and reduce pain.

Adult Flat Foot

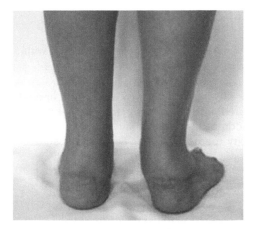

Figure 17.3c This patient's right hindfoot lies in a valgus position. The medial arch is flat, resulting in a planovalgus deformity.

In this clinical case the 'too many toes' sign is positive, resulting in almost all toes being visible. The tiptoe test will help determine if the hindfoot valgus is fixed or flexible. Test also for the strength of the tibialis posterior muscle.

Close inspection will reveal a transverse incision bilaterally. This is a Cincinnati incision and approach that is predominantly used in the child and especially for clubfoot surgery, as they allow for a circumferential soft tissue release of the subtalar joint in a single sitting.

In this patient, it will be important to also assess for Achilles contracture. The subtalar joint must first be reduced to a neutral starting position and ankle dorsiflexion assessed with the knee extended and then flexed (Silfverskiöld's test).

Key aspects in examining an adult patient with a flat foot:

1. Stand the patient and inspect from behind, looking at the calves, looking at the heels for alignment and looking for forefoot abduction with 'too many toes' when observed from the back.
2. Perform single heel rise test. The inability to perform up to 10 heel rises may indicate tibialis posterior tendon weakness.
3. Palpate along the course of the tibialis posterior tendon for tenosynovitis.

4. Examine the gastrocsoleus complex for tightness.
5. Evaluate subtalar mobility.
6. Test the tibialis posterior muscle.

Key Points

- Remember to do a Beighton score, especially with a flexible flat foot.
- Tarsal coalitions (calcaneonavicular or talocalcaneal) usually present in children and is associated with a non-correctable deformity, stiff hindfoot movements and peroneal spasticity (peroneal spastic flat foot). Less commonly, they present in adulthood. The differential diagnosis of a rigid flat foot in an adult is therefore tarsal coalition, muscle spasm or advanced arthritis.
- Tibialis posterior dysfunction occurs in older patients and is commonly classified using the Johnson and Strom criteria as modified by Myerson (Table 17.1).[22]

Table 17.1 Tibialis posterior dysfunction[22]

Stage	Characteristics
1	Tenosynovitis, medial pain/swelling, no flat foot, able to heel raise
2	Rupture, flat foot, flexible hindfoot, abducted forefoot, cannot heel raise
3	Rupture, flat foot, rigid hindfoot, rigid abducted forefoot, cannot heel raise
4	Rupture, flat foot, rigid hindfoot, rigid abducted forefoot, cannot heel raise, deltoid ligament compromise (talar tilt)

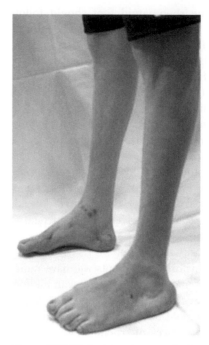

Figure 17.3d(i) Both legs have small calves and large, posterior longitudinal surgical scars and deformities affecting the feet. The deformity is most pronounced on the right side with midfoot cavus and hindfoot varus. There are multiple scars around the heel.

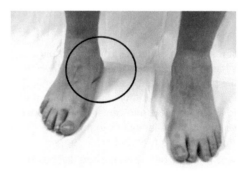

Figure 17.3d(ii) On inspection from the front, with pes cavus, the medial heel can be seen on the right foot. This is called the 'peek-a-boo' sign.

Adult Cavovarus Foot

The positive 'peek-a-boo' heel sign means that the heel is in varus. It is not seen on the normal foot nor with pes planus. It is a useful sign in identifying the subtle cavovarus foot.[23]

Scars give an indication as to the previous surgery the patient may have had. In Figure 17.3d(i), the scar over the first ray may be due to a dorsiflexion osteotomy +/− Jones transfer of extensor hallucis longus (EHL) to the first metatarsal neck. The posterior scar is likely due to tendoachilles or gastrocnemius lengthening to address ankle equinus. The anteromedial scars may be due to a posterior tibial tendon transfer to the dorsum of the foot to aid with weakness of the tibialis anterior.

The bilateral nature of the deformity suggests a congenital condition such as Charcot–Marie–Tooth (CMT) Type 1. Check the hands for interossei wasting.

A Coleman block test should always be conducted when faced with a cavovarus foot.

Key aspects in examining an adult patient with pes cavus:

1. Stand the patient and look at the deformity, realising that if the medial heel is visible from the front this indicates that the heel is in varus. Inspect the plantar aspect for callosities, especially over the first and fifth metatarsal heads.
2. Perform the Coleman block test to determine whether the cavovarus foot is forefoot driven or hindfoot driven.
3. Assess ankle movements for gastrocnemius contracture.
4. Assess subtalar joint movement to test for rigidity.
5. Perform relevant neurological examination.

Key Points

- The cavus is caused by a plantarflexed first ray due to peroneus longus overpowering a weak tibialis anterior. The varus is caused by tibialis posterior overpowering a weak peroneus brevis.
- The effect of peroneus longus compared to tibialis anterior is greater when the ankle is in

---

equinus. Therefore, in assessing these patients it is important to check for gastrocnemius contracture by dorsiflexing the ankle with the knee extended then flexed (Silfverskiöld's test).

- The Coleman block test is designed to show if the hindfoot varus deformity is correctable when the forefoot deformity (plantarflexed first ray and forefoot pronation) is eliminated. In normal conditions, the plantarflexed first ray and forefoot pronation need to be counteracted by hindfoot varus to allow the foot to rest level on the floor. Having the first ray off the block during the test eliminates the need for compensatory hindfoot varus. If the hindfoot varus corrects, it suggests that the cavus is forefoot driven and correction of the forefoot deformity via surgery or orthoses is all that is required. If the hindfoot does not correct, forefoot procedures will need to be supplemented with hindfoot osteotomy to correct the deformity.

Miscellaneous

Poliomyelitis

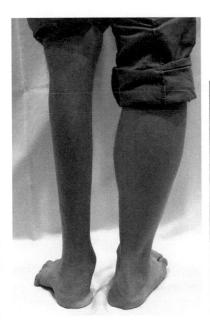
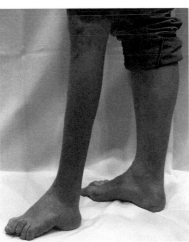

Figure 17.4a(i) This 65-year-old patient with a history of poliomyelitis in childhood has unilateral leg wasting with significant loss of calf musculature. Scars are present consistent with previous external fixation and foot and ankle procedures. The foot itself is small, and there is a cavus midfoot with claw toes. There will be callosities over the pressure points on the plantar aspect of the foot, including the heel pad and the metatarsal heads.

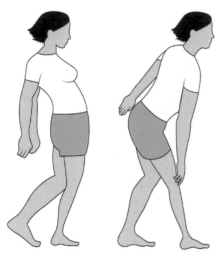

Figure 17.4a(ii) (*left*) Patient walking with a gluteus maximus lurch where the trunk is arched backwards to compensate for the weak gluteus maximus. (*right*) The 'hand–thigh gait' in a patient with quadriceps weakness. The hand is used to stabilise the knee in the stance phase.

Poliomyelitis is a viral disease that results in destruction of the anterior horn cells in the spinal cord and the motor nuclei in the brain stem, leading to muscle paralysis or weakness. These patients have lower motor neuron signs but with normal sensation.

Clinical examination findings will be manifested by the consequence of motor paralysis:

1. Muscle weakness.
2. Deformity. Unbalanced paralysis will lead to deformity at the joint; if this is prolonged, this deformity will be fixed.
3. Joint instability. Usually due to balanced paralysis.
4. Shortening of the limb. Due to lack of muscle activity stimulating bone growth. Shortening is also a result of joint contractures.
5. Vascular dysfunction. Cold, blue limbs.

The pattern of involved muscles varies between extremities and between patients, but characteristic features are seen as certain groups of muscles are affected more often. These are the ones that have their anterior horn cells in a small localised area of the spinal cord. As such, the deltoid, opponens pollicis, tibialis anterior and quadriceps muscles are commonly affected. Muscles such as the hamstrings are less affected because they have long columns of anterior horn cells at multiple levels.[24]

Because any muscle can be involved, all muscle groups must be tested for power and graded using Muscle Research Council (MRC) grading. It is important to differentiate grade 2 from grade 3 power. Usually, this will involve turning the patient on their side and eliminating the effect of gravity. The importance of assessing power in all muscle groups is that the examiner is able to identify the weak muscles and also to identify the grade 4/5 muscles that may be used for tendon transfer.

Gait can be affected by quadriceps involvement that results in weakness of knee extension. Deformities such as the equinus ankle (stepping on the floor will automatically force the knee into extension) or recurvatum of the knee can, to some degree, compensate for this quadriceps weakness. The patient will, however, adapt by walking with a hand placed just over the affected knee ('hand–thigh' or quadriceps gait), and leaning to the affected side to prevent collapse in the stance phase (Figure 17.4a(ii)).

The gait can also be influenced by the muscles around the hip. If the abductors are involved, the patient will have a Trendelenburg gait. If the hip extensors are involved, the patient will have a gluteus maximus lurch, where in stance phase, the trunk has to be bent backwards to prevent forward collapse of the trunk (Figure 17.4a(ii)).

Key Points

- The orthopaedic surgeon will mainly see these patients in the stage of residual paralysis. The lower limb is mainly affected. In the upper limb, the patient presents with difficulty of shoulder abduction, elbow flexion or extension and thumb opposition.

- In the spine, a scoliosis may occur. When examining these patients with scoliosis, it is important to assess the hip for an asymmetrical hip abduction contracture, which can result in a compensatory scoliosis.

- Hip deformities most commonly seen in polio are flexion, abduction and external rotation (often in combination). Adduction and internal rotation are less frequent. The flexion, abduction and external rotation can in part be caused by contracture of the iliotibial band. Ober's test is used to assess this.

- Hip adduction or abduction deformities will cause pelvic obliquity and a compensatory lumbar scoliosis. The pelvic obliquity can predispose to hip dislocation.[24]

- Foot and ankle equinovalgus and cavus deformity are the most common foot and ankle deformities. Because tibialis anterior is a dorsiflexor and invertor of the ankle, with paralysis, an equinovalgus deformity can develop. The equinus becomes worse because of contracture of triceps surae. Because of this, there is overactivity of the long toe extensors in an attempt to dorsiflex the ankle, resulting in toe hyperextension ('cock-up toes'). Overactivity of peroneus longus will result in a cavus deformity.

- Foot and ankle calcaneus and cavus deformity (Figure 17.4a(i)): The Achilles tendon can also be affected with weakness in function, leading to a calcaneus deformity with the hindfoot being dorsiflexed, resulting in weightbearing on the heel pad. If poliomyelitis was contracted in childhood, the foot would have developed in the absence of Achilles strength. As a result, the patient would also have plantarflexion of the forefoot, resulting in a high arch.

- The goal of treatment is to achieve a painless, plantigrade foot and maximise function of the lower limb. This may be achievable by orthoses and stretching in the early period. Surgery is indicated for correcting deformity, improving stability, addressing muscle imbalance and limb lengthening.

- Post-polio syndrome: In the years following polio infection, patients may develop slowly progressive muscle weakness in the muscles already involved. This is especially evident in the quadriceps and calf muscle,s but can occur in any muscle.

Key Points

- Plexiform neurofibromas are usually present from birth and present in 30–50% of patients with neurofibromatosis. They are benign tumours of the nerve sheath surrounded by fibrous tissue.
- Treatment consists of monitoring for malignant change. Malignant transformation can occur in 2–3%.
- Surgical excision is often unsuccessful due to difficult resection and incomplete clearance. Biologic therapies can be used for symptomatic lesions.
- The differential diagnosis of a soft tissue swelling in this region could be a lipoma, haematoma or even a quadriceps rupture. Straight leg raising should be a part of the clinical examination to rule out rupture and to see if this lump is fixed to the deeper structures.
- In general, red flag signs in a patient presenting with a soft tissue mass consist of size >5 cm (bigger than a golf ball), increasing in size, deep to the fascia and painful. In addition, look for a surgical scar to see if this a recurrent lesion.[25]

Soft Tissue Swelling

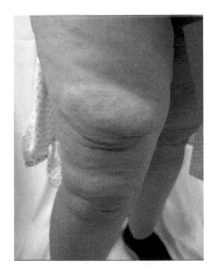

Figure 17.4b This patient has a large, diffuse skin-coloured swelling in the mid-thigh, which is rubbery but non-tender to palpation. This is a plexiform neurofibroma, which is pathognomonic of neurofibromatosis.

Further inspection of the above patient will reveal café-au-lait spots and potentially other features of neurofibromatosis. These plexiform neurofibromas are commonly cutaneous/subcutaneous and can affect the head, neck or limbs.

Trauma

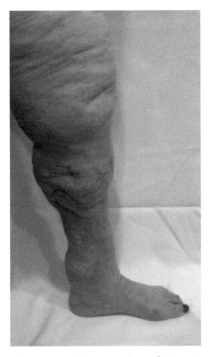

Figure 17.4c This patient has soft tissue signs in the lower half of their leg. There is a loss of calf muscle definition and a clear demarcation where a skin graft has been placed.

313

Proximally, pinhole scars are visible, indicating that this was secondary to trauma and external fixation of an open fracture. In any patient following lower limb trauma, leg alignment and leg length must be assessed.

The examination should proceed to assess the function of the ankle and, in particular, the power of plantarflexion of the ankle. Dorisflexion may also be restricted due to scarring.

As this patient may have had a skin graft and possibly a flap, the donor sites should also be examined. Assess the sensation over the graft and assess the distal neurovascular status as nerves, blood vessels and lymphatics may have been damaged.

Key Points

- The reconstructive ladder consists of direct closure, skin grafts, local and regional flaps, distant pedicle flaps and finally free flaps (microsurgical free-tissue transfer).
- Free flaps can be cutaneous, fasciocutaneous, musculocutaneous, or osteocutaneous.
- Flaps are used when skin grafts are not suitable (e.g. exposed joint, tendon, bone, implants).
- Free flaps are used for coverage in the distal third of the tibia. Latissimus dorsi, rectus abdominis and gracilis can be used for large defects, whereas the radial forearm can be used for smaller defects. Proximal tibial defects can be treated using medial or lateral gastrocnemius flaps. Soleus flaps can be used for the middle third.[26]

References

1. Thambyah A, Hee HT, Das De S, Lee SM. Gait adaptation in patients with longstanding hip fusion. *J Orthop Surg* 2003;**11**(2):154–158.

2. Beaule PE, Matta JM, Mast JW. Hip arthrodesis: current indications and techniques. *J Am Acad Orthop Surg* 2002;**10**(4):249–258. doi: 10.5435/00124635-200207000-00003.

3. Jain S, Giannoudis PV. Arthrodesis of the hip and conversion to total hip arthroplasty. *J Arthroplasty* 2013;**28**(9):1596–1602. doi: 10.1016/j. arth.2013.01.025.

4. Abram SGF, Beard DJ, Price AJ, BASK Meniscal Working Group. Arthroscopic meniscal surgery a national society treatment guideline and consensus statement. *Bone Joint J* 2019 Jun;**101-B** (6):652–659.

5. Caldas M, Braga G, Mendes S, Martins da Silveira J, Kopke R. Posterior cruciate ligament injury: characteristics and associations of most frequent injuries. *Rev Bras Ortop* 2013 Oct 22;**48**(5):427–431. doi: 10.1016/j.rboe.2012.09.010.

6. Skyhar MJ, Warren RF, Ortiz GJ, Schwartz E, Otis JC. The effects of sectioning of the posterior cruciate ligament and the posterolateral complex on the articular contact pressures within the knee. *J Bone Joint Surg Am* 1993 May;**75**(5):694–699. doi: 10.2106/00004623-199305000-00008.

7. Lobenhoffer P. Indication for unicompartmental knee replacement versus osteotomy around the knee. *J Knee Surg* 2017 Oct;**30**(8):769–773. doi: 10.1055/s-0037- 1605558. Epub 2017 Aug 25.

8. Wilson HA, Middleton R, Abram SGF, et al. Patient relevant outcomes of unicompartmental versus total knee replacement: systematic review and meta-analysis. *BMJ* 2019 Feb 21;**364**:l352. doi: 10.1136/bmj.l352.

9. Lobenhoffer P, Agneskirchner JD. Osteotomy around the knee vs. unicondylar knee replacement. *Orthopade* 2014 Oct;**43**(10):923–929. doi: 10.1007/s00132-014-3011-x.

10. Shivji FS, Foster A, Risebury MJ, Wilson AJ, Yasen SK. Ten-year survival rate of 89% after distal femoral osteotomy surgery for lateral compartment osteoarthritis of the knee. *Knee Surg Sports Traumatol Arthrosc* 2020;**29**(2):594–599. doi: 10.1007/s00167-020-05988-5.

11. Pandit H, Jenkins C, Beard DJ, et al. Mobile bearing dislocation in lateral unicompartmental knee replacement. *Knee* 2010; **17**(6):392–397.

12. MacDonald JH, Agarwal S, Lorei MP, Johanson NA, Freiberg AA. Knee arthrodesis. *J Am Acad Orthop Surg* 2006;**14**(3):154–163.

13. Kernkamp WA, Verra WC, Pijls BG, et al. Conversion from knee arthrodesis to arthroplasty: systematic review. *Int Orthop* 2016 Oct;**40**(10):2069–2074. doi: 10.1007/s00264-016-3150-2.

14. Lennox IA, Cobb AG, Knowles J, Bentley G. Knee function after patellectomy. A 12 to 48 year follow up. *J Bone Joint Surg Br* 1994 May;**76** (3):485–487.

15. Sutton FS Jr, Thompson CH, Lipke J, Kettlekemp DB. The effect of patellectomy on knee function. *J Bone Joint Surg Am* 1976 June;**58**(4):537–540.

16. Dodds A, Crowley R, Menz T, et al. Outcome following total knee replacement in patients with previous patellectomy. *Acta Orthop Belg* 2018;**84**:251–256.

17. Asadollah S, Sorial R, Coffey S, et al. Total knee arthroplasty after patellectomy. A meta-analysis of case-control studies. *Knee* 2017 March;**24**(2):191–196.

18. Nelitz M. Femoral derotational osteotomies. *Curr Rev Musculoskelet Med* 2018 Jun;**11**(2):272–279.

19. Herron ML, Kar S, Beard D, et al. Sensory dysfunction of the great toe in hallux valgus. *J Bone Joint Surg* 2004;**86**:54–57.

20. Fraissler L, Konrads C, Hoberg M, Rudert M, Walcher M. Treatment of hallux valgus deformity. *EFFORT Open Rev* 2016 Aug;**1**(8):295–302. doi: 10.1302/2058-5241.1.000005.

21. Brooks F, Hariharan K. The rheumatoid forefoot. *Curr Rev Musculoskelet Med* 2013 Dec; **6**(4):320–327. doi: 10.1007/s12178-013-9178-7.

22. Myerson MS. Adult acquired flatfoot deformity: treatment of dysfunction of the posterior tibial tendon. *Instr Course Lect* 1997;**46**:393–405.

23. Beals TC, Manoli A. The 'peek-a-boo' heel sign in the evaluation of hindfoot varus. *Foot* 1996;**6**:205–206.

24. Joseph B, Watts H. Polio revisited: reviving knowledge and skills to meet the challenge of resurgence. *J Child Orthop* 2015 Oct;**9**(5):325–338. doi: 10.1007/s11832-015-0678-4.

25. Nandra R, Forsberg J, Grimer R. If your lump is bigger than a golf ball and growing, think sarcoma. *Eur J Surg Oncol* 2015 Oct;**41**(10):1400–1405. doi: 10.1016/j.ejso.2015.05.017.

26. Steiert A, Gohritz A, Knobloch K, Krettek C, Vogt P. Damage control flap reconstruction. *Plast Reconstr Surg* 2009;**124**(3):1010–1011.

Chapter 18

Orthopaedic Cases in the Developing World

Charlene Chin See, Shashikanth Vokkaleri, Ravikumar Shankarlingegowda and Stanley Jones

Introduction

There are many similarities in orthopaedic pathology seen in developing countries compared to the more developed ones. This chapter will, however, show some examples of how presentation in orthopaedic clinics can differ throughout the world. These differences may be a reflection of geographical or environmental causes as well as economic or social factors. Consequently, we have subdivided this chapter into sections that may reflect these differences.

As a result of genetic transmission, certain congenital problems can be identified more commonly in some regions compared to others. Because of economic and environmental reasons, the presentation

and subsequent treatment of some conditions may be delayed or neglected. The volume of trauma cases may lead to associated fractures being commonly managed non-surgically. This can result in long-term sequelae in some cases.

The population now moves freely around the world. Hence, these conditions are no longer restricted to the developing world and therefore it is not uncommon for patients to present to orthopaedic clinics (and examinations) in the developed world with these clinical features.

Conditions That Present in Childhood

Blount's Disease

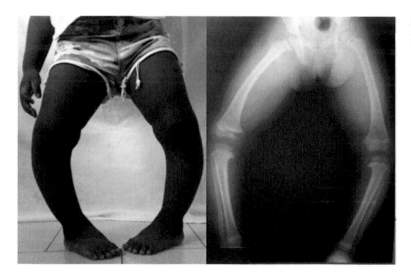

Figure 18.1a(i) Early onset Blount's disease in a 2-year-old with medial tibial metaphyseal beaking on radiographs.

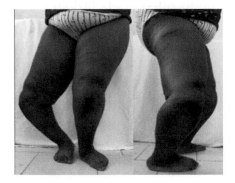

Figure 18.1a(ii) A 12-year-old with late onset Blount's disease.

In Blount's disease, abnormal endochondral ossification at the posteromedial portion of the proximal tibial physis leads to tibia vara, internal tibial torsion and procurvatum deformities. A lateral thrust is typically present on ambulation. This disease is more common in Hispanic and black populations and is bilateral (but not usually symmetrical) in 50%.[1,2]

A strong association has been identified between obesity and Blount's disease at any age. Recently, vitamin D deficiency has also been identified as a possible risk factor. Ask the parent at which age the child commenced walking (associated with early walking) and if there is a family history (familial predisposition).

Key Points

- Early onset or infantile disease (up to 4 years) can be distinguished from physiological varus by its progressive nature, asymmetry and radiographic changes. The metaphyseal–diaphyseal angle of Drennan ≥11° also predicts Blount's disease. Langenskiöld described six radiographic stages of progression, ranging from irregular tibial medial metaphyseal beaking to medial physeal bony bar formation.
- Late onset disease encompasses juvenile (4 to 10 years) and adolescent (>10 years) subgroups. Radiographic changes include widening of the proximal medial tibial physis and associated distal femoral varus deformity in approximately 30% of patients.[3]
- Management includes bracing (knee-ankle-foot orthosis) in the early stages of early onset disease, guided growth and hemiepiphysiodesis (temporary and permanent), medial plateau elevation, acute or gradual correction via proximal tibial and fibular osteotomies and epiphysiolysis.[1,2,3]

Haemophilic Arthropathy

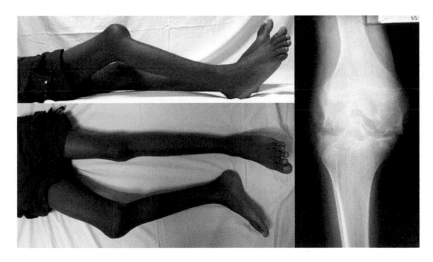

Figure 18.1b A 15-year-old with haemophilic arthropathy of both knees and hips with flexion contractures of the right hip and knee and limb length inequality. Plain radiograph of the right knee shows classic features of severe haemophilic arthropathy.

Haemophilia is an X-linked, autosomal recessive disorder. It results in diminished coagulation Factor VIII (haemophilia A) or Factor IX (haemophilia B or Christmas disease).

Patients present with pain and swelling of the affected joint. Peri-articular muscle atrophy ensues with recurrent haemarthrosis, leading to joint subluxation. The joints most affected are the knees, ankles and elbows. Contractures also occur at the affected joints due to recurrent inflammation.

Key Points

- Intra-articular haemarthrosis and subsequent haemosiderin deposition results in a cycle of synovial proliferation and hypertrophy, synovitis and cartilage destruction via iron deposition and up-regulation of inflammatory cytokines. There is often a rapid progression to degenerative joint disease if inappropriately managed.[4,5]
- Radiographic changes noted as the disease progresses are increased soft tissue space, juxta-articular osteopenia, epiphyseal widening and irregularity with erosions, cyst formation and sclerosis. Squaring of the femoral condyles occurs in affected knees.
- The current standard of care for haemophilic arthropathy includes prophylaxis and 'on-demand' treatment with appropriate factors, analgesia, physiotherapy, synovectomy (chemical, radionucleotide, arthroscopic or open) and arthroplasty.[4,5,6]
- Other clinical sequelae include intramuscular haematoma and pseudotumour formation. Compressive neuropathy and compartment syndrome are possible complications. Angular deformities and limb length discrepancy also occur.[6]

X-Linked Hypophosphataemic Rickets

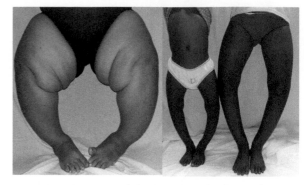

Figure 18.1c(i) X-linked hypophosphataemic rickets in an aunt and two nieces. They present with the more common genu varum.

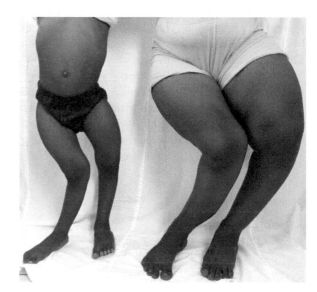

Figure 18.1c(ii) A mother and son also with X-linked hypophosphataemic rickets. They both have genu valgum on the right side in addition to left-sided genu varum, creating 'windswept' knees.

Children typically present with clinical features of coxa vara, genu vara (most common) or valgum. There is also internal tibial torsion and short stature. Windswept deformity of the knees is also common. Delayed ambulation may also be the reason for presentation. Costochondral junction enlargement ('rachitic rosary'), radioulnar joint enlargement and frontal bossing can occur.

Key Points

- X-Linked hypophosphataemic rickets (XLH) is a genetic disorder manifesting in childhood in which there is increased renal tubular phosphate wasting and decreased vitamin D production. There is impaired osteoid matrix mineralisation, leading to osteomalacia.
- Blood investigations will show low serum phosphate and vitamin D and elevated alkaline phosphatase. Increased urinary phosphate is also evident. Radiographs assist in the differentiation of rickets from other causes such as physiological genu varum, Blount's disease and skeletal dysplasias. The physes are widened and irregular, and adjacent metaphyseal deformities can be seen.
- Remember leg length discrepancy is to be assessed by measuring each limb in segments or by using blocks to stand on.
- Treatment with calcitriol and phosphate supplementation should commence immediately and continue until cessation of growth. Osteoclasis is only recommended after medical treatment is instituted for pain, gait abnormalities and progressive deformities.[7,8]

Sickle Cell Disease

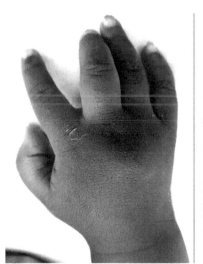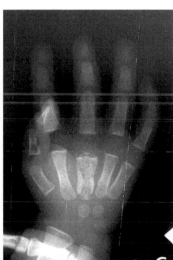

Figure 18.1d(i) Initial presentation of sickle cell disease (SCD) in a 9-month-old infant with swelling of the right hand. This is sickle cell dactylitis, affecting the middle metacarpal.

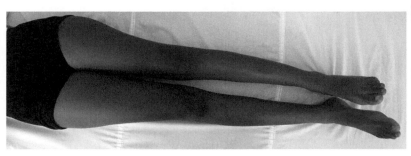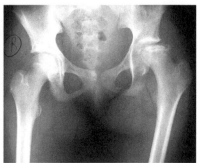

Figure 18.1d(ii) Osteonecrosis of the left hip due to SCD with subsequent limb length inequality in an 11-year-old.

Sickle cell disease (SCD) is an autosomal recessive disorder, most frequently occurring in children from 10 weeks to 6 years of age. Dactylitis is one of the first clinical features of SCD and is considered a prognostic indicator of the expected severity of SCD.[9,10]

The prevalence of osteonecrosis of the femoral head (ONFH) in SCD is low in children and gradually increases to 50% in adults greater than 35 years. The head of the humerus is also prone to osteonecrosis. Patients may be asymptomatic or present with pain (typically in the groin in ONFH) and decreased range of motion at the affected joint. Limb length discrepancy and joint contractures are chronic sequelae.[11]

Other orthopaedic manifestations of SCD in both children and adults include osteomyelitis (which must be differentiated from acute vaso-occlusive crises with bone infarction) and septic arthritis. Chronic leg ulceration can occur in the region of the malleoli and tend to appear 'punched out'.[10] Decreased bone mineral density leads to fractures (including vertebral collapse). Delayed skeletal maturation is also more frequent in patients with SCD.[12]

Key Points

- The cause of the osteonecrosis is hypothesised as vascular congestion with associated thrombosis and stasis. Intraosseous pressures increase secondary to medullary hyperplasia, leading to bone infarction.
- The natural history of osteonecrosis secondary to SCD is progression to osteoarthritis. No treatment has been proven to halt progression, as the underlying pathophysiology is not addressed. Treatment options aim to decrease pain and improve function and depend on the stage of osteonecrosis. These range from core decompression with or without the use of bone graft to arthroplasty. The latter is the accepted treatment of severe osteonecrosis.[11]
- Dactylitis is typically self-limiting, with improvement within 1 week. Superimposed osteomyelitis can occur and will delay resolution of symptoms.
- Dactylitis also occurs in spondyloarthropathies, psoriatic arthritis and other inflammatory arthritides.[9]

Osteogenesis Imperfecta

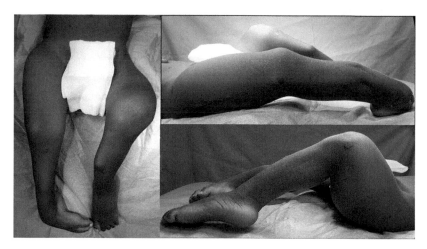

Figure 18.1e A 6-year-old with bilateral lower limb deformities secondary to osteogenesis imperfecta and multiple pathological fractures.

Clinical features of osteogenesis imperfecta include blue sclerae, dentinogenesis imperfecta, hearing impairment and pulmonary and cardiac abnormalities. Orthopaedic manifestations include short stature, bone fragility, bowing of long bones, scoliosis, basilar invagination and ligamentous laxity.

> **Key Points**
>
> - Osteogenesis Imperfecta (OI) is a genetic disorder of defective type 1 collagen synthesis and modification secondary to mutations in *COL1A1* and *COL1A2* genes.
> - Medical treatment is not curative. Bisphosphonates have proven efficacious in the reduction of fractures and deformities and in the improvement of height. Other emerging therapies include denosumab (RANK-L inhibitor), teriparatide (recombinant parathyroid hormone) and growth hormone.
> - Physical therapy and exercise are beneficial in improving bone mass and muscle function in mild cases. Intramedullary rodding is used to prevent fractures but can also be used for fracture treatment and deformity correction.[13]

Juvenile Idiopathic Arthritis (JIA)

Juvenile idiopathic arthritis (JIA) encompasses multiple inflammatory diseases in which arthritis (in at least one joint) occurs for greater than 6 weeks in children less than 16 years.

The majority of patients are rheumatoid factor negative. Systemic forms will have one or more joints affected, fever and one or more of the following: an associated rash, generalised lymphadenopathy, hepatosplenomegaly or serositis. JIA is further classified based on the number of joints affected (oligoarticular, polyarticular).

> **Key Points**
>
> - The management is multidisciplinary and incorporates the use of NSAIDs, disease-modifying antirheumatic drugs and biologic agents. Physical and occupational therapy may also be beneficial.
> - Surgical interventions aim to decrease pain (with synovectomy), correct deformities and definitively treat severe arthritis.[14]

Neurofibromatosis

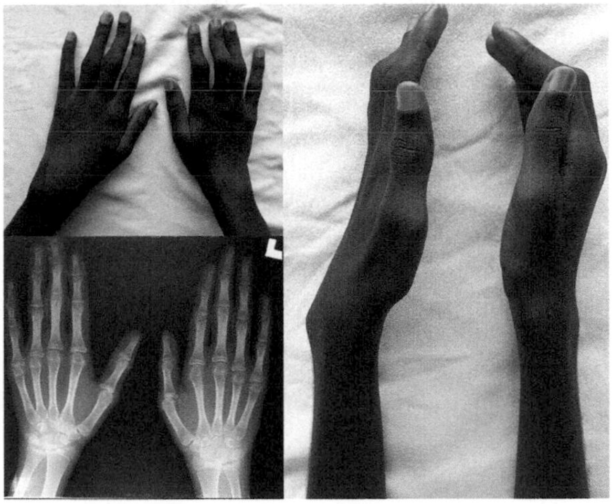

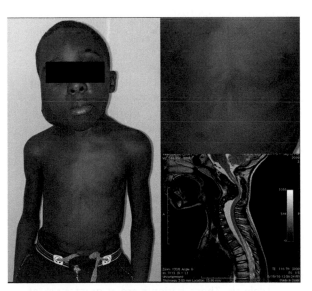

Figure 18.1f A 12-year-old with juvenile idiopathic arthritis with wrist deformities due to collapse of both proximal carpal rows and Boutonniere deformity of second to fourth digits bilaterally. Radiographs also show generalised osteopenia.

Figure 18.1g A 10-year-old with neurofibromatosis type 1 and traumatic central cord syndrome secondary to a fall. Cervical kyphoscoliosis and a large right cervical plexiform neurofibroma with spinal cord compression were noted. Café-au-lait patches and smaller neurofibromata were identified on the trunk.

Three well defined forms of neurofibromatosis exist: type 1 (Von Recklinghausen's disease, NF1), type 2 (NF2) and Schwannomatosis.[15]

NF1 is an autosomal dominant disorder caused by the NF1 gene on chromosome 17. It is the most common type and has specific clinical diagnostic criteria across multiple organ systems.

Two or more of the following clinical features will confirm the diagnosis:

- Two or more Lisch nodules
- Two or more neurofibromas or one plexiform neurofibroma
- Optic glioma
- Axillary or inguinal freckling
- Six or more café-au-lait macules greater than 5 mm in diameter in prepubertal patients and greater than 15 mm in post-pubertal patients
- A distinctive bone lesion
- First degree relative with neurofibromatosis

The common orthopaedic manifestations are short stature, anterolateral tibial bowing and congenital tibial pseudarthrosis, spinal deformities (including scoliosis, kyphosis and spondylolisthesis), hemihypertrophy (unilateral segmental hypertrophy), osteopenia and osteoporosis.

> **Key Points**
>
> - Café-au-lait spots are usually the first identifying features. These arise in infancy as macular areas of hyperpigmentation. Skin-fold freckling appears soon after. Freckling can be identified within the axillae, inguinal region, eyelids, breast folds and neck. Neurofibromas present in late childhood as two types: cutaneous and plexiform. The latter are at risk of transformation to malignant peripheral nerve sheath tumours.
> - Up to one-quarter of patients with NF1 have scoliosis, usually of the thoracic spine. Scoliosis is termed dystrophic when the curves are short, sharply angulated and severe. The rate of progression is greater than that of idiopathic scoliosis. These patients are at greater risk of neurological complications and warrant earlier surgical intervention. Apart from earlier presentation, non-dystrophic curves have features similar to idiopathic scoliosis.[15,16]

Hemihypertrophy

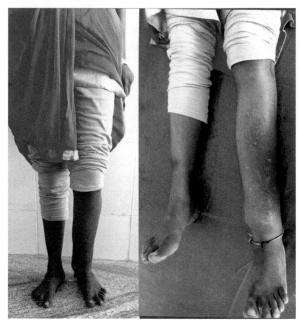

Figure 18.1h A 19-year-old with hemihypertrophy of the left leg and anterolateral bowing of the tibia secondary to neurofibromatosis.

Asymmetry of both sides of the body greater than what can be attributed to normal variation (considered as greater than 5% of growth discrepancy) is termed hemihypertrophy. This may be classified as total and limited, or syndromic and non-syndromic (isolated).

Clinical evaluation must aid the identification of any cause or associations of hemihypertrophy. Anthropometric measurements including limb circumferences must be serially documented. The skin must be assessed for lesions that would suggest neurofibromatosis or vascular disorders. The presence of hypertension may suggest renal or adrenal disease. Dysmorphic features may be present in syndromic cases. Abdominal and neurological examinations must be performed. Limb length discrepancy and pelvic obliquity can lead to non-structural scoliosis.[17]

> **Key Points**
>
> - The aetiology of hemihypertrophy is unknown and, except for the variant 'idiopathic congenital hypertrophy', is rarely identifiable at birth. Causes include:

Syndromic

- ○ Beckwith–Wiedemann syndrome
- ○ Proteus syndrome
- ○ Klippel–Trenaunay–Weber syndrome

Non-syndromic

- ○ Neurofibromatosis
- ○ Lymphangiomatosis
- ○ Haemangiomas
- ○ Arteriovenous fistulae

- An increased incidence of embryonal tumours, such as Wilms' tumour and hepatoblastoma, have been documented in isolated hemihypertrophy and particularly in Beckwith–Wiedemann syndrome. [17]

Post-trauma Presentations

Trauma may be treated non-surgically or in fact not treated at all, thereby resulting in some of the complications seen following fractures such as malunion, non-union and infection. In the younger patient, growth plate problems may occur if damaged. Post-traumatic arthritis is a consequence of inadequately treated intra-articular fractures.

Physeal Arrest

In this patient, clinical examination should include assessment of deformities while standing. Limb length discrepancy is best evaluated by the placement of blocks under the shortened limb to obtain a level pelvis. Gait analysis is also useful, as a valgus thrust may be seen.

Examination of adjacent joint mobility and stability, rotatory abnormalities and peripheral neurovascular status can be performed when supine. True and apparent limb length must be assessed. True leg length must be measured in segments. [18]

Key Points

- Proximal tibial physeal injuries are rare, accounting for approximately 0.5–3% of all physeal injuries. High-velocity injuries impart an increased risk of physeal arrest.
- Surgical options include physeal bridge resection and tissue interposition (if more than two years of growth remain and the affected area is less than 50%), corrective osteotomies and physeal manipulation in the ipsilateral or contralateral limb. [18]

Deformities of the Distal Humerus in Children

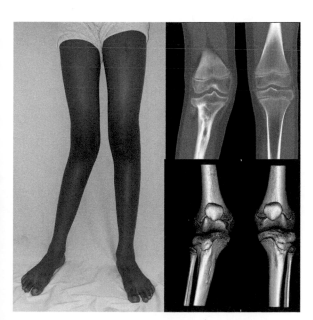

Figure 18.2a An 11-year-old with valgus deformity of the right tibia secondary to proximal tibial physeal arrest due to penetrating trauma.

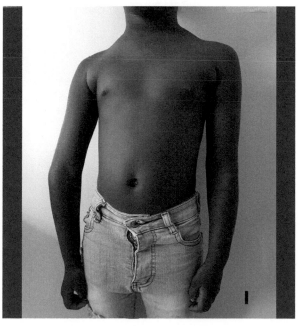

Figure 18.2b(i) Gunstock deformity of the right elbow secondary to malunited supracondylar fracture of the distal humerus.

323

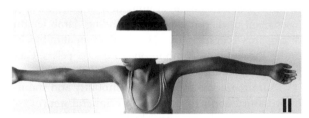

Figure 18.2b(ii) Accentuation of hyperextension as part of left cubitus varus deformity in a 12-year-old, also due to a malunited supracondylar fracture.

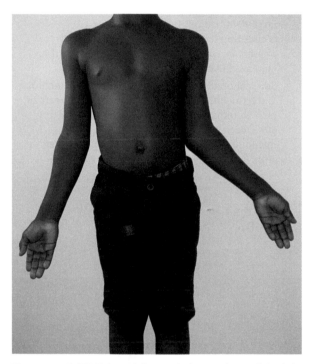

Figure 18.2b(iii) Valgus deformity (cubitus valgus) of the left elbow secondary to a lateral condyle fracture of the distal humerus.

Cubitus varus commonly occurs secondary to malunion or physeal arrest in extension-type supracondylar fractures. It is frequently due to unrecognised or inadequately reduced fractures and is less likely to be secondary to underlying physeal disturbance from the fracture itself. Comminution or impaction of the medial column of the distal humerus increases the risk of varus deformity.[19] Cubitus valgus is much less common in supracondylar fractures than in lateral condylar fractures.[20]

Key Points

- Cubitus varus is multiplanar and was previously considered a purely cosmetic problem. However, increased internal rotation predisposes to tardy ulnar nerve palsy and varus deformity, altering the elbow biomechanics. This can lead to posterolateral instability. An extension deformity is also present. The normal carrying angle is therefore absent on full extension.

- Lateral condyle fractures can also lead to cubitus varus deformity due to lateral overgrowth and is more common in minimally or nondisplaced fractures. The deformity is less severe than cubitus varus secondary to supracondylar fractures.

- Lateral condylar non-union and lateral physeal arrest are the proposed mechanisms for cubitus valgus. Continued medial condylar growth creates the valgus deformity. Secondary tardy ulnar nerve palsy can also occur in rare instances.[20]

- Corrective osteotomies can be performed to correct both deformities. Osteotomy and distraction osteogenesis with circular external fixators can also be performed.[21]

Cervical Nerve Root Injury

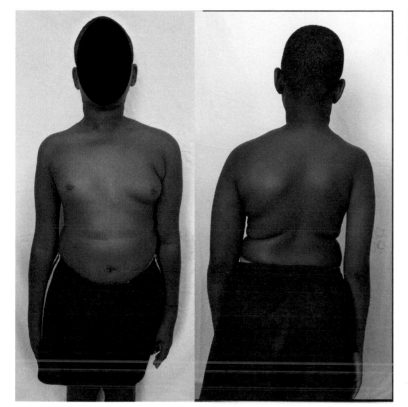

Figure 18.2c A 12-year-old with long-standing traumatic right cervical nerve root avulsions (C3–C8) with significant periscapular and proximal arm muscle wasting.

This is essentially a preganglionic injury to the brachial plexus; therefore, the child will have weakness of the rhomboids and the serratus anterior as well as weakness related to the myotomes. This child (Figure 18.2c) did not have a Horner's syndrome probably because T1 root was not involved (T1 lies near to the sympathetic ganglion and chain).

Key Points

- Examination of C3 root lesions is as follows: Reduced sensation at the temporal area, the lower pinna, the posterior cheek and the lateral aspect of the neck. There is no detectable motor weakness for C3 lesions. The best place to test for C3 is the side of the neck.
- Examination of C4 root lesions is as follows: Reduced sensation in a band over the spine of the scapula, mid-deltoid and clavicle. The only motor deficit is slight weakness of the trapezius muscle on shrugging.
- It is important to distinguish preganglionic (proximal to dorsal root ganglion) from postganglionic (distal to dorsal root ganglion) injuries of the brachial plexus, as this affects treatment options.[22]

Neglected Elbow Dislocation

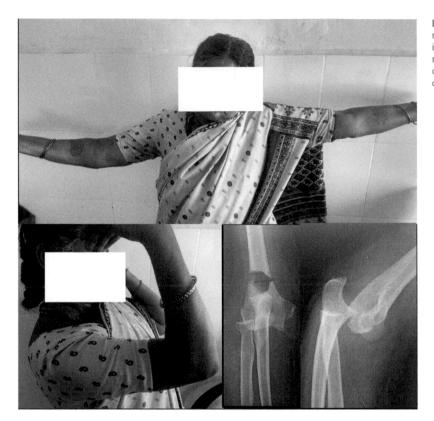

Figure 18.2d A 45-year-old with neglected right elbow dislocation. The initial elbow dislocation was incompletely reduced some months prior. She has since complained of pain, stiffness and deformity of the right elbow.

Examination reveals alteration in the bony three-point relationship of the medial and lateral epicondyles and tip of the olecranon. This isosceles triangle relationship is broken in a chronic dislocated elbow but is maintained in a malunited supracondylar fracture.

The range of motion will be restricted in both flexion and extension. The ulnar nerve especially is likely to be stretched.

Key Points

- Elbow dislocations can be either simple or complex, with associated fractures. Posterolateral dislocation is the most common type. The injury progresses from lateral to medial.
- Simple dislocations are treated with closed reduction and, once stable, can be managed with a short period of immobilisation in a sling and proceed to graduated range of motion.[23]
- Neglected elbow dislocations lead to a loss of the functional range of motion, with limitations in all movements. Dislocations less than 3 months can be treated with open reduction and ligament reconstruction. Hinged external fixation and arthroplasty are options for dislocations of longer duration.[24]

Volkmann's Ischaemic Contracture

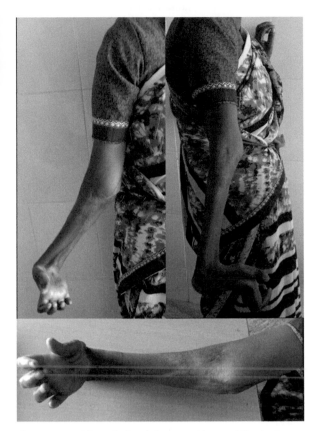

Figure 18.2e This right-hand-dominant 38-year-old had open reduction and internal fixation of their right radius and ulna, which was complicated post-operatively by compartment syndrome and Volkmann's ischaemic contracture (VIC). Flexion contractures of wrist and fingers and gross wasting of muscles of forearm and hand are evident. There is decreased sensation in their hand. Volkmann's sign is positive (see below).

Muscle ischaemia and necrosis in acute compartment syndrome lead to the clinical features of Volkmann's ischaemic contracture (VIC). This can be secondary to fractures (particularly supracondylar fractures of the distal humerus), tight circumferential bandages, burns, snake bites and vascular injury.

Necrosis occurs after 4 hours of ischaemia and is preceded by myofibroblast proliferation, leading to contraction of affected muscles. Peripheral neuropathy secondary to ischaemia and compression within the osteofascial compartment can lead to chronic pain, loss of sensation or paraesthesia and further motor paralysis.[25]

The fixed length of the forearm muscles leads to finger flexion, with active wrist extension and passive finger extension only being possible with wrist flexion. This is termed **Volkmann's sign.**

Key Points

- The severity of VIC was classified by Seddon and then modified by Tsuge:
  - Type 1 (Mild): Flexor digitorum profundus involvement with contractures of two to three fingers. Minimal loss of sensation.
  - Type 2 (Moderate): Deep flexor compartment and some superficial flexors are affected, resulting in contractures of all digits and wrist. Sensation is also partially affected or absent.
  - Type 3 (Severe): All flexors and some extensors are affected, with loss of sensory and motor function leading to a claw-type deformity of the hand.
- VIC can be initially treated conservatively in mild cases, focusing on improvement of range of motion and muscle function. Surgical intervention can be performed in all (including refractory mild) cases. This involves release or excision of fibrotic tissue and reconstruction for lost function.[26]

Non-union

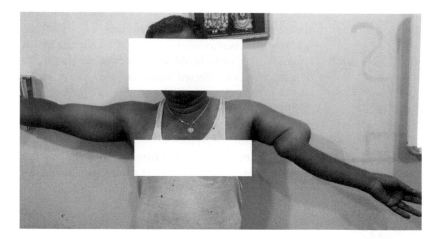

Figure 18.2f A 50-year-old with a non-union of the left humerus after initial open reduction and plate and screw fixation. There are multiple scars with deformity, shortening of the arm and mobility at the non-union site. No neurovascular deficit is present. All nerves need to be examined but in particular the radial nerve.

Patients with fracture non-union present with pain and increased mobility at the fracture site. Of note, this differs from pseudarthrosis, which is not associated with pain.[26]

Key Points

- Non-unions are due to a poor mechanical environment (such as inadequate immobilisation), biological factors (affecting blood supply) and general factors (including age, nutrition, diabetes and cigarette smoking). These factors need to be looked at in the history and examination.
- The principle of treatment is to identify and address all underlying mechanical and biological issues. This includes débridement to excise infected bone and soft tissue and antibiotic coverage if necessary, stable fracture fixation and bone grafting (particularly in avascular non-unions). Adjunctive therapy with bone morphogenic protein is being investigated. Low-intensity pulsed ultrasound is currently recommended to improve healing, particularly in acute fractures.[27]

Problems Related to Infection

Infection remains a problem with managing orthopaedic problems in the developing world. The causes of this are multifactorial, ranging from the increased incidence of open injuries to the delay in presentation.

Necrotising Fasciitis

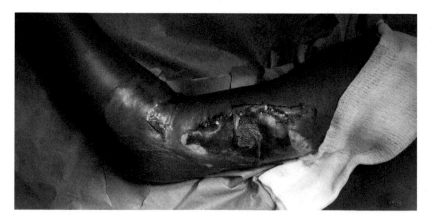

Figure 18.3a Right arm and proximal forearm of a 19-year-old with necrotising fasciitis secondary to an abrasion.

Patients typically present with a triad of severe pain, swelling and fever with progressive bullae (with serous fluid) formation and crepitus. Skin sloughing then occurs. The classic 'dishwater' exudate may be present.[28]

Finger probe test will be positive. This is performed under local or general anaesthesia. A 2 cm incision is made down to the deep fascia. A finger is placed through the hole down to the fascia and meets little resistance and therefore penetrates it. This is a positive result, as the subcutaneous tissue is normally adherent to the fascia. Lack of bleeding and a 'dishwater fluid' ooze is also typical.[29]

Key Points

- Necrotising fasciitis (NF) is an infectious disorder involving the fascia, subcutaneous tissue and skin. Bacterial angiothrombotic invasion occurs and can progress to liquefactive necrosis.[28]

- The mechanism of infection varies widely and includes penetrating and blunt trauma and post-surgical infections. Polymicrobial infections are most common and are classified as type 1 NF. Type 2 or monomicrobial NF is commonly caused by Group A *Streptococcus* or *Staphylococcus aureus*. *Vibrio* species have been separately grouped as type 3.[28,29]

- Management involves early diagnosis and appropriate treatment. Aggressive surgical debridement and early commencement of appropriate antibiotic coverage are important and will also reduce its significant morbidity.[29]

Sequelae of Septic Arthritis in Children

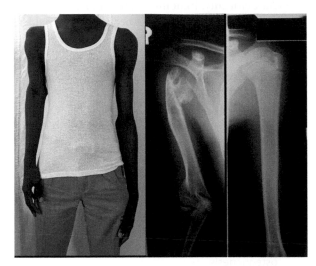

Figure 18.3b A 13-year-old with upper limb length inequality (8 cm shortening of the right humerus) secondary to neonatal septic arthritis of the right shoulder and subsequent physeal injury with deformity of the humeral head. The patient had decreased abduction and forward flexion but maintained a functional range of motion, with adaptation of scapulothoracic function.

The majority of cases (80%) of septic arthritis in children occur in the hip and knee, while only 4% occur at the shoulder. The most common causative organism is *Staphylococcus aureus*, followed by Group A *Streptococcus* and *Enterobacter* species.[30]

Presentation later on is either due to recurrent infection, joint destruction, limb length inequality or angular deformity. Joint instability is more common in hip septic arthritis but can also occur in the shoulder.

Chronic osteomyelitis, though rare in the developed world, is still associated with significant morbidity worldwide.

The hallmark of chronic osteomyelitis is necrotic bone (sequestrum) with or without new bone formation (involucrum). The clinical features include increasing pain, sinus tract formation and low-grade fever.

Key Points

- Majority of growth (80%) of the humerus occurs in the proximal physis.
- Delay in diagnosis, the onset of infection at an early age and microbial characteristics all have prognostic effects.
- Unlike septic arthritis of the hip, significant complications from shoulder septic arthritis are rare and mainly cosmetic.
- Surgical intervention is indicated only if there is functional limitation.[31] This includes joint stabilisation via arthrodesis and humeral lengthening, preferably via distraction osteogenesis.
- Due to its rarity, there are no clinical guidelines for the management of these complications.[32]

Key Points

- Treatment is mainly surgical and involves debridement of sequestrum and surrounding devitalised soft tissue. Antibiotic therapy, local and systemic, is also recommended.
- Once infection is controlled and a viable soft tissue envelope remains, bony defects can be reconstructed with bone grafts (vascularised or non-vascularised) and bone transport techniques.[33]

Chronic Osteomyelitis

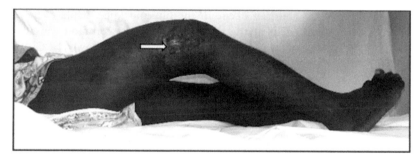

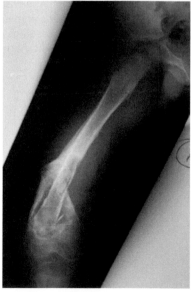

Figure 18.3c(i) Chronic osteomyelitis of the right femur with a lateral sinus (arrow). Flexion and varus deformity along with shortening of the distal femur is secondary to malaligned pathological fracture. Involucrum and sequestrum are also evident on plain radiographs

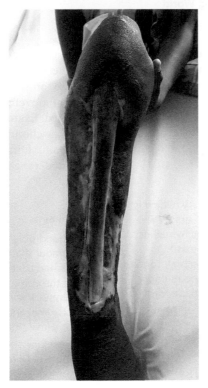

Figure 18.3c(ii) Exposed tibia showing sequestrum post-decompression of acute osteomyelitis and fasciotomies for compartment syndrome.

Late Presentation of Tumours

Sometimes there is a later presentation of tumours than would be seen in the developed world. There are multiple reasons for this, e.g. socioeconomic, cultural and accessibility. Some countries have little or no screening programmes or longer waiting times for appointments, which leads to patients presenting at a more advanced stage of illness. Some examples are presented here.

Secondary Chondrosarcoma

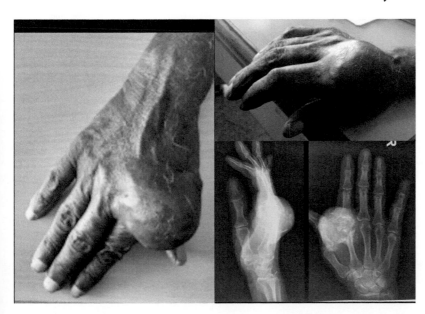

Figure 18.4a A 62-year-old diagnosed with secondary chondrosarcoma of the right hand after presenting with pain and a well-defined mass for many years, which gradually increased in size. The mass was irregular and immobile, appearing to arise from bone.

Chondrosarcoma is a cartilage-producing, primary malignant tumour of bone, which usually affects individuals aged 40–75 years and has a male preponderance.

Clinical manifestations of malignant transformation in a benign cartilaginous lesion include new onset pain in the absence of fracture, enlarging soft tissue mass and greater than 50% cortical erosion on plain radiographs.

Key Points

- Chondrosarcoma is classified as primary (which is further classified into low grade, high grade, dedifferentiated, clear cell and mesenchymal) or secondary. The latter arises from pre-existing benign cartilage lesions such as osteochondroma (<1% risk), enchondromas (1% risk) and multiple hereditary exostoses (1–10% risk). Patients with Ollier's disease and Maffuci syndrome have a significantly higher risk (25–30% and up to 100%, respectively) of developing chondrosarcoma.

- The most common locations of primary chondrosarcoma are pelvis, proximal femur and scapula. They usually metastasise to lungs. The prognosis is dependent on the grade of the tumour. Wide surgical excision is the recommended method of management, as these tumours are usually resistant to chemotherapy and radiotherapy.[34]

Chondroblastoma

In this patient (Figure 18.4b), by palpating the swelling, the examiner will notice a bony consistency. Because of the location, the ulnar nerve and the range of movement of the elbow joint will need to be examined. Examine the regional lymph nodes.

With chondroblastoma, most patients present with pain. Other symptoms include swelling and decreased range of motion. Joint effusions may be present.

Key Points

- Chondroblastoma is a benign cartilage-forming tumour that is more common in males in the second to third decade of life. The majority occur in the epiphysis of long bones but can cross the physis. The most common locations are the proximal and distal femur, proximal humerus and proximal tibia.

- Histology shows chondroblasts in a cobblestone pattern. Differential diagnoses include giant cell tumour and osteomyelitis.

- The gold standard of treatment is intralesional curettage and bone grafting. Local recurrence can occur and is more likely in the skeletally immature. Benign pulmonary metastases have been described.[35]

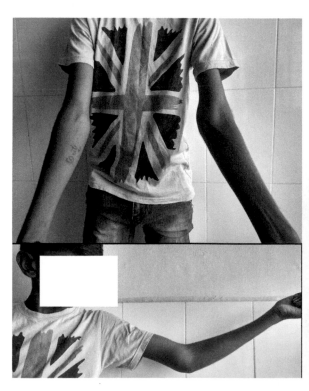

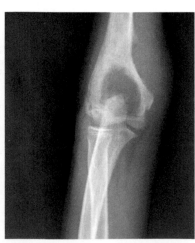

Figure 18.4b A 14-year-old with left elbow swelling and restriction of elbow movement. There is no evidence of neurovascular compromise. The radiograph shows a geographic-type lucent lesion in the epiphysis of the left distal humerus representative of a chondroblastoma.

Multiple Hereditary Exostosis

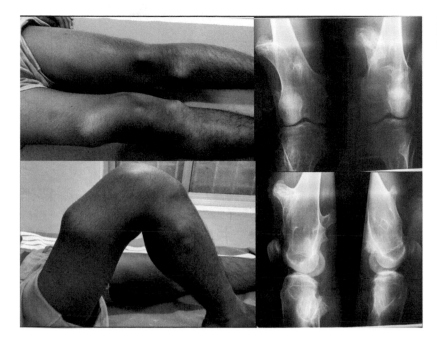

Figure 18.4c A 22-year-old with multiple broad-based exostoses involving both distal femora and proximal tibiae.

Examine the bony lumps. Multiple bony lumps around the knee are suggestive of hereditary multiple exostosis (HME). These may also be present around the proximal humerus, wrist and ankle.

Patients are either asymptomatic or present with pain, decreased range of motion or, rarely, features of neurovascular compression or entrapment. Some deformities that can occur are shortening of the ulna, bowing of the radius, ulnar deviation of the hand, limb length discrepancies, varus or valgus deformities of knee, ankle deformities and short stature.

> **Key Points**
>
> - Multiple hereditary exostosis (MHE) is an autosomal dominant condition with variable penetrance. Males are slightly more affected. *EXT1* on chromosome 8 and *EXT2* on chromosome 11 are tumour suppressor genes affected in this condition.
> - The exostoses are cartilage capped and either pedunculated or, in the majority of cases, sessile (broad based). Deformities arise due to disorganised endochondral ossification, particularly in the paired bones.
> - Other complications of exostoses are bursitis, arthritis, spinal cord compression and, in 10% of patients with MHE, malignant transformation into chondrosarcoma.[36]

Neglected Presentations

In this section, we present examples of some clinical conditions that leads to severe deformity if medical attention is not sought early and then followed by early diagnosis and treatment.

The Neglected Clubfoot

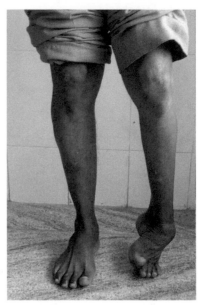

Figure 18.5a(ii) A 15-year-old with unilateral neglected club foot. There is equinocavovarus deformity with callosities on the lateral aspect of the foot. Note the smaller foot compared to the other side.

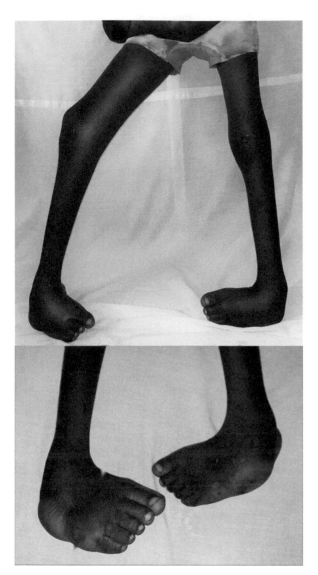

Figure 18.5a(i) An ambulant 8-year-old with bilateral neglected clubfeet (congenital talipes equinovarus (CTEV)). Callosities are present on the dorsolateral aspect of both feet due to abnormal loading with ambulation. There is also wasting of the muscles of both legs. In addition, there is an untreated developmental dysplasia of the left hip, leading to limb length inequality and wasting of the muscles in the thigh.

Congenital talipes equinovarus (CTEV), which has had inadequate or no initial treatment within infancy or early childhood, is considered 'neglected'.[37]

In severe deformities, with a rigid cavus and equinus deformity, the patient will ambulate on the dorsal and lateral border of the foot, leading to callosities and bursae formation and contraction of the medial soft tissues. Plastic deformation of the bones of the feet occur to allow adaptation to abnormal axial loading. Ulcerations can arise. Pain is due to the abnormal pressures applied on the skin, subcutaneous tissues and joints, particularly the ankle and midtarsal joints.

Key Points

- The goal of treatment is to create a plantigrade foot that will allow pain-free ambulation on the sole and in a shoe without modifications. Flexibility is also desirable but difficult to achieve.
- Due to variations in deformity, multiple surgical procedures, including soft tissue releases and osteotomies, have been described. Surgical interventions must be tailored to each patient. Fusion will most likely be the choice at late presentation.[38]

Pes Cavus

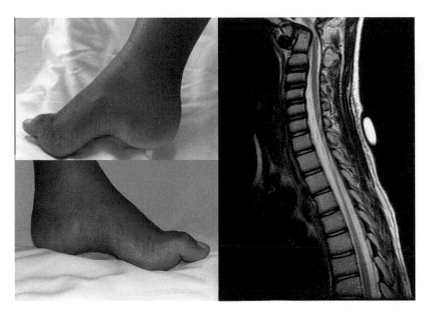

Figure 18.5b Progressive quadriparesis and bilateral rigid pes cavus and equinus deformity in a 10-year-old. This was a case of delayed presentation. Magnetic resonance imaging (MRI) showed an os odontoideum with spinal stenosis. Patient was unable to perform a Coleman block test.

Any patient who presents with a progressive pes cavus should be assumed to have an underlying neurological problem, and thus a complete neurological examination must be performed.

Key Points

- Neuromuscular conditions (especially Charcot–Marie–Tooth disease) are the most common cause of pes cavus. It can also be idiopathic, traumatic or secondary to clubfoot deformity.
- This is due to an imbalance between intrinsic and extrinsic muscles of the foot and ankle, particularly weak tibialis anterior and peroneus brevis and strong tibialis posterior and peroneus longus.
- The deformity can be rigid or flexible, and forefoot or hindfoot driven. The Coleman block test will differentiate between the two. Late presentation is likely to demonstrate a fused hindfoot and associated toe clawing.[39]
- Os odontoideum is a smooth ossicle that is not continuous with the body of the second cervical vertebra or a shortened odontoid peg. Patients present with features of vertebrobasilar ischaemia and spinal instability. This finding can be incidental.[40]

Knee Osteoarthritis

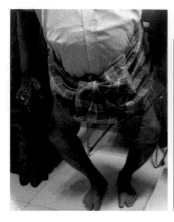 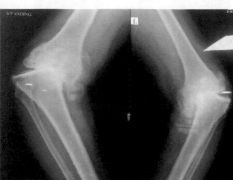

Figure 18.5c This 65-year-old complained of pain and worsening deformity of both knees. There are varus and flexion deformities bilaterally secondary to osteoarthritis.

A patient who presents with such advanced knee osteoarthritis will walk with a varus lurch. There will be a fixed flexion deformity and reduced range of movement. The patella will maltrack. It is likely that the medial collateral ligament (MCL) will be contracted and the lateral collateral ligament (LCL) lax. The anterior cruciate ligament (ACL) is likely ruptured, while the posterior cruciate ligament (PCL) may be contracted if flexion deformity is present.

Because of the altered limb alignment, the other joints in the lower limb and lumbar spine can also be affected. Therefore, the patient may complain of back pain or arthralgia in other joints.

Key Points

- Severe coronal plane (varus/valgus) deformity requires a thorough pre-operative assessment of associated deformities (sagittal or rotational) and ligamentous laxity.

- For the varus knee, the posteromedial corner is usually contracted. Therefore, performing the following releases can be done sequentially: medial osteophyte excision, deep MCL and posteromedial capsule, semimembranosus tendon and PCL (especially if flexion deformity is present) and, if necessary, the superficial MCL. Tibial reduction osteotomy can also be performed in severe cases such as this one.

- For the varus knee with flexion contracture, posterior-stabilised cruciate sacrificing total knee arthroplasty (TKA) is recommended, as the PCL is likely to be released due to its contribution to the flexion deformity. More constrained devices, including constrained non-hinged (with a high central tibial post) and the highly constrained hinged TKA, will be necessary if there is significant ligamentous deficiency.

- Bone defects can be addressed with bone cement, bone graft (supplemented with screw fixation) and metal wedges. Longer tibial stems can also be considered to improve stability.[41,42]

Scoliosis

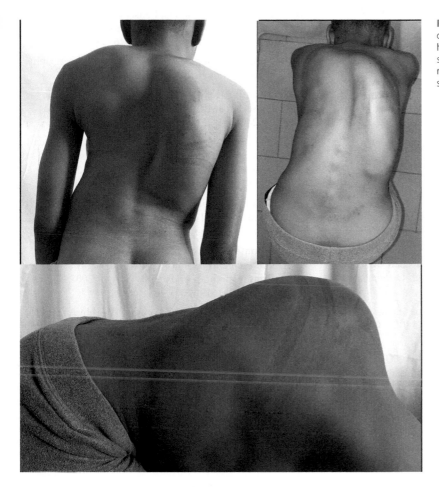

Figure 18.5d This child with congestive cardiac failure and severe pulmonary hypertension was referred at age 8 after a spine deformity was noted on a chest radiograph. The patient has a congenital scoliosis.

Now at 15 years, this patient (Figure 18.5d) has intermittent shortness of breath with minimal exercise tolerance, back pain and a rigid kyphoscoliosis deformity of the thoracolumbar spine with a right rib prominence that is exaggerated on performing Adams forward bend test. There is a high likelihood that with this degree of deformity, there will be some neurological deficit that is picked up on examination of the lower limbs and on testing the abdominal reflexes.

Key Points

- Congenital kyphoscoliosis can present with severe curvatures. There is also an association with congenital cardiac and urogenital abnormalities, and some syndromes. Spinal cord anomalies are identified in 40% of patients.[43,44]

- Congenital kyphosis is not amenable to bracing. Patients presenting early (before 5 years of age) and with less severe curves (Cobb angle less than 55°) can be treated with prophylactic hemiepiphysiodesis or posterior in situ fusion to decrease deformity progression and aid further correction. Performing the latter in the young can, however, leads to the crankshaft phenomenon in which anterior vertebral bodies continue to grow.[43]

- Severe cases in older children are difficult to treat. In all procedures, spinal cord monitoring is necessary due to the high risk of injury. They require mobilisation of the spine via corrective osteotomies (resections) and releases (usually anterior). Shortening of the spine (spinal column resection) via hemivertebra excision, vertebral body decancellation, pedicle excision and

337

immediate or staged removal of the posterior laminae may be necessary to achieve balance. Both posterior and anterior instrumentation can be utilised along with anterior strut grafts to improve stability.[43,44]

References

1. Sabharwal S. Blount disease. *J Bone Joint Surg Am* 2009;**91**(7):1758–76.

2. Sabharwal S. Blount disease: an update. *Orthop Clin* 2015;**46**(1):37–47.

3. Birch JG. Blount disease. *J Am Acad Orthop Surg* 2013;**21**(7).

4. Raffini L, Manno C. Modern management of haemophilic arthropathy. *Br J Haematol* 2007;**136**(6):777–787.

5. Luck JV Jr, Silva M, Rodriguez-Merchan CE, et al. Hemophilic arthropathy. *J Am Acad Orthop Surg* 2004;**12**(4):234–245.

6. Rodriguez-Merchan EC. Musculoskeletal complications of hemophilia. *HSS J* 2010;**6**(1):37–42.

7. Sharkey MS, Grunseich K, Carpenter TO. Contemporary medical and surgical management of X-linked hypophosphatemic rickets. *J Am Acad Orthop Surg* 2015;**23**(7):433–442.

8. Pavone V, Testa G, Gioitta Iachino S, et al. Hypophosphatemic rickets: etiology, clinical features and treatment. *Eur J Orthop Surg Traumatol* 2015 Feb 1;**25**(2):221–6.

9. Healy PJ, Helliwell PS. Dactylitis: pathogenesis and clinical considerations. *Curr Rheumatol Rep* 2006;**8**(5):338.

10. Serjeant GR. The natural history of sickle cell disease. *Cold Spring Harb Perspect Med* 2013;**3**(10):a011783.

11. Kamath AF, McGraw MH, Israelite CL. Surgical management of osteonecrosis of the femoral head in patients with sickle cell disease. *World J Orthop* 2015;**6**(10):776.

12. Osunkwo I. An update on the recent literature on sickle cell bone disease. *Curr Opin Endocrinol Diabetes Obes* 2013;**20**(6):539–546.

13. Franzone JM, Shah SA, Wallace MJ, Kruse RW. Osteogenesis imperfecta: a pediatric orthopedic perspective. *Orthop Clin* 2019;**50**(2):193–209.

14. Bovid KM, Moore MD. Juvenile idiopathic arthritis for the pediatric orthopedic surgeon. *Orthop Clin* 2019;**50**(4):471–488.

15. Woodrow C, Clarke A, Amirfeyz R. Neurofibromatosis. *Orthop Trauma* 2015;**29**(3):206–210.

16. Feldman DS, Jordan C, Fonseca L. Orthopaedic manifestations of neurofibromatosis type 1. *J Am Acad Orthop Surg* 2010;**18**(6):346–357.

17. Leung AK, Fong JHS, Leong AG. Hemihypertrophy. *J R Soc Promot Health* 2002;**122**(1):24–27.

18. Escott BG, Kelley SP. Management of traumatic physeal growth arrest. *Orthop Trauma* 2012;**26**(3):200–211.

19. Vaquero-Picado A, González-Morán G, Moraleda L. Management of supracondylar fractures of the humerus in children. *EFORT Open Rev* 2018;**3**(10):526–540.

20. Tejwani N, Phillips D, Goldstein RY. Management of lateral humeral condylar fracture in children. *J Am Acad Orthop Surg* 2011;**19**(6):350–358.

21. Piskin A, Tomak Y, Sen C, Tomak L. The management of cubitus varus and valgus using the Ilizarov method. *J Bone Joint Surg Br* 2007 Dec;**89**(12):1615–1619.

22. Noland SS, Bishop AT, Spinner RJ, Shin AY. Adult traumatic brachial plexus injuries. *J Am Acad Orthop Surg* 2019;**27**(19):705–716.

23. Elzohairy MM. Neglected posterior dislocation of the elbow. *Injury* 2009;**40**(2):197–200.

24. Jupiter JB, Ring D. Treatment of unreduced elbow dislocations with hinged external fixation. *J Bone Joint Surg Am* 2002;**84**(9):1630–1635.

25. Khan F, Cheema TA, Bhatti ZI. Volkmann's ischaemic contracture: post circumferential contracture of the forearm. *Prof Med J* 2014;**21**(3).

26. Pettitt DA, McArthur P. Clinical review: Volkmann's ischaemic contracture. *Eur J Trauma Emerg Surg* 2012;**38**(2):129–137.

27. Nandra R, Grover L, Porter K. Fracture non-union epidemiology and treatment. *Trauma* 2016;**18**(1):3–11.

28. Stevens DL, Bryant AE. Necrotizing soft-tissue infections. *N Engl J Med* 2017 Dec 6;**377**(23):2253–2265.

29. Narayan N, McCoubrey G. Necrotizing fasciitis: a plastic surgeon's perspective. *Surgery (Oxford)* 2019 Jan 1;**37**(1):33–37.

30. Brown DW, Sheffer BW. Pediatric septic arthritis: an update. *Orthop Clin North Am* 2019;**50**(4):461–470.

31. Bos CF, Mol LJ, Obermann WR, Tjin a Ton ER. Late sequelae of neonatal septic arthritis of the shoulder. *J Bone Joint Surg Br* 1998 Jul;**80**(4):645–650.

32. Pawar UM, Bapat MR. Management of sequalae of neglected septic shoulder. *Indian J Orthop* 2009 Jan;**43**(1):90.

33. Panteli M, Giannoudis PV. Chronic osteomyelitis: what the surgeon needs to know. *EFORT Open Rev* 2016;**1**(5):128–135.

34. Fiorenza F, Abudu A, Grimer RJ, et al. Risk factors for survival and local control in chondrosarcoma of bone. *J Bone Joint Surg Br* 2002;**84**(1):93–99.

35. Xu H, Nugent D, Monforte HL, et al. Chondroblastoma of bone in the extremities: a multicenter retrospective study. *J Bone Joint Surg Am* 2015;**97**(11):925–931.

36. Stieber JR, Dormans JP. Manifestations of hereditary multiple exostoses. *J Am Acad Orthop Surg* 2005;**13**(2):110–120.

37. Dimeglio A, Canavese F. Management of resistant, relapsed, and neglected clubfoot. *Curr Orthop Pract* 2013;**24**(1):34–42.

38. Penny JN. The neglected clubfoot. *Tech Orthop* 2005;**20**(2):153–166.

39. Rosenbaum AJ, Lisella J, Patel N, Phillips N. The cavus foot. *Med Clin* 2014;**98**(2):301–312.

40. Rozzelle CJ, Aarabi B, Dhall SS, et al. Os odontoideum. *Neurosurgery* 2013;**72**(Suppl 3):159–169.

41. Rossi R, Cottino U, Bruzzone M, et al. Total knee arthroplasty in the varus knee: tips and tricks. *Int Orthop* 2019;**43**:151–158.

42. Mullaji AB, Padmanabhan V, Jindal G. Total knee arthroplasty for profound varus deformity: technique and radiological results in 173 knees with varus of more than 20. *J Arthroplasty* 2005 Aug 1;**20**(5):550–561.

43. Arlet V, Odent T, Aebi M. Congenital scoliosis. *Eur Spine J* 2003 Oct 1;**12**(5):456–463.

44. Noordeen MH, Garrido E, Tucker SK, Elsebaie HB. The surgical treatment of congenital kyphosis. *Spine* 2009 Aug 1;**34**(17):1808–1814.

Index